Springer
Tokyo
Berlin
Heidelberg
New York
Barcelona
Hong Kong
London
Milan
Paris
Singapore

N. Matsui, Y. Taneda, Y. Yoshida (Eds.)

Arthroplasty 2000

Recent Advances in Total Joint Replacement

With 165 Figures, Including 13 in Color

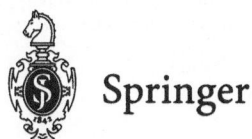 Springer

Nobuo Matsui, M.D.
Professor and Chairman
Department of Orthopaedic Surgery
Nagoya City University Medical School
1 Kawasumi, Mizuho-cho, Mizuho-ku
Nagoya 467-8601, Japan

Yoichi Taneda, M.D.
Associate Professor
Department of Orthopaedic Surgery
Nagoya City University Medical School
1 Kawasumi, Mizuho-cho, Mizuho-ku
Nagoya 467-8601, Japan

Yukio Yoshida, M.D.
Assistant Professor
Department of Orthopaedic Surgery
Nagoya City University Medical School
1 Kawasumi, Mizuho-cho, Mizuho-ku
Nagoya 467-8601, Japan

ISBN-13: 978-4-431-68429-9   e-ISBN-13: 978-4-431-68427-5
DOI: 10.1007/978-4-431-68427-5

Library of Congress Cataloging-in-Publication Data

Arthroplasty 2000 : recent advances in total joint replacement / N. Matsui, Y. Taneda, Y. Yoshida (eds.).
    p. ; cm.
    Includes bibliographical references and index.

    1. Total hip replacement—Congresses. 2. Arthroplasty—Congresses. 3. Hip joint—Surgery—Congresses. 4. Knee—Surgery—Congresses. 5. Total knee replacement—Congresses. I. Title: Recent advances in total joint replacement. II. Title: Total joint replacement. III. Matsui, Nobuo. IV. Taneda, Y. (Yoichi), 1949– V. Yoshida, Yukio.
    [DNLM: 1. Arthroplasty, Replacement, Hip. 2. Arthroplasty, Replacement, Knee. 3. Hip Prosthesis. 4. Knee Prosthesis. WE 855 A787 2001]
    RD549 .A745 2001
    617.5'810592—dc21

                                                                2001020427

Printed on acid-free paper

© Springer-Verlag Tokyo 2001
Softcover reprint of the hardcover 1st edition 2001

Typesetting, printing, and binding: Best-set Typesetter Ltd., Hong Kong
SPIN: 10784680

Preface

Several million people in the United States have received total joint arthroplasties for osteoarthritis, rheumatoid arthritis, or other joint diseases in the past 30 years. About 100 000 patients in Japan and 350 000 patients in the United States undergo joint replacement surgery every year. Of these patients, 98% are freed from pain and disability and obtain good quality of life after surgery. In the 21st century, about 30% of the population will be over 65 years old, and osteoarthritis will be one of the major problems in the orthopedic field. More and more reconstructive surgery will be necessary to relieve joint disability.

In 1938, Phillip Wiles in Britain developed the first total hip arthroplasty (THA), but poor-quality material resulted in low durability. In 1963, John Charnley, also in Britain, developed the epoch-making low-friction hip joint using high-density polyethylene and bone cement, thereby prolonging the survival of artificial joints by approximately 20 years. In the past 40 years, total joint arthroplasty has made remarkable progress thanks to new knowledge of materials for artificial joints based on biomechanics, and on surgical experience and improved technique.

The development of total knee arthroplasty (TKA) has lagged slightly behind that of total hip arthroplasty, but nowadays good clinical outcomes have been reported from many facilities. Forty years have passed since Charnley's development of THA, but longevity of the artificial joint is a goal that has not yet been totally attained, regardless of the improvement of quality control in new materials.

Friction wear of polyethylene in the artificial joint cannot be avoided. Small polyethylene particles within 10 microns are caught by macrophages, which release inflammatory mediators such as cytokines and proteases, leading to osteolysis and causing loosening of artificial joints. However, ultra-high molecular weight polyethylene (UHMWPE) strengthened by gamma irradiation under oxygen-free conditions has been developed and used effectively.

Recently, combinations of ceramic or zirconia heads for UHMWPE acetabular components and metal-on-metal or ceramic-on-ceramic THA have been developed to address the problem of polyethylene wear particles that lead to bone absorption around artificial joints and subsequent loosening. Further studies in these fields are expected.

This book deals with recent developments in total joint arthroplasty, as reported at the 30th annual meeting of the Japanese Society for Replacement Arthroplasty held

February 8–11, 2000, in Nagoya, Japan. At that meeting, guest speakers from many overseas countries and specialists of total joint arthroplasty in Japan presented papers that focused on the following topics: problems of wear and loosening, revision THA and TKA, metal-on-metal and ceramic-on-ceramic interfaces for THA, posterior cruciate ligament retention or resection in TKA, and TKA for Charcot joint. Papers on these as well as such current topics as cross-linked UHMWPE, custom hip prostheses, and computer-assisted surgery in THA are collected in this volume to provide up-to-date information and knowledge on joint arthroplasty surgery that will be valuable to all orthopedic surgeons.

Nobuo Matsui

Contents

Part 7 Current Topics in Total Knee Arthroplasty

Part 8 PCL Resection Versus PCL Retention in Total Knee Arthroplasty

Part 9 Total Knee Arthroplasty for Charcot Joint

List of Contributors

Akagi, M.   219
Amino, H.   3, 35
Asano, T.   219
Boerner, M.   119, 137
Clarke, I.C.   3, 35
Edidin, A.A.   211
Epinette, J.-A.   19, 189, 211
Good, V.   3, 35
Hagio, K.   157
Haraguchi, K.   111, 157
Hattori, Y.   91
Hiroshima, S.   247
Hua, J.   91
Iguchi, H.   91, 151
Imai, Y.   81
Iwamoto, Y.   75
Jacobs, J.J.   41
Jingushi, S.   75
Kaneda, E.   219
Kawakubo, M.   145
Kawanishi, T.   91, 151, 239
Kawate, K.   99
Kester, M.A.   211
Kim, T.S.   229
Kobayashi, A.   247
Kobayashi, M.   239
Koyama, T.   157
Koyanagi, T.   145
Lahmer, A.   119, 137
Lee, S.-B.   111
Liu, H.-C.   165
Maloney, W.J.   41
Masuda, K.   229

Masuda, S.   3
Mata, T.   219
Matsui, M.   111
Matsui, N.   91, 151, 239
Matsumura, A.   81
Moriya, H.   229
Nagatani, Y.   239
Nakahodo, K.   129
Nakamura, N.   157
Nakamura, T.   219
Nakashima, Y.   75
Nakata, K.   111
Natsume, Y.   99, 105
Nelsen-Freund, E.M.   41
Nishihara, S.   129, 157
Nishii, T.   111, 129, 157
Noguchi, Y.   75
Ochi, T.   111, 129, 157
Ohashi, H.   81
Ohdera, T.   247
Ohmura, T.   99
Ohzono, K.   111, 129, 157
Oneda, Y.   105
Oonishi, H.   3, 35
Sakai, T.   111, 129, 157
Sasama, T.   129
Sato, Y.   129
Shuto, T.   75
Sugano, N.   111, 129, 157
Suzuki, M.   229
Takahashi, M.   145
Tamai, H.   229
Tamai, S.   99

Part 1 Current Topics in Total Hip Arthroplasty

Cross-Linked UHMWPE on Alumina Total Hip Arthroplasty

HIRONOBU OONISHI[1], IAN C. CLARKE[2], VICTORIA GOOD[2], HIROKAZU AMINO[3], and SHINGO MASUDA[3]

Summary. The clinical wear rate of cross-linked polyethylene cups (RCH 1000) irradiated in air with 100 Mrad (clinical use, 1971–1978) decreased to 18%. Tensile strength and elongation decreased, but deterioration did not progress, and the toughness greatly increased in retrieved 100-Mrad polyethylene (PE). The degree of oxidation after 18 years slightly increased. In the hip simulator test using 30% bovine serum as lubricant, cross-linked cups irradiated with 50–150 Mrad did not show detectable wear. Wear of ultrahigh molecular weight polyethylene (UHMWPE) irradiated with 6.5 Mrad (Aeonian) decreased to 3% by the hip simulator test without deterioration of physical properties. Oxidation caused by free radicals produced by gamma-ray sterilization was extremely low.

Key words. Wear, Physical characteristics, Cross-linked polyethylene, Hip simulator, Clinical result

Introduction

To alleviate polyethylene (PE) wear problems, either the total hip prosthesis (THP) needs to be developed using either a non-PE system or the material properties of the present ultrahigh molecular weight polyethylene (UHMWPE) must be dramatically improved. Realizing this fact in 1970, we gamma-irradiated PE (RCH 1000; molecular weight, 10^6) with doses up to 100 Mrad to improve the PE properties. Initial wear-screening tests with cylinder-on-flat specimen geometry demonstrated that the wear resistance improved up to the 100-Mrad dose. The clinical study began in 1971 and continued until 1978 [1–6].

The objective of this study was to investigate the dose response of megaradiation on the wear performance of UHMWPE to improve PE wear resistance dramatically, using bovine serum as the lubricant in a multichannel hip simulator model.

[1] Department of Orthopaedic Surgery, Artificial Joint Section and Biomaterial Laboratory, Osaka-Minami National Hospital, 2-1 Kidohigashi-machi, Kawachinagano, Osaka 586-8521, Japan
[2] Orthopaedic Department, Loma Linda University Medical Center, Loma Linda, CA, USA
[3] Kyocera Corporation, Kyoto, Japan

3

Cross-Linked Polyethylene

It is well known that the sterilization of a PE component with gamma irradiation in air causes the mechanical properties of PE to deteriorate and increases the wear rate. On the other hand, in 1970 we gamma-irradiated PE (RCH 1000) with doses up to 100 Mrad in air to improve the PE properties. The molecular weight of RCH 1000 was 10^6 and that of UHMWPE, which is used at present, is $5-6 \times 10^6$. In an early stage, Charnley used RCH 1000, which was called high-density polyethylene (HDP); however, RCH 1000 was UHMWPE. Initial wear-screening tests with cylinder-on-flat specimen geometry demonstrated that the wear resistance improved to 50% of the nonirradiated value up to the 100-Mrad dose [1–6].

The clinical study was from 1971 until 1978. The color of the PE cup changed to brown. As the PE cup was irradiated in ambient air, there was a surface oxidized layer. As the company that performed the gamma radiation went bankrupt, we had to discontinue using the cross-linked PE cup.

The clinical wear rate of the gamma-irradiated cross-linked PE cup decreased to 20% of the nonirradiated one on radiography, and on the retrieved cup, even 29 years after operation, there was no visible wear of the cup and all the bone-implant interfaces were well maintained. When the retrieved irradiated cup was observed with SEM, the weight-bearing lesion was very smooth. On the other hand, nonirradiated cups showed scratching, delamination, flaking, and a folding phenomenon.

The physical and chemical changes of retrieved samples were examined. High-dose gamma irradiation decreased tensile strength and elongation, but changes in characteristics over time did not differ between the retrieved samples and stored samples, and deterioration did not progress rapidly in the body. The degree of oxidation of a PE cup exposed to 100 Mrad was, after 18 years, only slightly higher than that of the surface of a nonirradiated PE cup after the same period of time. In other words, the oxidation of nonirradiated PE progressed rapidly. However, the oxidation of irradiated PE progressed very slowly. After a long period of use or storage, residual free radicals attributable to gamma-ray irradiation scarcely affected the progression of oxidation and deterioration.

A small-punch test for PE cups was performed by Kurtz [7]. By these tests, ductility, ultimate strength, and toughness can be characterized (Fig. 1). In this test, small test pieces (core diameter, 5–6 mm; thickness, 0.5 mm) were extracted from the surface, subsurface, and interior. A small-punch biaxial test was performed using these extracted small test pieces. Uniaxial tests (for example, tensile test) were inadequate over a large range of stress and strain on shape and the function of THP. The biaxial test is very sensitive to Mrad dose and aging.

Comparisons of biaxial mechanical strength in surface, subsurface, and interior of a retrieved 100-Mrad PE cup and 3-Mrad UHMWPE were performed, and the 100-Mrad PE cup showed tight distribution of mechanical strength. As a result, the 100-Mrad PE cup can be considered excellent in terms of both wear resistance and mechanical properties (Fig. 2).

FIG. 1a,b. Comparison of uniaxial (a) and biaxial (b) specimens. Core diameter, 5–6 mm; thickness, 0.5 mm

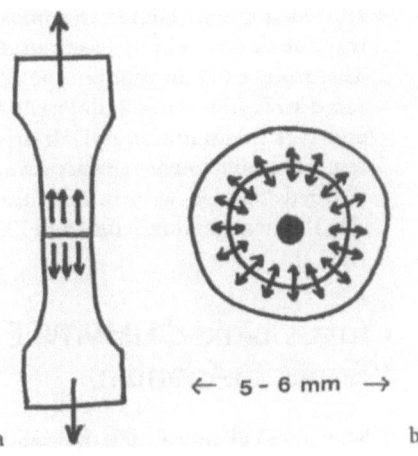

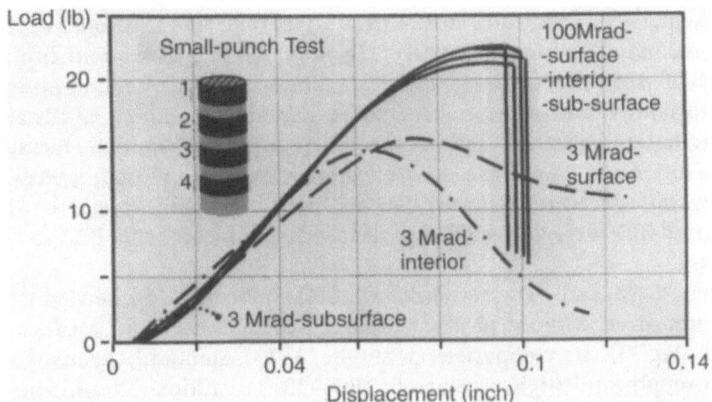

FIG. 2. Comparison of toughness of 3 Mrad and 100 Mrad retrieved polyethylene (PE) by small-punch test. 1, surface; 2, subsurface 1; 3, subsurface 2; 4, interior

Cross-Linked UHMWPE

Our recent wear test results of cross-linked PE with high-dose gamma irradiation are discussed next. For the contemporary gamma-irradiated PE THR, the molecular weight of UHMWPE has been changed from 10^6 to $5–6 \times 10^6$. The PE material and its processing evolved.

The objective of this study was to investigate the dose response of high-dose gamma radiation on the wear performance of UHMWPE in a hip simulator model [8–12]. The PE bar stock was gamma irradiated by 50, 100, or 150 Mrad in air and then annealed under vacuum at 110°C for 2h to remove free radicals. The bars were sectioned and machined to eliminate any surface "skin" effects. Three wear cups and three soak-control cups were used. The matching femoral heads were 26 mm Al_2O_3. This study used an orbital-type 12-station hip simulator with cam rotation synchronized with hip-joint loading. The Paul load profile was used with 2 kN peak loading and 0.2 kN minimum at 1-Hz frequency. The wear cups were mounted below the femoral heads to ensure adequate lubrication exposure with 30% bovine serum.

No detectable wear was demonstrated in the gamma-irradiated PE cups, and for the non-gamma-irradiated PE cups, the volumetric wear averaged 57.1 mm^3/Mc [11,12].

Cross-Linked UHMWPE Clinically Used at Present (Aeonian)

The physical properties of high-dose gamma-irradiated PE do not satisfy ASTM (American Society for Testing and Materials) and FDA (U.S. Food and Drug Administration) standards. Consequently, lower-dose gamma-irradiated PE has been used throughout the world.

At present, we use clinically cross-linked UHMWPE that is gamma irradiated with lower doses, named Aeonian (Kyocera, Kyoto, Japan). The Aeonian cup is made as follows. GUR-1050 sheet is irradiated with 4 Mrad in N_2 gas, and annealed at 110°C for 12 h to remove free radicals. The cup is made by machining and is sterilized by gamma radiation with 2.5 Mrad in N_2 gas. Consequently, Aeonian is irradiated with a total of 6.5 Mrad. When the dose of gamma rays was too high, tensile strength and elongation decreased. However, in the biaxial mechanical test, the "toughness" of 100-Mrad PE increased in comparison with nonirradiated PE after long-term clinical use.

For the ASTM and FDA standards of UHMWPE, it is desired that wear resistance is improved without physical property changes. Aeonian satisfies the ASTM standard (Fig. 3). In comparison with the ASTM standard, Aeonian has higher impact strength and higher values by 20%–30% in ultimate tensile strength and yield strength. In our wear study by hip simulator, Aeonian demonstrates a 97% reduction in PE wear (Fig. 4). Reduction of PE wear and no property change contributes to the long-term clinical result. However, because the creep deformity of lower-dose gamma-irradiated PE does not decrease, if a thinner PE cup is used, the wear rate will increase. Consequently, the thinner PE cup should not be used. Moreover, dramatic improvement in the wear of lower-dose gamma-irradiated PE has not been yet obtained from long-term clinical results but only obtained from hip simulator tests.

Because great improvement in wear and much higher toughness of high-dose gamma-irradiated PE (100 Mrad on RCH 1000) was found after long-term clinical use (Fig. 2), however, it could be assured that the optimum dose will exist at more than 20 Mrad. The toughness of nonirradiated PE decreased greatly after long-term clinical use. If the wear rate decreases to less than 10%, longevity of PE will be more than 100 years at least.

Aeonian is GUR 1050 that does not contain calcium stearate and is made by compression molding; its molecular weight is 6 million. The swell ratio is 15, which

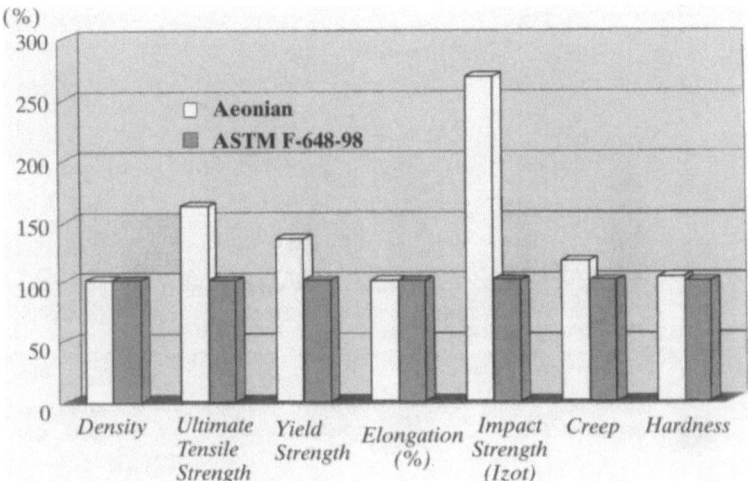

FIG. 3. Comparison of physical and chemical properties of Aeonian and ASTM (American Society for Testing and Materials) standard

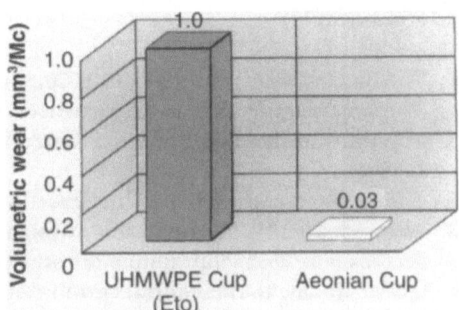

FIG. 4. Wear of Aeonian cup by hip simulator

is the lowest. Low swell ratios show increased cross-linking, and high swell ratios show lower levels of cross-linking. The swell ratio of ram extrusion is higher than that of compression molding. In consequence, compression molding is preferred to ram extrusion.

When PE is sterilized by gamma rays, even in nitrogen gas, oxidation and free radical formation are expected. However, from our long-term clinical results, we need not expect this because, the increment of oxidation in vivo was extremely low (Fig. 5).

Furthermore, we performed an aging test of oxidation on UHMWPE sterilized with 2.5 Mrad in N_2 gas and on Aeonian. The aging test was done in air at 80°C. As a result, the degree of oxidation was extremely low in both types of UHMWPE. Consequently, we need not expect oxidation in UHMWPE after sterilization with gamma rays in N_2 gas.

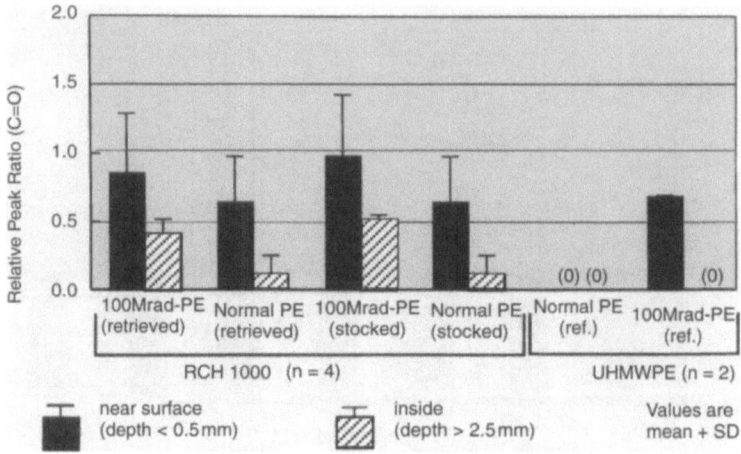

FIG. 5. Oxidation of RCH 1000 PE cup with 100 Mrad irradiation and without irradiation retrieved from patients as and stocked on the shelf. Oxidation was measured by FTIR (Fourier Transform Infrared Spectroscopy)

Conclusions

1. The clinical wear of PE (RCH 1000; molecular weight, 10^6) cups irradiated with 100 Mrad gamma rays in air decreased to 20%; after a long period of clinical use, physical and chemical properties scarcely changed and oxidation increased slightly in vivo.
2. The toughness of RCH 1000 increased when irradiated with 100 Mrad.
3. Wear of UHMWPE (molecular weight, $5-6 \times 10^6$) irradiated with 6.5 Mrad decreased to 3% by hip simulator test without deterioration of physical properties.
4. Oxidation due to free radicals produced by gamma-ray sterilization was extremely low.

References

1. Oonishi H, Igaki H, Takayama Y (1988) Wear resistance of gamma-ray irradiated UHMWPE socket in total hip prostheses: wear and long term clinical results. In: 3rd world biomaterials congress transactions, April 21–25, 1988, Kyoto, Japan, p 588
2. Oonishi H, Igaki H, Takayama Y (1989) Wear resistance of gamma-ray irradiated U.H.M.W. polyethylene socket in total hip prosthesis: wear test and long term clinical results. In: MRS international meeting on advanced materials, vol 1. Materials Research Society, Tokyo, pp 351–356
3. Oonishi H, Tsuji E (1990) SEM observation on the clinically used gamma-irradiated reinforced HDP socket in total hip replacement. In: Heimke G, Soltes Z, Lee AJC (eds) Clinical implant materials advances in biomaterials, vol 9. Elsevier, Amsterdam, pp 379–384
4. Oonishi H, Takayama Y, Tsuji E (1992) Improvement of polyethylene by irradiation in artrificial joints. Radiat Phys Chem 396:495–504

5. Oonishi H, Takayama Y, Tsuji E (1992) In vivo and in vitro wear behavior on weight-bearing surfaces of polyethylene sockets improved by irradiation in total hip prosthesis. Surf Modif Technol V:101–105

6. Oonishi H, Saito M, Kadoya Y (1998) Wear of high-dose gamma irradiated polyethylene in total joint replacement: long term radiological evaluation. In: 44th annual meeting, ORS, March 16–19, 1998, New Orleans, LA, USA, pp 97–17

7. Kurtz SM, Foulds JE, Jewett CW, et al (1998) Small punch test for characterization of aged UHMWPE after gamma-sterilization in air and nitrogen. In: 44th annual meeting, ORS, March 16–19, New Orleans, LA, USA, p 361

8. Oonishi H, Ishimaru H, Kato A (1996) Effect of cross-linkage by gamma irradiation in heavy doses to low wear polyethylene in total hip prostheses. J Mater Sci Mater Med 7:753–763

9. Oonishi H (1995) Clinical results of total hip prostheses in combination with an alumina head and a cross-linked UHMWPE socket (in Japanese). Orthop Surg Traumatol 38:1255–1264

10. Oonishi H, Kuno M, Tsuji E, et al (1997) The optimum dose of gamma irradiation: heavy doses to low wear polyethylene in total hip prostheses. J Mater Sci Mater Med 8:11–18

11. Clarke IC, Good V, Williams P, et al (1997) Simulator wear study of high dose gamma-irradiated UHMWPE cups. Trans Soc Biomater 20:71

12. Oonishi H, Clarke IC, Good V, et al (1999) Low wear effect of high-dose gamma-irradiated crosslinked polyethylene in total hip prostheses. In: Joint arthroplasty. Springer, Tokyo, pp 97–108

The Difficult Primary Total Hip Arthroplasty

TIE-LIANG ZHANG and JIAN-HUA YU

Summary. Between 1995 and 1999, 12 difficult primary total hip arthroplasties were performed on 7 patients (7 hips) with failed initial treatment of traumatic dislocation of the hip and 5 patients (5 hips) with untreated congenital dislocation of the hip. The arthroplasties were performed in the position of the true acetabulum in all patients who had either congenital or posttraumatic dislocation of the hip. After a mean follow-up of 24 months, 11 hips showed considerable improvement concerning pain, gait, and mobility based on Harris' score, except that 1 had sciatic nerve injury due to overlengthening of the limb. Although it is technically demanding and presents a difficult surgical problem, total hip arthroplasty is a reasonable treatment option and satisfactory solution for patients who present with either failed treatment of traumatic fracture and dislocation of the hip or painful neglected congenital dislocation of the hip.

Key words. Total hip arthroplasty, Traumatic dislocation of the hip, Congenital dislocation of the hip, True acetabulum, Acetabular fracture

Introduction

Total hip arthroplasty is an established surgical procedure for the treatment of many hip disorders and has broad indications. However, total hip arthroplasty in posttraumatic dislocation of the hip associated with deficiency of the acetabular rim and neglected congenital dislocation of the hip in adults still presents a difficult surgical problem. In posttraumatic dislocation, acetabular reconstruction can involve contained or segmental bone deficiencies or a combination. Central fracture dislocations of the hip can result in acetabular discontinuty and often are associated with a variety of bone defects. In congenital dislocation, there are many considerations related to specific anatomic pathology including excess narrowing of the medullary canal of the femur, excessive anteversion of the femoral neck, malorientation and dysplasia of the acetabulum, and soft tissue contractures. All of these can be challenging reconstructive problems. In this study, the authors present their preliminary experience in these difficult primary total hip arthroplasties.

Department of Orthopaedic Surgery and Traumatology, Tianjin Hospital, No. 406, Jie Fang Road, Tianjin, People's Republic of China

Materials and Method

From 1995 to 1999, 12 hips in 11 patients (7 men and 4 women) were subjected to total hip arthroplasty at The Department of Orthopaedic Surgery and Traumatology, Tianjin Hospital. The reasons for total hip arthroplasty were posttraumatic subluxation or dislocation in 7 patients (7 hips) and untreated congenital dislocation of the hip in 5 patients (5 hips). The ages of the patents at the surgery ranged from 30 to 50 years, with an average of 39.5 years.

In the posttraumatic subluxations or dislocations, three hips were associated with posterior wall fracture of the acetabulum, four with comminuted posterior wall fracture of the acetabulum; three patients received nonoperative treatment and four patients underwent initial operative treatment including open reduction and internal fixation with lag screws. The reasons for the secondary total hip arthroplasty were malunion in four hips and hardware failure in the other three hips. In congenital dislocation of the hip, two femoral heads still had some contact with the area of the true acetabulum, one was above the roof of the original acetabulum, and the other two were articulated with the wing of the ilium.

Preoperative plain radiographs were used for selection of acetabular and femoral component size and length. Conventional CT including three-dimensional reconstructions was used for assessment of bone loss in posttraumatic dislocations of the hip with acetabular fractures and for evaluation of the orientation of the femoral neck and the size and width of the true acetabulum in neglected congenital dislocations.

The Kocher–Langenbeck incision, which provides ample circumferential visulization of the peripheral acetabuar rim, was used in all the patients in this series. Patients were placed in the lateral position, and two padded posts were held against the anterior superior iliac and sacrum to maintain the patient perpendicular to the operative table so that the pelvic position could be assessed during placement of acetabular prostheses.

In congenital dislocation of the hip, the anterior wall of the acetabulum was generally thin but the posterior wall usually was thicker. When the acetabulum exposure was completed and the center of the true acetabulum was located, widening and deepening the narrow and shallow aceabulum should be started by reaming toward the posterior wall. Once the true acetabulum was prepared, a trial reduction was attempted to accurately assess the potential magnitude of reduction before the placement of the plastic socket. If the reduction was difficult or impossible, it could be facilitated by shortening of the femur by cutting the femoral neck at the upper limit of the lesser trochanter to prevent overlengthening of the limb.

In fracture dislocation of the hip, posterior structural rim defects were restored by use of an autogenous graft taken from the removed femoral head. Morselized cancellous graft was used for cavity-contained defects in the dome and medial wall of the acetabulum. When reconstruction of the superoposterior rim of acetabulum was employed, internal fixation with lag screws was routinely applied for structural graft fixation.

In this series, the resected femoral heads were applied as grafts in six hips for either acquired or developed deficiency in the upper and posterior wall of the acetabulum. A morselized cancellous graft was employed in three hips for defects in the dome and medial wall of the acetabulum. Shortening of the femur by cutting the femoral neck at the upper limit of the lesser trochanter was performed in two hips with higher congenital dislocations. Total or partial release of the iliopsoas tendon from the lesser trochanter was performed on one hip each to obtain reduction.

Results

The mean duration of follow-up was 24 months (range, 6–48 months). The Harris hip score system [1] was used to evaluate the clinical results. The Harris score improved from an average of 34.5 to 85 based on pain, function, and mobility. All the femoral heads were positioned from the false to the true acetabulum in congenital dislocation,, and the lengthening of the limbs ranged from 3 to 5 cm. Although the activities of some of these patients were still restricted postoperatively, all the patients regained their ambulatory ability and returned to a relatively normal lifestyle. There was no evidence of loosening on the radiographs at the final follow-up study. One patient, who had a high congenital dislocation of the hip and was the first case of this series, developed sciatic nerve paralysis resulting from overlengthening of the limb. After the acetabulum and femur had been routinely prepared and the trial components been implanted, the reduction was found rather difficult and total release of the iliopsoas tendon from the lesser trochanter was performed. The lengthening of the limb in this patient was as much as 5 cm. The patient recovered from the sciatic nerve symptoms in 6 months, except for weakness of dorsum flexion of the toe.

Case Reports

Case 1

A 42-year-old man with an acetabular fracture had undergone open reduction and internal fixation in a rural hospital 2 years earlier. The preoperative radiographs showed malreduction and delayed union of the fracture with a bone defect in the posterior rim of the acetabulum (Fig. 1). Reconstruction of the acetabulum with the resected femoral head was performed during the surgery and stabilized by two lag screws. For the poor bone stock in the acetabular side, a cemented acetabular component and cementless stem were used for replacement (Fig. 2). The patient regained his ambulatory ability in 8 weeks without pain or inequality of the lower limbs. This total hip replacement produced excellent results.

Case 2

A 45-year-old woman had high congenital dislocation of the hip. Preoperative radiographs showed that the femoral head was completely dislocated and articulated with the wing of the ilium (Fig. 3). Total hip replacement with a cementless acetabular component and cemented femoral component was performed. The femoral head was positioned down from the false to the true acetabulum. Instead of soft tissue release, the femoral neck was shortened by bone cutting at the level of the lesser trochanter to obtain reduction (Fig. 4). The limb was eventually lengthened about 4 cm, and the patient has had excellent functional results.

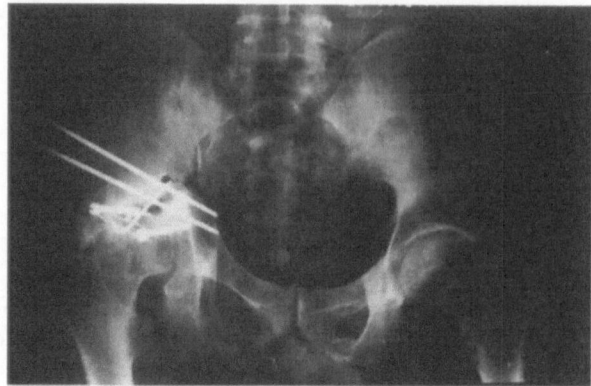

FIG. 1. Malreduced and delayed union of acetabular fracture with a bone defect of the acetabular rim

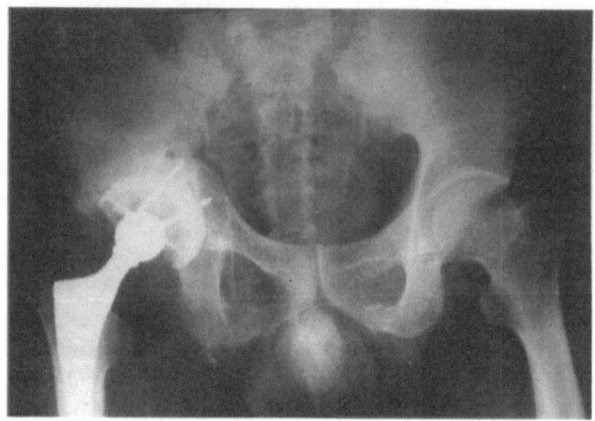

FIG. 2. Total hip arthroplasty with a cemented acetabular component and cementless femoral component was performed. A bone graft using resected femoral head was done and stabilized with two screws to reconstruct the acetabular defects

FIG. 3. High congenital dislocation of the hip. The femoral head is articulated with the iliac wing

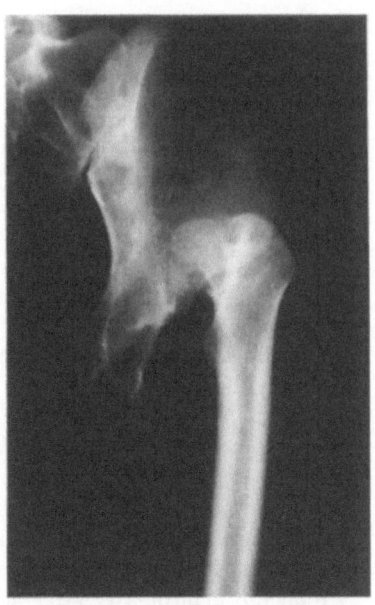

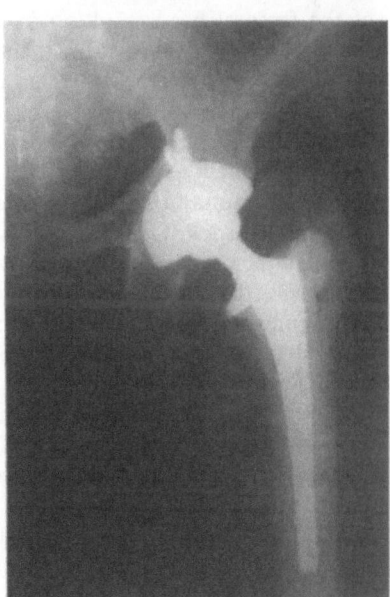

FIG. 4. Hybrid total hip arthroplasty was performed after shortening of the femoral neck by bone cutting at the level of the lesser trochanter

Discussion

As experience with routine total hip arthroplasty has increased, surgeons have become enthusiastic about reconstructing joints that have abnormalities in the proximal femur and acetabulum secondary to development and congenital or posttraumatic disorders. Although it is technically demanding, total hip arthroplasty is currently considered a reasonable treatment option and satisfactory solution for patients who present with either symptomatic posttraumatic arthritis of the hip, subluxation or dislocation of the hip following acetabular fracture, or painful neglected congenital dislocation of the hip [2].

The choice of surgical approach in posttraumatic dislocation of the hip depends on many factors including the previous treatment approach and the need to remove metal implants. However, the Kocher–Langenbeck exposure is sufficient in most instances in which the posterior hardware requires removal. When a previous posterior approach to the hip has been employed, it is critical to document the past history and present state of the sciatic nerve as part of the preoperative plan, and the sciatic nerve should be routinely identified and carefuly protected during the arthroplasty [3].

Total hip arthroplasty after acetabular fracture is most commonly indicated in patients with symptomatic posttraumatic arthritis and dislocation or subluxation of the femoral head resulting from failed initial osteosynthesis for restoration of function and relief of pain [4]. Total hip arthroplasty has an important role in the management of acetabular fractures in late reconstruction following failed non-operative or operative treatment with symptomatic posttraumatic arthritis, avascular necrosis of the femoral head, nonunion, or malunion. Because of the technical difficulties of achieving stability of the acetabular component, initial management of an acetabular fracture with primary total hip arthroplasty is rarely indicated. In general, total hip arthroplasty should be reserved for the late salvage of hips in which initial treatment of the acetabular fracture has failed.

In neglected congenital dislocation of the hip, the true acetabulum is usually too narrow and atrophic, and the proximal femur has an increased anteversion and narrow femoral canal. Transposition of the femoral head down from the false to the true acetabulum is a relatively risky procedure and presents a difficult surgical problem. However, an increased number of studies agree that arthroplasty should be done in the position of the true actetabulum for several reasons. First, the iliac bone at the level of the false acetabulum is very thin and cannot support the cup of the prosthesis. Furthermore, the abductor muscles of the hip in this position are lax and insufficient, resulting in a Trendelenburg sign. Finally, the leg length discrepancy would remain unchanged and cause limping and back pain [5]. Nevertheless, overlengthening of the leg resulting from reduction of the femoral head from the false to the true acetabulum may cause stretching of the sciatic nerve and lead to sciatic nerve paralysis. Dunn and Hess advocated that the lengthening of the leg to 7–8 cm did not lead to nerve injuries [6]. In this series, however, the lengthening of 5 cm actually caused the sciatic nerve injury; this may due to the difference between Asians and Occidentals in stature.

In our opinion, there is no indication to attempt to release the iliopsoas tendon from the lesser trochanter and medial gluteus to achieve reduction. The tension of the iliopsoas tendon and medial gluteus has an important role in prevention of excessive stretching of the sciatic nerve during the reduction. If lengthening of the leg is estimated to be more than 4 cm during trial reduction, an bone cutting at the level of the lesser trochanter or removing bone from the superior wall of the true acetabulum by reaming should be performed. If the reduction is extremely difficult, only in this circumstance can the transposition of the femoral head to true acetabulum be achieved without a risk of sciatic nerve injury. It is often necessary to remove a segment of bone at the level of the lesser trochanter instead of releasing the iliopsoas tendon from the lesser trochanter to obtain reduction.

Component selection is at the discretion of the surgeon. If possible, the authors generally prefer to use a noncemented acetabular and a cemented femoral component for the patients in this series who are relatively young and at a higher level of activity. In congenital dislocation of the hip, a small straight femoral component should be selected because the femoral canal usually is narrow.

References

1. Harris WH, Crothers O, Oh I (1977) Total hip replacement and femoral head bone grafting for severe acetabular deficiency in adults. J Bone Joint Surg 59A:752–759
2. Border LS, Greenky SS (1991) The difficult primary total hip replacement: acetabular problems. In: Steinberg ME (ed) The hip and its disorders. Saunders, Philadelphia, pp 1007–1018
3. Jimenez MJ, Tile M, Schenk RS (1997) Total hip replacement after acetabular fracture. Orthop Clin North Am 28:435–446
4. Romaness DW, Lewallen DG (1990) Total hip arthroplasty after fracture of the acetabulum. J Bone Joint Surg 72B:761
5. Symeonides P, Pournaras J, Petsatodes G, et al (1997) Total hip arthroplasty in neglected congenital dislocation of the hip. Clin Orthop 341:55–61
6. Dunn HK, Hess WE (1976) Total hip reconstruction in chronically dislocated hips. J Bone Joint Surg 58A:838–845

A Radiographic Study of Noncemented Femoral Implants

Jean-Alain Epinette

Summary. Any artificial joint deeply modifies the nature of bony metabolism and its biomechanical behavior. Noncemented implants cause the host bone to be in direct relationship with the metallic content: over years, radiographic changes will occur, related to often poorly known principles. This study presents the results of 136 HA-coated Omnifit stems of which 58 stems could be assessed clinically and radiologically with a minimum of 10-year+ follow-up. Based upon this particular study, we were happy to confirm that proximal fixation was assured as the result of the bioactive coating. The final conclusion concerned the lack of lesser results over years as the Engh score was 17.1 at 2 years and up to 19.4 at 10 years. Of this global score, fixation was 6.7 at 2 years, up to 7.9 at 10 years, and stability was 10.4 at 2 years, up to 11.4 at 10 years. In such a way, 100% of the cases in this series had a "bony ingrowth confirmed." The problem, then, is determining, for some of the bony patterns, if it is a matter of a normal simple biomechanical adaptation to the bony physiology or whether these patterns are forerunners of a prosthetic failure.

Key words. Hydroxyapatite, Omnifit stem, Total hip replacement, Radiographic patterns, Engh's classification

Introduction

Bone is a living structure. From the time implants are no longer embedded in a cement mold, there is a closer bone–implant contact, and they begin to respond directly to the fixation requirements where the flexible bone is fitted onto a stiff implant. The type of implant, of course, but also the femoral anatomic shape—with its axes, flexibility, curves, and spongy cortical components—as well as the age of the subject, their functional performance, and the pathological aspect necessitating a prosthetic replacement, all contribute to the number of elements to be considered toward the long-term success or failure of arthroplasties [1].

The different phases of this successful or unsuccessful fixation onto the implant in relation to the host bone can only be closely studied through X-rays. Data from the

Orthopaedic Surgery, Clinique Medico-Chirurgicale, 62700 Bruay-Labuissière, France

X-ray studies very often precede clinical data, and they certainly give the most convincing prognosis. Although you still have the task of deciphering the radiographic patterns correctly and differentiating simple bony reactions, which are the result of successful biomechanical anchorage leading to a lasting fit, from other patterns that could represent the forerunners of the next prosthetic failure. It would be of great help if we had a score that can be assessed quickly, simply, and reliably so as to follow up our implants efficiently.

Great merit is attributed to Charles Engh and Philippe Massin for having differentiated "noncemented" implants for the first time with radiographic findings [2]. It was mainly a matter of proving that there is some reality in fitting back in a bony structure. Their works mainly entail a systematized comparison of histological data of retrieved implants in relation to their radiographic findings. As for femoral components, they were able to define a certain number of criteria relating to direct or indirect modifications linked to the reaction of the bone–implant couple. These fundamental works have paved the way for new knowledge of radiographic signs for implants that are directly embedded in a host bone and have helped us to better understand this prosthetic implantation.

The analysis of the numerical score by Engh, in his mind, comprises an anatomopathological diagnostic essay using radiographic pictures. A complementary approach could be proposed whereby a monitored X-ray of any other noncemented prosthetic type is viewed (with or without hydroxyapatite [HA]), defining the fixation criteria of the bone in relation to the prosthetic stem, whether it is derogatory or not. The result of such a process would help us to come up with a perfect fit, guaranteeing an ideal prognosis or guaranteeing a movement of all the intermediates toward signs of a failure in the coexistence of the bone–implant, which would lead in a rather long term to a clinical failure. In the long run, it would amount to the radiographic rendering of the compensated or uncompensated "neutral status" theory offered by Schneider and the Swiss School almost 20 years ago [3].

Material and Methods

Our experience of approximately 5000 noncemented prosthetic stems has a history of 15 years, with a systematized radioclinical comparison of results that were first obtained from "porous" implants (microstructured titanium, macrostructures, porous coating, and also fibermesh). Then, from 1986, these were followed by implants with a hydroxyapatite (HA) coating [5]. The often too unreliable results obtained from our first "porous" models led us to a high percentage of revisions and gave us important anatomic findings that helped us to better understand our failures. Ever since implantations have been done with bioactive implants, a computerized analysis of radiographic data has been followed up under the aegis of the Orthopaedic Research and Imaging Center in Arthroplasties (CRDA) located in Bruay, North France. The present study reports the results of 134 HA-coated Omnifit stems (Osteonics, Allendale, NJ, USA) implanted by the author at the Clinic of Bruay-Labuissière, France, from May 1987 to December 1988. Of this number, 26 were dead of an unrelated cause, 30 were unable to attend a clinical examination at the doctor's office and had a phone interview, 14 could not undergo a clinical assessment due to another significant disabling

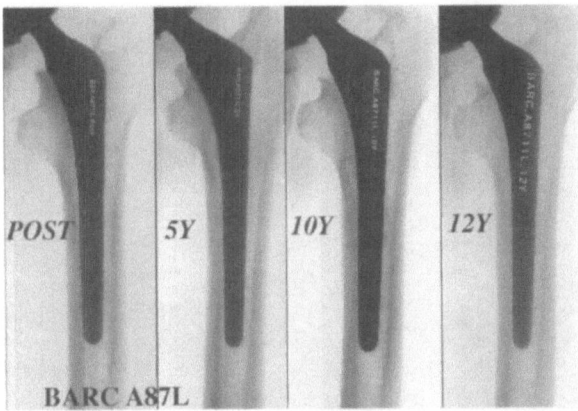

FIG. 1. Typical radiographic follow-up at 12 years shows excellent long-lasting fixation. Y, years

problem, 2 were lost to follow-up, 4 were revision cases, and finally 58 stems could be assessed clinically and radiologically with a minimum of 10-year+ follow-up.

Clinical data and related X-rays are systematically recorded as a prospective study in our outcomes studies software, called OrthoWave, which allows us to store at the same time data, clinical scores, radiological assessments, and digitized films (usually preop, postop, and further at 2, 5, 7, 10, and 12 years) dedicated to a specific patient (Fig. 1). A statistical modulus, StatWave, provides us with statistics. An image cataloger, Call Image, makes global radiographic study powerful and easy to use [4].

Description of Radiographic Patterns

We would like to make precise definitions of each radiographic pattern to help with better understanding of results and to make clear discussion regarding the evolution of X-ray findings over 10 years and thus the explanations that should be given. The description of the different evaluating parameters regarding different zones of the femur are in keeping with the rules set down by Gruen, whereby he divides 14 zones into sectors, 7 of which consider front views and the other 7 profile effects [6].

Reactive Lines Versus Lucencies

The reactive lines, as described by Engh, are distinctly different from lucent lines. As we understand it, a lucent line is a clear bordering line adjoining either the stem or the cement, with a rather large gap (1, 2, or 3 mm or more) on the metal–cement or the cement–bone interface or even on the metal–bone interface. This gap, which is filled with connective tissue, is still a sign of loosening and a break-up in contact on that interface. It is still a derogative sign. The reactive line, on the other hand, is defined as a thin compact line separated from the metal part of the implant by approximately 1 mm, with a bony tone that is identical on both sides of the ossification line or the endosteal sclerosis (Fig. 2). The explanation varies

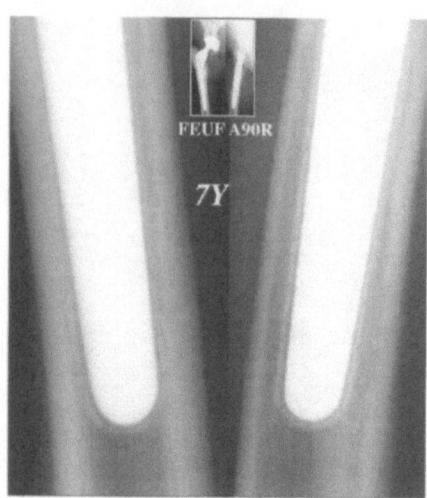

FIG. 2. Typical reactive line onto noncoated areas at the midpart of the stem

according to its location, but it always corresponds to a necessary fit between the stem and the flexibility of the bone, without having to transfer the bone–implant directly from the constraint lines [7]. There is no gap on the metal interface, as is the case with lucent lines.

The presence of this reactive line coming into contact with a surface where a fixation is supposedly possible is still derogative because it causes an absence of cohesiveness between this prosthetic part and the adjoining bony segment, whereby a harmonious rendering of the lines of force is nonexistent at this stage. Nevertheless, finding them in contact with the "smooth" parts of the implant is quite normal. The presence or absence of these lines in zones where fixation is not possible depends mainly on the shape of the medullary canal and how the stem fits, as well as the flexibility gradient of the femoral shaft, which differs according to the individual as regards their age and morphotype.

We have seen a particular case in which the reactive sclerosis line was observed at the upper part of the back of the stem and at the top end of zone 1. This line starts at the back of the stem, about 2 mm away from the upper rear angle, and a curve is drawn up to the beginning of the cervix of the greater trochanter. We understood it to be a common reaction to the flexibility of the greater trochanter "towed" by the muscular gluteal fan, and therefore leading a flexible gradient away from the constraint lines that come from the underlying femoral shaft. This reaction takes place frequently and is not a derogative sign for us. However, it can mean the beginning of osteolytic-type modifications that demand a special kind of monitoring (Fig. 3).

Endosteal Bone Formation

This sign was described by Engh as the "bony bridges" and the "spots welds." These are zones where there are spot welds and bony bridges, leaving a space between the metal and the cortical periphery. The explanation is subject to discussion, but we may understand that it involves an effort made by the bone at that stage to fit itself and to

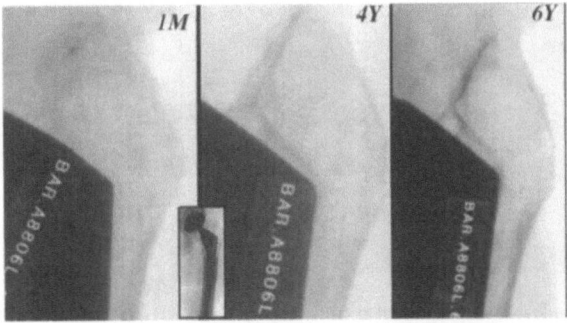

FIG. 3. Reactive line onto zone 1A may lead to osteolytic cysts over the years

encourage the stability of the implant by creating a hard endosteal bone where the soft spongy bone is usually present.

We have encountered these formations regularly just under the HA coating zone, at the very beginning of the smooth part, where there is a tendency to expand distally by a "flow," thus hardening the bony segment (bony densification). These spots hardly stand out at the lowest part of the HA coating and never stand out at the top part where the transfer of the lines of force is carried out preferentially. This fact leads us to believe that these ossifications do not materialize the transfer of constraints, but on the other hand materialize a difference in flexibility that the bone tries to compensate by becoming harder. We have sometimes encountered these ossifications with a stemlike point, and they respond to the same process on the nosological border with the pedestal sign.

These endosteal bone formations are not initially of a prognostic nature, neither beneficial nor derogative. Their presence generally depends on the distance that separates the cortical bone from the metallic implant and also on the flexible or hard nature of the bony structures. If these reactions seemed favorable to Engh because they marked an osteocondensation induced by the porous coating, we will identify them as being a "neutral" accompanying sign, except when they are isolated in zone 4. In that case, it can be considered a test for the femoral shaft to be stabilized distally, which proves to be derogative because it is contrary to the principle of the proximal stabilization of the implants whose top third part is coated.

Pedestal

This sign is extremely important because it explains perfectly the reaction of the femur in relation to the stem at the crucial spot where there is a distal transition of the "bone bearing" and "implant" and the "free bone." Let us remind ourselves that Engh described the pedestals as dense ossification zones adjoining the tip of the stem, with a tone that is identical to the cortical bone, having a sharp edge like the bottom of an egg cup turned upside-down, which explains how it got its name (Fig. 4a). The pedestal is said to be "stable" if the bony condensation is in direct contact with the metal from the distal part of the stem; it is said to be "unstable" if the pedestal is separated from the stem by a lucent line (Fig. 4b).

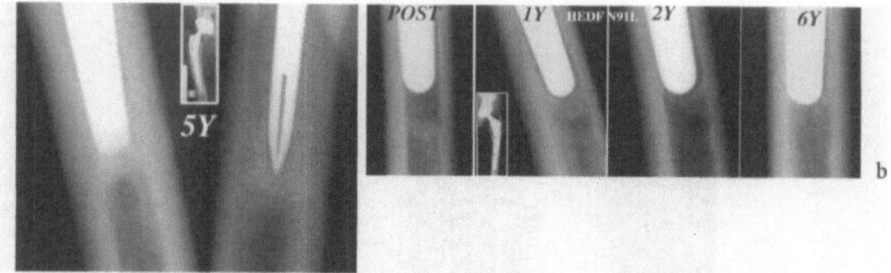

FIG. 4. **a** Stable pedestal at the tip of a noncemented non-HA-coated stem, indicating a distal fixation. **b** Temporary unstable pedestal at 1 year in a very active young woman, having undergone a HA Omnifit stem. Thanks to a secondary stable proximal HA fixation, this pedestal surprisingly disappears at 2 years, with a satisfactory result at 6 years. HA, hydroxyapatite

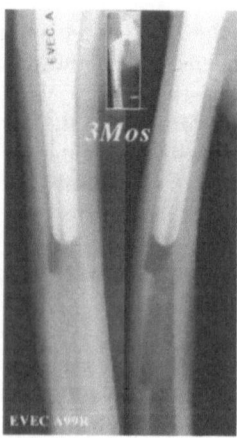

FIG. 5. Endosteal bony formation as a "healing" of the reaming procedure. This specific pattern is not to be confused with a pedestal

The presence of a pedestal always explains an accepted (stable pedestal) or insufficient (unstable pedestal) distal fixation. We encounter these almost systematically in all our noncemented stems without hydroxyapatite, and we have considered that as being the best sign of failure of proximal stabilization because this pedestal is generally associated with a line of widespread sclerosis, lining at least the proximal part and sometimes the whole part.

The main problem is differentiating the pedestal, which is derogative as a rule in the case of proximal fixation, from an endosteal ossification with a stemlike point or even from a simple "healing" of the distal abrasion caused by reaming (Fig. 5). We believe that a real pedestal should have a sharp edge with an adjoining bone. "Hemipedestals" would carry the same definition, operating as half the bottom of an egg cup between one of the lateral parts of the tip of the stem with the corresponding part of the endomedullary cortex, which is often closer than the diametrically opposite cortex.

Periosteal Bone Reactions

Many interpretations have been rendered concerning the diaphyseal remodeling of the bony segment bearing an implant for rather a long period of time. It concerns the remodeling of the cortex without periostitis or without a reaction from the adjoining nonrigid parts. Making it stand out is sometimes difficult because there are different rotations on different films displaying an oval-shaped femur with uneven cortical walls, calling for a close, comparative study. True "thickening of the cortex" in reality is very easily recognized because very often in the second year a "bumpy" steady arching appears, thus breaking the continuity of the whole curve on the femur, and progressively requiring constant checks. The explanation has for a long time been derogative, and we may believe that it is a process provoking an irritation of the bone as a reaction to the metallic contact of the prosthetic edge of the stem, which could be the cause of the well-known "thigh pains."

Our experience throughout the years has led us to offer a different interpretation, which will need to be corroborated by statistical research covering a long period of time.

It is not a question of an "irritative" reaction of the bone when it comes into contact with the stem. These remodelings are indeed found in the absence of a bone–cortex contact, and on the other hand, it is exceptional to encounter such a remodeling in the presence of a bone–metal contact, except in zone 3, which we discuss later because this is a specific zone.

These periosteal bone reactions are encountered in 25%–30% of the cases, preferentially in zone 5 (Fig. 6).

We were never confronted with thigh pains, either spontaneous or provoked by palpation. We consider these remodelings as having an additional fixation sign of the carrier bone to its new biomechanical conditions of a bone bearing an implant, according to a similar condition where there is remodeling of a bony postfracture healing. They appear around the second year, which corresponds to the time when

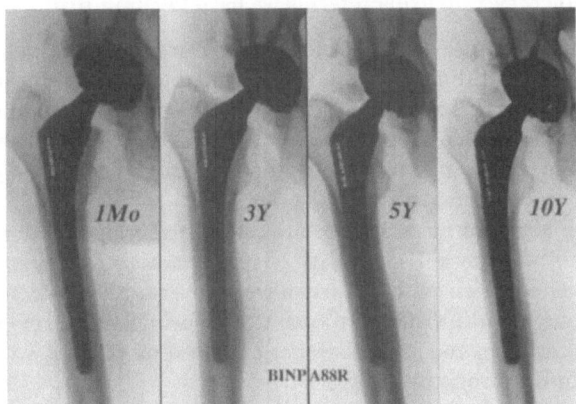

Fig. 6. Remodeling over years onto zone 5 of a HA-coated stem as a typical "cortical thickening"

the flexibility of the bone begins to recuperate after the "sideration" phase following the prosthetic implantation. These remodelings develop over a period of 1–2 years before stabilizing. Throughout the years we have not observed, in a precise way, a ceding of the remodeling zones that appear to have been definitely acquired, but this phenomenon calls for specific and more complete research to be done at a later date.

There is a particular case of cortical thickening being isolated in zone 3. In the light of our experience, it concerns the start of loosening due to a varus tilt, compared with the cortical contact, and being accompanied by contemporary or preceding, by a few months, real thigh pain. In developed cases, we encounter not a hypertrophy but rather a calcar atrophy: all the stems that bear this sign had to be taken out eventually because of pain and instability. Conversely, we could consider the isolated cortical thickening in zone 5 as a "neutral" sign of a simple fixation to the constraints from the pressure of the inner femoral walls. However, the overall or circular remodeling show a great bony fixation reaction and could constitute the beginning of a warning sign. From our experience with porous or HA implants, cortical remodeling isolated in zone 3 is nevertheless still derogative and can be the beginning of a varus loosening and thigh pains.

Calcar Remodeling: Resorption Versus Hypertrophy

The calcar is a very distinctive surgical zone because it is located at the upper inner end of the bony femur, where the bony structure continues with the inner part of the prosthetic cervix. Modifications brought to the structure and to the bone system at this stage have stirred up a number of controversies. In fact, this zone, destined for the femur that does not bear an implant, corresponds to the preferential axis passage of the lines of force, from the diaphyseal shaft to the acetabular zone. The substitution by a prosthetic stem cervix will cause major modifications in the distribution of the lines of force and partly in the calcar zone, according to the laws of Wolf.

Whether or not we agree with the collar supporting itself on the calcar at the bottom of the prosthetic cervix, in general terms we have to admit that:

A partial atrophy means a "bypass" of the constraint lines coming directly from the metaphyseal zone of the stem in the pelvis, via the prosthetic cervix. Some people refer to it as internal "stress shielding," which is correct in a biomechanical sense, but without the derogative connotation of stress shielding related to the greater trochanter. Engh makes a favorable sign of the proximal fixation of the prosthetic stem with a moderate atrophy of the calcar.

However, a major atrophy has always been a rather strong sign of overturn of the varus stem, the bony atrophy corresponding to real osteolysis resulting from excess constraint. We generally encounter it when we go over cases of old stems, with a fixation that is clearly insufficient, in a context of associations, atrophy of the calcar remodeling cortex in zone 3, a chamber of dorsal mobilization (cemented stems) and with a rather strong unsealing.

Special mention must be made of the small atrophies "dripping," so-called scalloping of the calcar (Fig. 7), at the point where the metal from the inner zone of the stem and the upper inner end of the calcar meet. We generally encounter this after 3 to

FIG. 7. Scalloping of the calcar in a bilateral case at 5 years as a reaction to polyethylene (PE) debris

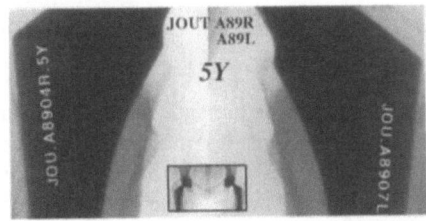

4 years, and we believe that these small osteolysis zones must be related to the wearing-away remains of the polyethylene that are deposited on the lowest part of the joint space.

On the whole, the remodeling of the calcar mainly depends on the type of fixation used to fit the stem into the femoral shaft, which will influence the method of transfer of loads to its upper level. The parameters would be therefore the conformation of the canal (cylindrical or in funnel form), the presence or absence of a collar, the type of proximal or distal fixation, and above all whether the prosthetic stem is correctly stabilized. A considerable atrophy or, on a higher level, a hypertrophy, could be a forerunner of a prosthetic failure.

The "dripping" osteolysis of the calcar, which is the usual scalloping spoken of by North American authors, is to be included in the osteolysis and cavitation setting, and also forms a derogative sign that could eventually open the door to widespread granulomas resulting from remains (PE, metal, or other).

Bony Osteolysis (Lysis), Cavitation, and Widespread Granulomas

If we except septic osteolyses, the widespread endocanal osteolyses correspond to granulomas whose origins are commonly related to macrophagic inflammatory reactions, following the resorption of cement or polyethylene particles or even of both. We evoked this possibility during our calcar study. Some publications reporting the shedding of apatite cristal particles are right now of no interest, because the observations made in these reports took only a very limited number of observations into consideration, and could assume either the implant being badly sustained with a certain loosening and the creating of tearing-away forces at the surface, or a poor initial coating.

One may differentiate proximal progressive lysis, which may be called "creeping osteolysis" on the one hand, located at the proximal aspect of the femur, and the distal osteolysis on the other hand, in which may be assumed a pathway for debris through a fibrous layer all around the stem. These osteolyses always have a natural derogative nature, and we should differentiate the moderate stable cavitations and the widespread extensive or multifocal osteolyses. Anyway, osteolysis remains an enigma, as particles are not only to be taken into account. New means of development for osteolysis are currently being studied, as the lytic bony response to some kinases belonging to the joint fluid, or different levels of personal ability to set up or not a lytic reaction against particle shedding.

The Loss of Bone Density in the Greater Trochanter (Stress Shielding)

The loss of bone density in the greater trochanter is a symptom that has become very common because it concerns long uncemented stems in press fit with porous metal (of the Lord or Judet type). For these prosthetic types there is a preferential transfer of the lines of force directly from the femoral diaphysis to the level of the femoral component, and even through there, there is a shunt of the entire upper metaphyseal part, mainly affecting the greater trochanter area. The opposite pictures of osteoporosis that came with a thinning-out of the cortical walls were common for madreporic implants of the Judet or Lord type. We have never encountered them in our implants with hydroxyapatite coating with a metaphyseal fixation.

Even the question of this sign's validity is subject to controversy, and the problem is finding out if this "stress shielding" is only an accompanying sign not having any real clinical value, and especially when painless, or if on the other hand it shows a failure in the mutual relationship between the carrier bone and the prosthetic stem that can later lead to the failure of arthroplasties. In any case, apart from the developed caricatural pictures, the very basis for the loss of bone density in the upper metaphyseal area still remains difficult to diagnose on standard radiographic negatives. The development of densitometric methods (DEXA, etc.) should enable us to have a more precise analysis and better knowledge of this type of bony reaction.

Results

The main radiographic schemes regarding HA-coated stems and host femoral bone were studied based upon 58 cases operated on in 1987 and 1988 in which we obtained complete radiographic follow-up with a minimum of 10 years.

1. Calcar atrophy: In 64% of cases, the calcar zone did not experience any atrophy whereas 30% was moderate and 6% was marked. We had no hypertrophy in this series. Engh considered a moderate atrophy as a good sign of proximal fixation and some stress shielding in the calcar zone. Perhaps we have to consider that HA proximate coated stems may provide an optimal transfer of force at the proximal aspect of the femur without any change in more than 60% of cases. Conversely, we had no hypertrophy and certainly no distal fixation with this stem, which should confirm the success of proximal fixation. We certainly must pay attention to the neck angle of the femur: a valgus in this neck may lead to more important forces being transmitted to this calcar zone.

2. Lines onto the HA-coated aspect of femur: We had no lines in 43% of cases. A reactive line was observed in 57% of cases onto zone 1A and as the greater trochanter. We had no cases of reactive line onto any other HA-coated zone and additionally no case of lucent line anywhere in this area. We demonstrated that it is normal to have no line onto coated zones except in zone 1A, and we suggest this reactive line is following a conflict of elasticity between the greater trochanter and the shaft itself. This reactive line must be taken into consideration because it can be a gateway for osteolysis, and we had several cases of limited lyses down the previous reactive line.

3. Lines onto noncoated zones: These findings were very interesting to point out over the years. During the first years of follow-up postoperatively, we had more than two-thirds of reactive lines onto noncoated zones. At 10 years+, 69% of cases did not show any reactive line; only 19% had lines under 50% and 12% had lines over 50%. No case showed any lucent line. We may explain this phenomenon if we consider that reactive lines onto noncoated zones are the witness of a conflict of elasticity between the elastic bone and the rigid metallic stem. That idea may explain that, at the beginning, we had a majority of reactive lines. Over the years, the shaft becomes more rigid, and we can point out an endosteal ossification filling down the medullary canal progressively starting from the upper part of noncoated zones onto zones 2 and 6. This endosteal ossification takes place around the stem, and thus the reactive line disappears. This result may suggest that in such a way a long-lasting fixation can be ensured.

4. Cortical thickening: We discussed this radiographic change, and we may address these patterns as a reaction of bone facing strength and stretching forces. We had no cortical thickening in 38% of cases, an isolated cortical thickening onto zone 5 in 45%, a circular napkin-ring cortical thickening in 15% of cases, and finally 2% of cases onto zone 3. We may consider that the cases without any cortical thickening belong to a rigid femur or nonactive older patients. Conversely, isolated cortical thickening onto zone 5 has to be considered as a normal reaction, especially in heavy patients or elastic bones. We have no clear explanation for circumferential napkin-ring cortical thickening; maybe there are some difficulties for bone to adapt its transfer of load around the stem. Finally, the unique case of cortical thickening onto zone 3 had neither thigh pain nor abnormal patterns at the proximal aspect, especially neither line nor cortical hypertrophy or severe atrophy. We must remain cautious on this case, despite the clinical results, which remain so far excellent. Once again we confirm that there was no significant relationship between a cortical thickening and any metallic contact at the tip of the stem.

5. Changes at tip: This pattern was considered as a critical pattern by Engh. As a matter of fact, we must take care for the right description of this distal ossification. We often saw this endosteal ossification filling down the shaft and reaching the tip of the stem (Fig. 8). In such a way, bone formation is irregular and is not to be confused with the clearly defined limits of the pedestal. Based upon our 10-year+ study, no tip experienced any change in 34% of cases defined as "mute tips." Endosteal ossification was reported in 60% of cases, whereas a stable pedestal can be addressed in 6% of cases. We had no unstable pedestal in this series. We have to confirm that the 6% of stable pedestals had no other significant abnormal pattern and the clinical results are good. Theoretically, this stable pedestal proves a distal fixation without any proximal fixation. In our cases, proximal fixation was assured in this case, and we had no explanation for this specific change at the tip.

6. Osteolysis: Osteolysis is certainly the most critical concern in radiographic analysis. We were happy to confirm in this HA series that no femoral lysis was evidenced in 50% of cases. A limited osteolysis onto the calcar zone, described as "scalloping," was shown in 28% of cases. In an additional 22% of cases, this osteolysis was more important all around the proximal part of stem and may later on cause problems of fixation (Fig. 9). Conversely, 0% of distal lysis was observed. In all these cases of proximal lysis, the clear area filled by fibrous tissue was surrounded by a very dense

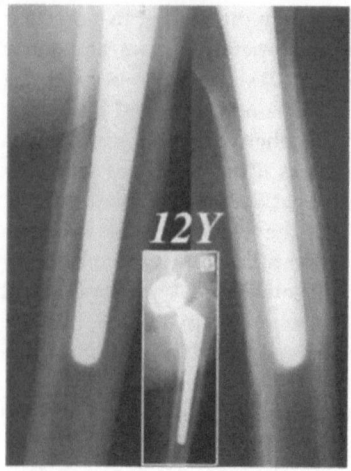

FIG. 8. Endosteal ossification filling down the medullary canal over years and reaching the tip of the stem at 12 years. This bone remodeling often replaces the preexisting reactive line

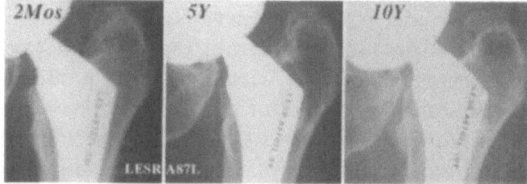

FIG. 9. Severe proximal osteolysis at 10 years that may make the stem become loose with time. We expect that ceramic/ceramic bearing surfaces will decrease the rate of these lytic lesions

bony formation, and we could confirm the seal provided by an intimate contact between bone and metal resulting from the bioactive interface.

In a further study, we will make systematic comparison between the wearing of the polyethylene liner and osteolysis. To date, we have had no significant relationship between these two phenomenona and we may suggest, as do other authors, that the lytic reaction to polyethylene debris is very different according to different types of patients. Nevertheless, these figures may confirm that polyethylene wear remains a very great problem and may lead to extensive lytic reactions and a potential loosening of the stem. We started 2 years ago using ceramic-on-ceramic bearing surfaces, and comparison between lytic lesions in the polyethylene group versus the ceramic group over the years will be of major interest.

Conclusion

Systematic studies of the radiographic scheme at 10 years of follow-up in noncemented stems are fruitful and may help us to a better understanding of the behavior of bone over years when a metallic stem has been inserted. Some patterns are not clearly defined, and we have many difficulties to address: some specific reactions considering the tremendous number of parameters related to the stem itself, the shape of femur, the quality of bone, and the patient themselves. We remain certain that a better knowledge of radiographic schemes will assure a better knowledge of success or failure in prosthetic replacement. Further studies are to be carried out, and thus we must consider radiographic analysis as fundamental [3].

Based upon this particular study, we were happy to confirm that proximal fixation was assured by means of bioactive coating. We must pay attention to endosteal ossification, and we will have to confirm this scheme regarding the elasticity of bone. Some additional biomechanical studies are suggested. Finally, the main problem for long-lasting good results in femoral fixation belongs to cup and not stem as regards osteolysis caused by polyethylene debris. Perhaps new bearing surfaces will solve this potential disaster. The final conclusion was about the lack of lower results over years as the Engh score was 17.1 ± 4.0 at 2 years and up to 19.4 ± 4.0 at 10 years. Of this global score, fixation was 6.7 at 2 years, up to 7.9 at 10 years, and stability was 10.4 at 2 years, up to 11.4 at 10 years. In such a way, 100% of cases in this series had a "bony ingrowth confirmed."

Whatever the case may be, and whatever the method of evaluation used, we need to be very alert and attentive to the results on our X-rays, for only they can give us precise information on the outcome of our implants. The problem will then be determining, for some of the bony patterns, if it is a matter of a normal simple biomechanical adaptation to the bony physiology, or whether the patterns are forerunners of a prosthetic failure.

References

1. D'Antonio JA, Capello WN, Jaffe WL (1992) Hydroxyapatite-coated hip implants. Multicenter three-year clinical and roentgenographic results. Clin Orthop 285:102–115
2. Engh CA, Massin P (1989) Cementless total hip arthroplasty using the anatomic medullary system: results using a survivorship analysis. Clin Orthop 249:141–158
3. Epinette JA, Geesink RGT, AGORA Group (1995) Radiographic analysis of noncemented hip implants: the ARA scoring system. In: Cahiers d'enseignement de la SOFCOT (Hydroxyapatite coated hip and knee arthroplasty; English volume), vol 51. Expansion Scientifique Française, Paris, p VII
4. Epinette JA, Manley MT (1997) Outcome studies and computerized follow-up in knee arthroplasty. In: Cahiers d'enseignement de la SOFCOT (Unicompartmental knee arthroplasty, English volume), vol 61. Expansion Scientifique Française, Paris, pp 111–117
5. Geesink RGT, DeGroot K, Klein CPAT (1987) Chemical implant fixation using hydroxyapatite coatings. Clin Orthop 225:147–170
6. Gruen TA, McNeice GM, Amstutz HC (1979) "Modes of failure" of cemented stem-type femoral components: a radiographic analysis of loosening. Clin Orthop 141:17–27
7. Manley MT, Kay JF, Uratsuji M, et al (1987) Hydroxyapatite coatings applied to implants subjected to functional loads. In: 13th annual meeting of the Society for Biomaterials, New York, p 210

Part 2 Total Hip Arthroplasty with Nonpolyethylene Surfaces

Wear of Alumina-on-Alumina Total Hip Prosthesis: Effect of Diametrical Clearance and Lubricant on Hip Simulator Test

Hironobu Oonishi[1], Ian C. Clarke[2], Victoria Good[2], Masaru Ueno[3], and Hirokazu Amino[3]

Summary. The wear test of an alumina-on-alumina total hip prosthesis (THP) was performed on a hip simulator by using saline and 90% bovine serum, respectively; 28-mm alumina/alumina acetabular cups with matching femoral heads were tested. The out-of-roundness was less than 2μm, the surface roughness was less than 0.02μm, and crystal size was 1.4μm on average. The diametrical clearances were 10–20μm when saline was used as lubricant, and the clearances were 20–30μm, 60–70μm, and 90–100μm when using 90% bovine serum. The wear trends were biphasic, "run-in," and "steady-state" phase. "Run-in" wear rates in the case of saline and 90% bovine serum were 0.08 and 0.27 mm^3/million cycles, respectively; "steady-state" wear rates in the case of saline and 90% bovine serum were 0.0015 and 0.004 mm^3/million cycles, respectively; and "run-in" and "steady-state" wear rates in 90% bovine serum were threefold higher than those in saline. Alumina-on-alumina wear was extremely low in diametrical clearance between 10 to 100μm in both saline and bovine serum.

Key words. Wear, Alumina-on-alumina THP, Hip simulator, Diametrical clearance, Lubricant

Introduction

It has been reported in Europe that the wear rate of alumina-on-alumina total hip prostheses (THP) is much lower than that of ultrahigh molecular weight polyethylene (UHMWPE) on metal or alumina [1–5]. We have reported the same results in simulator tests [6]. The effect of the lubricant and diametrical clearance in the wear test is great, in general [7–9]. The objectives of this study were to investigate the effect of the lubricant and diametrical clearance in the wear of alumina-on-alumina THP.

---

[1] Department of Orthopaedic Surgery, Artificial Joint Section and Biomaterial Research Laboratory, Osaka-Minami National Hospital, 2-1 Kidohigashi-machi, Kawachinagano, Osaka 586-8521, Japan
[2] Orthopaedic Department, Loma Linda University Medical Center, Loma Linda, CA, USA
[3] Kyocera Corporation, Kyoto, Japan

TABLE 1. Lubricant and diametrical clearance results

Lubricant	Saline	90% bovine serum with additives (sodium azide and EDTA)
Diametrical clearance (μm)	10–20	20–30
		60–70
		90–100

Materials and Methods

We tested 28-mm alumina acetabular cups with matching femoral heads (Bioceram; Kyocera, Kyoto, Japan) in a multichannel hip simulator. Spherical deviation was fixed at 2 μm. The average grain size of alumina was 1.4 μm, and surface finish was controlled to a roughness of less than 0.02 μm.

Hip simulator wear test protocols have evolved as summarized in FDA guidelines. This study used an orbital-type SWM 12 station hip simulator (Shore Wesern, Monrovia, CA, USA) with cam rotation synchronized with hip joint loading. The Paul load profile was used with 2 kN peak loading and 0.2 kN minimum at 1 Hz frequency. The wear cups were mounted below the femoral heads to ensure adequate lubrication exposure. Fluid evaporation during test was corrected by adding additional lubricant. Lubricant bulk temperatures were monitored, but not controlled, and varied from 32° to 36°C on average. The simulator room parameters averaged 20.5°C and 48% humidity.

As lubricants, saline and 90% bovine serum were used, and the effect of these two different lubricants in wear were compared. The bovine serum (Hyclone, Ogden, UT, USA) was used at 90% concentration with additives ethylenediaminetetracetic acid (EDTA) and sodium azide (Sigma, St. Louis, MO, USA). When using 90% bovine serum as lubricant, the diametrical clearances were 20–30 μm, 60–70 μm, and 90–100 μm. The test duration was 14 million cycles. In the case of saline, the diametrical clearance was 10–20 μm and the test duration was 3 million cycles (Table 1).

Wear was determined by the weight loss method. The heads were weighed with the taper cone to avoid metal transfer during the removal process. Volumetric wear rates (linear regression) were calculated using a specific density (Al_2O_3, 3.97 mg/mm^3).

Results and Discussion

For 90% bovine serum, there was no significant difference between three groups of different clearances. Figure 1 shows the wear trend from 0 to 14 million cycles and indicates linear regression treatments for "run-in" phase and "steady-state" phase. One liner (HL 384) is shown for comparison with linear regression ($n = 9$). Figure 1 shows that the alumina liners transitioned from "run-in" phase to "steady-state" phase beginning at 0.45 million cycles and completed by 0.69 million cycles. So, clearly alumina-on-alumina has to be treated as a biphasic wear response. The run-in phase for alumina liners averaged 0.27 mm^3/million cycles (Fig. 2) and the steady-state phase averaged 0.0042 mm^3/million cycles (Fig. 3). This result represented a 64.5-fold difference between the first half-million cycles and beyond the first half-million cycles.

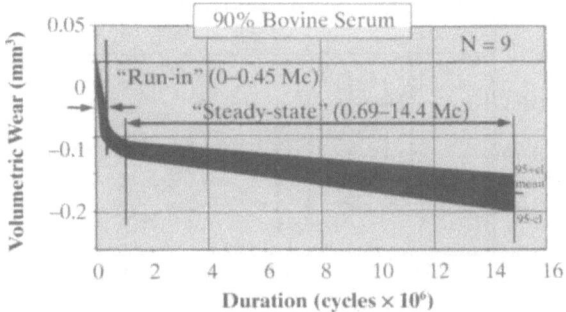

FIG. 1. Wear trend from 0 to 14 million cycles and linear regression treatments for "run-in" phase and "steady-state" phase using 90% bovine serum as lubricant

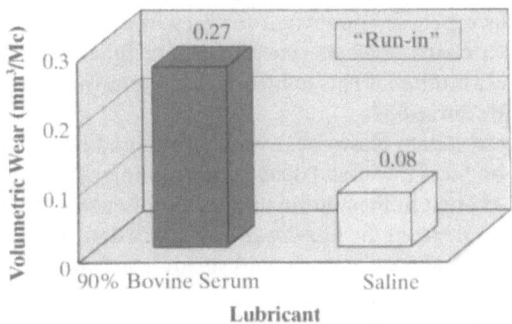

FIG. 2. Comparison of alumina-on-alumina "run-in" wear rate using 90% bovine serum and saline, respectively, as lubricant

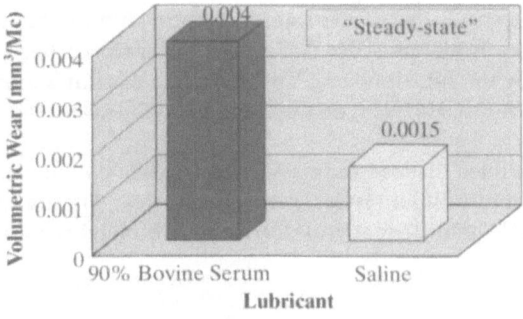

FIG. 3. Comparison of alumina-on-alumina "steady-state" wear rate using 90% bovine serum and saline, respectively, as lubricant

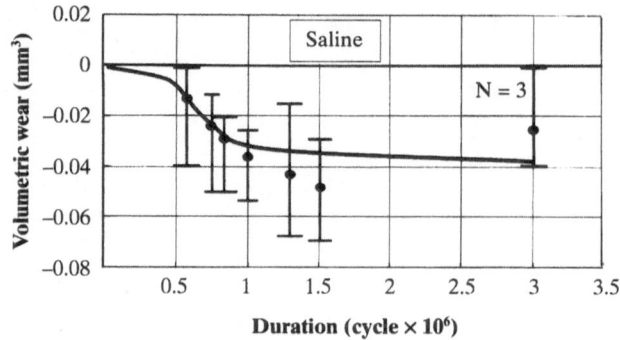

FIG. 4. Wear trend from 0 to 3 million cycles and linear regression treatments for "run-in" phase and "steady-state" phase using saline as lubricant

We always run a Co-Cr ball to check for "systemic errors" in our hip simulator process. This step is especially important for very low wear rate alumina-on-alumina implants. The Co-Cr control ball was cleaned and weighed sequentially with ceramic wear liners but never mounted. This control ball also showed a slight weight loss (with negative slope) with duration.

As low as the steady-state phase wear was for alumina liners (0.00420 mm³/million cycles), the Co-Cr ball was lower at 0.00095 mm³/million cycles and represented about 25% of the "wear" evident in the alumina liners. In other words, the alumina wear was real and distinguishable from the non-wear Co-Cr ball data. In comparison of alumina liners with individual and group run-in and steady-state wear rates, the ranking three groups had no significant difference.

Figure 4 shows the wear trend in the case of using saline from 0 to 3 million cycles. The diametrical clearance was 10–20 μm. This case also showed a biphasic wear response at run-in and steady-state as in bovine serum. The run-in phase for ceramic liners averaged 0.08 mm³/million cycles and the steady-state phase averaged 0.0015 mm³/million cycles (Figs. 3, 4). Figures 3 and 4 show the comparison of run-in and steady-state wear rate in bovine serum and saline. Both wear rates, run-in and steady-state, were three times higher in bovine serum than those in saline.

Incidentally, the steady-state wear rates of 28-mm alumina-on-alumina, UHMWPE on 22-mm alumina head, and UHMWPE on 22-mm Co-Cr head were compared in saline lubricant by the hip simulator. The wear rate of alumina-on-alumina was 500 times less than that of UHMWPE on Co-Cr and 330 times less than that of UHMWPE on alumina.

It could be concluded that as steady-state wear rates in bovine serum and saline were 0.004 and 0.0015 mm³/million cycles, respectively, wear of alumina-on-alumina was extremely low in adequate diametrical clearances in both lubricants, bovine serum and saline.

Conclusion

- Alumina-on-alumina wear was biphasic, with a run-in and steady-state phase.
- Run-in and steady-state wear rates of alumina-on-alumina in 90% bovine serum were three times higher than that in saline.
- Alumina-on-alumina wear was extremely low in diametrical clearance between 10 and 100 μm in both saline and bovine serum.

References

1. Boutine P (1972) Arthroplastie totale de hanche per prothese en alumine frittee. Rev Chir Orthop 58:229–246
2. Boutin P, Blanquaert D (1981) Le fronttement Al/Al en chirurgie de la hanche: 1205 arthroplasties totales. Rev Chir Orthop 67:279–287
3. Heimke G, Griss P (1981) Five years experience with ceramic-metal-composite hip endoprostheses. II. Mechanical evaluations and improvements. Arch Orthop Trauma Surg 98:165–171
4. Sedel L (1997) The tribology of hip replacement. In: Kenwright J, Duparc J, Fulford P (eds) European instructional course lectures, vol 3. Martin Dunitz, Paris, pp 25–33
5. Sedel L, Kerboull L, Christel P (1990) Alumina-on-alumina hip replacement: results and survivorship in young patients. J Bone Joint Surg 72B(4):658–663
6. Oonishi H, Nishida M, Kawanabe K, et al (1999) In vitro wear of Al_2O_3/Al_2O_3 implant combination with over 10 million cycles duration. In: 45th annual meeting, ORS, February, Anaheim, CA, USA, p 50
7. McKellop H, Hosseinian A, Clarke I, et al (1996) In vitro and in vivo wear of total joint replacements. In: Transactions, AAOS 63rd annual meeting, Atlanta, GA, Paper no. 11, 1996
8. Clarke IC, Dai QG, Brahm A, et al (1995) Effects of serum and water lubrication of PTFE/CoCr Implants. In: "Trans ORS", San Diego, CA, USA, p. 240
9. Good V, Clarke IC, Anissian L (1997) A wear analysis of hip prosthesis: lubricant choice for clinical/wear validation. In: AAOS, February, San Francisco, CA, USA

Ceramic Bearing Surfaces in Total Hip Arthroplasty

Edward M. Nelsen-Freund[1], Joshua J. Jacobs[1], and William J. Maloney[2]

Summary. The major long-term complication of modern total hip arthroplasty is osteolysis secondary to polyethylene wear debris. Ceramic articulations have the potential of decreasing the generation of particulates by improved adhesive, abrasive, and fatigue wear properties. High loosening rates and fracture of the ceramic material complicated early systems. Modern component designs, in addition to ceramic manufacturing processes, have addressed these issues. Laboratory wear data have shown significant improvements compared to metal-on-polyethylene. Wear results from clinical studies have been less dramatic and are dependent on technique as well as component positioning. Osteolysis has been reported infrequently. A successful outcome can be achieved when current ceramic total hip systems are used with appropriate attention to surgical technique.

Key words. Alumina, Zirconia, Alternate bearing, Wear, Osteolysis

Introduction

Rates of initial fixation of modern total hip arthroplasty components, both cemented and cementless, have dramatically improved over earlier designs. Most current systems give excellent short- and medium-term results. As such, attention has focused on prevention of the major long-term complication of total hip arthroplasty, namely periprosthetic osteolysis with secondary component loosening. It is recognized that polyethylene wear debris is a major cause of this process. Because of this, much research has been focused on developing alternate bearing surfaces, with the goal of improving on the 0.1-mm/year wear rate accepted for metal-on-polyethylene articulations. Alternate bearing couples include metal-on-metal, ceramic-on-ceramic, and ceramic-on-polyethylene.

The use of ceramic materials as a bearing surface in total hip arthroplasty was introduced in 1970 [1]. These components were ceramic-on-ceramic articulations made of

[1] Department of Orthopaedic Surgery, Rush-Presbyterian-St. Luke's Medical Center, 1725 W. Harrison St., Suite 1063, Chicago, IL 60612, USA
[2] Department of Orthopaedic Surgery, Washington University School of Medicine, St. Louis, MO, USA

alumina oxide. Early designs included use of an epoxy resin to secure the ceramic femoral head to the stainless steel stem, but clinical results were limited by dissociations at this junction. In addition, ceramic use has been complicated by fracture of both the prosthetic femoral head and the acetabulum.

Newer ceramic designs have addressed these complications. Improved ceramic quality has decreased the rate of component fracture, while modern head–neck junctions have decreased the rate of dissociation. In addition, newer manufacturing processes have addressed the problems with zirconia oxide, namely its biodegradability and radioactivity, and this material is now being used clinically [2]. This chapter reviews basic wear mechanisms and properties of ceramics, as well as the laboratory and clinical results of ceramic use as a bearing material.

Wear in Total Joint Arthroplasty

As previously stated, the main theoretical benefit of ceramic material use in joint replacements is that of decreased wear compared to metal-on-polyethylene or metal-on-metal articulations. Three main mechanisms of wear can occur: adhesive, abrasive, and fatigue wear [3,4].

Adhesive wear occurs when a bond forms between two surfaces with subsequent shearing loss of material; this can occur from the surface of polyethylene, and the naturally occurring oxide surface of metallic articulations, as well as from ceramic surfaces. This process is inversely related to the wettability of a surface. Highly wettable materials maintain a water layer at the surface, thus reducing adhesive wear. Wettability varies directly with the ionic character of a substance. Polyethylene, being a highly nonpolar solid, has a low surface energy and low wettability. The oxide film on the surface of metallic components is highly wettable, but also is thin and susceptible to shearing and abrasive forces. Ceramics are manufactured to be homogenous products and are highly polar, maintaining a water layer at the surface, which decreases adhesive forces.

Abrasive wear occurs when a roughened object articulates with a bearing. Although modern femoral heads are highly polished, they still possess irregularities that lead to abrasive wear of the counterbearing. A second type of abrasive wear can also occur when a third body is introduced. Hard third bodies from retained bone, polymethylmethacrylate cement, or the oxide films shed from metallic components can become entrapped in the articulation, leading to abrasion of both components and accelerated wear.

Fatigue wear results from local strain gradients exceeding the cohesive strength of a substance. The softer material in a bearing couple is most often affected, typically polyethylene. This type of wear manifests as vertical fissuring and delamination and can accelerate abrasive wear secondary to the increased surface irregularities as well as via third-body mechanisms. Metal alloys and ceramics are relatively immune to this type of wear mechanism when coupled with polyethylene; however, when articulating with similar hard counterbearings, fatigue wear may occur.

Summarizing the foregoing, ultrahigh molecular weight polyethylene is a soft, nonwettable substance that is relatively susceptible to adhesive, abrasive, and fatigue wear. The newer cross-linked polyethylenes should be less susceptible to damage, but this remains to be proven in clinical trials. Metallic components are hard and highly wettable secondary to surface oxidation, but this layer is thin and still susceptible to adhesive wear; this occurs whether opposed to a polyethylene or metal counterbearing. Finally, ceramics are hard and highly wettable, making them theoretically the most resistant of these materials to wear.

Physical and Chemical Properties of Ceramics

Zirconia oxide (ZrO_2) and alumina oxide (Al_2O_3) are inert, stable, dense, and hard ceramics [5]. As stated, these materials are highly wettable secondary to their hydrophilic nature. In addition, a surface protein monolayer develops in vivo that also helps decrease adhesive and abrasive wear of the implant [6].

Hardness is a measure of a material's resistance to scratching. Alumina ceramics have been shown to resist abrasive forces 30 to 40 times greater than those causing comparable damage to titanium-aluminum-vanadium and chrome-cobalt alloys [7]. In addition, ceramics are also stiffer than the metal alloys currently in use in total joint arthroplasties. Because of this property, components made of ceramics are more resistant to deformation and are better able to maintain congruence, effectively enabling a distribution of forces over a larger area and decreasing wear. In addition, machining of ceramic components must be more exact to maintain sphericity as well as clearance ($10-50\,\mu m$) [6]. Finally, ceramics are more brittle than other materials currently used. This brittleness results in a decreased resistance to fracture, which is catastrophic when occurring in vivo. Not only is revision mandatory in this situation, but retained ceramic fragments can lead to accelerated third-body wear of the revision articulation.

Although zirconia has been shown to have greater compressive strength, fracture toughness, and bending strength compared to alumina [2], both are still susceptible to brittle fracture, which has restricted their use to femoral heads and acetabular components. Zirconia has not been used to manufacture acetabular components because the wear properties of zirconia-on-zirconia are inferior [8].

Implant Fracture

The manufacturing of ceramic implants is highly technical. Microstructure, purity, density, and stress state affect the quality of the component. Factors implicated in ceramic component fracture include poor material quality, large grain size, small head size, residual internal stress, and taper problems [9–11]. In addition, intraoperative component positioning has been shown to be very important. Malpositioning of the femoral or acetabular components can lead to impingement, edge loading, and subsequent fracture, in addition to accelerated wear.

There are multiple reports of ceramic component fracture in the literature [12–22]. Frequency of this event ranges from a low of 1 in 1763 to a high of 9 in 130 [9,15,23–25]. As already stated, revision in this situation is mandatory, with problems arising from the difficulty in removing all retained ceramic material. Any ceramic left behind can cause severe and rapid third-body wear of both polyethylene and metal alloy components [26]. Revision of nonmodular acetabular components is recommended to remove the ceramic material embedded in the plastic and prevent wear of the replacement head. Callaway et al. [14] reported on 184 cases using ceramic femoral heads in combination with a high-density polyethylene counterbearing. An incidence of fracture of 2.2% was observed at 5 to 9 months postoperatively. The authors were unable to determine etiology but did note femoral trunion damage. Because of this, they recommended early revision to prevent damage to the trunion and avoid necessary femoral component revision. In addition, they recommended revising to a metallic head, as imperfections in the trunion would lead to stress risers, predisposing to recurrent fracture of a ceramic head.

The manufacturing process of ceramics has been improved to address these problems. Alumina heads of less than 28 mm are no longer produced. The use of 22-mm zirconia heads has recently been reported [2]. Design of the taper has also improved with a better understanding of criteria to avoid unacceptable stresses in the head. Quality control has been improved by ISO standards first adopted in 1979 and revised in 1994.

Wear of Ceramic Bearings

The major theoretical advantage of ceramic use in total hip arthroplasty relates to improvements in wear. Yearly wear rates averaging 0.1 mm or more are generally accepted for metal-on-polyethylene articulations, with younger active patients having higher wear rates and older sedentary patients having lower wear rates. Analysis of ceramic bearings has included in vitro wear testing as well as evaluation of clinical specimens both in situ and ex vivo after revision or death.

Laboratory wear testing of ceramics has shown a dramatic improvement in wear performance over metal-on-polyethylene bearings. Wear of ceramic-on-ceramic designs has been reported to be between 0.025 and 10 µm per year [27]. This is, at worst, an order of magnitude better than the accepted average rate for metal-on-polyethylene. The wear of ceramic-on-polyethylene has also been intensively studied. Oonishi [28] has reported lower wear comparing alumina to other metals, while McKellop et al. [29] reported similar wear rates between alumina and cobalt chrome heads. Lancaster et al. [30] performed reciprocating pin-on-plate tests to compare stainless steel, cast cobalt chrome, alumina ceramic, and zirconia ceramic against polyethylene. These authors found that all four of these materials had similar wear rates when similar surface roughness was obtained. Although this may be true initially, the intrinsic susceptibility of metal alloys to the adhesive wear mentioned previously can eventually increase the roughness of the femoral head and lead to accelerated abrasive wear. This situation is less applicable to ceramics given their hardness, wettability, and lack of surface oxidation.

Clinical retrieval studies at both autopsy and revision have also been performed, although information from the latter must be interpreted carefully as this is obtained from poorly functioning implants. Walter [31] reported on 48 alumina–alumina implants retrieved at revision surgery for loosening, fracture, or infection. Significant surface damage of the implants was noted. They also found a correlation between cup position and wear rate, with cups positioned in 60° of abduction showing significantly higher wear rates than those positioned at 45°. This result underscores the importance of surgical technique with ceramics and their unforgiving nature. Other retrieval studies [32,33] have shown similar results with respect to unexpected in vivo damage of the ceramic articular surface.

Clinical studies of in situ component wear can be more difficult. Although wear measurements of ceramic and metallic femoral heads in clinical studies vary, most agree that ceramics offer at least some wear advantage. Wroblewski et al. [34] examined the wear rate of 22.225-mm ceramic heads against a cross-linked polyethylene counterbearing. A prospective study of 17 patients (19 hips) was performed in addition to wear simulator studies. A rapid penetration rate was demonstrated in the first 1–2 years in the clinical specimens. After this, wear averaged 0.022 mm/year. Wear simulator studies demonstrated a similar high initial penetration rate, with linear wear decreasing to 0.06 mm/year after 5 simulated years. A review of reported clinical wear rates for alumina-polyethylene articulations by Dowson [35] demonstrated a 50% reduction in wear when compared to metal alloy heads. Jazrawi et al. [36] recently reported their wear data on 60 alumina-on-alumina hips followed for 10–12 years. Wear in this cohort averaged 0.016 mm/year.

Osteolysis

As stated previously, the major theoretical advantage of ceramic use in joint replacement is that of decreased wear and subsequent generation of less wear debris. Resultant osteolysis has been reported infrequently. Shih et al. [37] reported 8 cases of osteolysis in a series of 134 (6% incidence) Mittlemeir Autophor (Richards, Memphis, TN, USA) ceramic implants. All implants were inserted without cement and were followed for 7–11 years. Femoral loosening was observed in 7 of the 8 cases at revision surgery, all of which were revised. Numerous macrophages with ceramic as well as metal debris were observed on histologic examination of the periarticular soft tissues. Both types of particles likely played a role in the osteolysis development.

Lerouge et al. [38] compared the membranes of 18 loose metal–polyethylene articulations with those from 12 loose cemented alumina–alumina articulations. The cellular infiltrate was similar in the two groups. In the cemented ceramic-on-ceramic hips, it was noted that alumina particles made up only 12% of the total particle load. Zirconia dioxide, which was used in the cement as a radiopaque substance, was the predominant particle observed. The authors proposed that the zirconia from the fragmented cement was the etiology underlying the biological reaction.

Yoon et al. [39] reported on a series of uncemented alumina-on-alumina total hip replacements using threaded all-ceramic acetabular components. A high rate of socket loosening allowed the authors to examine the periarticular tissues, including that around well-fixed femoral components. Focal femoral osteolysis was seen. Ceramic wear debris was noted with an average particle size of 0.7 μm. The osteolysis seen in this study supports the theory that this type of process can be initiated by ceramic wear debris.

Clinical Results of Ceramic Bearings

Ceramic implant designs vary widely. When evaluating failure rates for these implants, it is important to determine the cause, whether from failure of the bearing, including wear and fracture, or from loosening of the component. Mahoney and Dimon [40] reported a high failure rate with the Autophor (Richards) prosthesis. At revision surgery, in vivo damage to the ceramic bearing was noted, along with histological evidence of wear debris and foreign-body reaction in the periarticular soft tissues. Despite this, the high failure rate reported is more likely related to implant design, rather than wear of the ceramic bearing and the resultant biological reaction to particulate debris. Reports by O'Leary et al. [41] and Garcia-Cimbrelo et al. [42] have described similarly high failure rates with the Autophor prosthesis.

Other studies of both ceramic-on-polyethylene and ceramic-on-ceramic designs have reported more favorable results. Sedel et al. [43] reported on 86 alumina-on-alumina implants with an 83% follow-up. Both the acetabular and titanium femoral implants were cemented. The articulation was designed as a matched pair with a 32-mm ceramic head. Survivorship at 10 years based on revision was 98%, although 4 hips had radiographic signs of impending failure.

A prospective analysis of an alumina-on-alumina total hip replacement is presently being conducted by D'Antonio et al. (unpublished data). The acetabular component is modular with the metal shell having been previously used successfully with a polyethylene liner. The design includes a recessed ceramic liner to minimize impingement. At 1–2 years, no problems with fracture or with the modular acetabular junction have been encountered.

Conclusion

The use of ceramic articulations in total hip arthroplasty is attractive, given the improvements in wear that can be seen in comparison to classic metal-on-polyethylene articulations. Previous problems with implant fracture can be minimized with improved manufacturing. In addition, many of the high failure rates seen with early prostheses were related to component design and not specifically to the ceramic material. With proper implant design, ceramic manufacture, and appropriate attention to intraoperative component positioning, a successful outcome can be achieved.

References

1. Boutin PM (1972) Arthroplastie totale de al hanche par prothese en alumine fritee. Rev Chir Orthop Reparatrice Appar Mot 58:3
2. Yamamuro T (1998) Zirconia ceramic for the femoral head of a hip prosthesis. In: Sedel L, Cabanela ME (eds) Hip surgery material and developments. Martin Duntz, London, pp 41–44
3. Davidson JA (1993) Characteristics of metal and ceramic total hip bearing surfaces and their effect on long-term ultra high molecular weight polyethylene wear. Clin Orthop 294:361–378
4. Litsky AS, Spector M (1994) Biomaterials. In: Simon SR (ed) Orthopaedic basic science. American Academy of Orthopaedic Surgeons, Rosemont, IL, pp 466–467
5. Drummond JL, Lenke JW (1998) In vivo and in vitro aging of dense alumina. Adv Ceram Mater 3:159
6. Lerouge S, Yahia LH, Sedel L (1998) Alumina ceramic in total joint replacement. In: Sedel L, Cabanela ME (eds) Hip surgery material and developments. Martin Duntz, London, pp 31–40

7. Clarke IC, Willmann G (1994) Structural ceramics in orthopedics. In: Cameron HU (ed) Bone implant interface. Mosby, St. Louis, pp 203–252
8. Sudanese A, Toni A, Catteno GL, et al (1989) Alumina vs. zirconia oxide: a comparative wear test. In: Oonishi H, Aoki H, Sawai K (eds), Bioceramics 1, Proceedings of the 1st international symposium on ceramics in medicine, Kyoto, Japan, pp 237–240
9. Plitz W, Griss P (1981) Clinical, histomorphological and material related observations on removed alumina-alumina hip joint components. In: Weinstein A, Gibbons C, Brown G, et al (eds) Implant retrieval: material and biologic Analysis. NBS special publication 601. U.S. Department of Commerce, New York, pp 131–156
10. Heimke G, Griss P (1981) Five years' experience with ceramic-metal-composite hip endoprostheses. II. Mechanical evaluations and improvements. Arch Orthop Trauma Surg 98:165–171
11. Nizard R, Sedel L, Christel P, et al (1992) Ten-year survivorship of cemented ceramic-ceramic total hip prostheses. Clin Orthop 282:53–63
12. Simon JA, Dayan AJ, Enrique E, et al (1998) Catastrophic failure of the acetabular component in a ceramic-polyethylene bearing total hip arthroplasty. J Arthroplasty 13(1):108–113
13. Burckhardt A, Berberat C (1993) How safe are ceramic heads as hip endoprostheses? Arch Orthop Trauma Surg 112:215–219
14. Callaway GH, Glynn W, Ranawat CS, et al (1995) Fracture of the femoral head after ceramic-on-polyethylene total hip arthroplasty. J Arthroplasty 10(6):855–859
15. Fritsch EW, Gleitz M (1996) Ceramic femoral head fractures in total hip arthroplasty. Clin Orthop 328:129–136
16. Higuchi F, Shiba N, Inoue A, et al (1995) Fracture of an alumina ceramic head in total hip arthroplasty. J Arthroplasty 10(6):851–854
17. Holmer P, Nielsen PT (1993) Fracture of ceramic femoral heads in total hip arthroplasty. J Arthroplasty 8(6):567–571
18. Hummer CD, Rothman RH, Hozack WJ (1995) Catastrophic failure of modular zirconia-ceramic femoral head components after total hip arthroplasty. J Arthroplasty 10(6):848–850
19. Krikler S, Schatzker J (1995) Ceramic head failure. J Arthroplasty 10(6):860–862
20. Michaud RJ, Rashad SY (1995) Spontaneous fracture of the ceramic ball in a ceramic-polyethylene total hip arthroplasty. J Arthroplasty 10(6):863–867
21. Peiro A, Pardo J, Navarrete R, et al (1991) Fracture of the ceramic head in total hip arthroplasty. J Arthroplasty 6(4):371–374
22. Pulliam IT, Trousdale RT (1997) Fracture of a ceramic femoral head after a revision operation. J Bone Joint Surg 79A(1):118–121
23. Griss P (1981) Results of alumina/alumina ceramic THR: the Lindenhof experience with 6 year follow-up. Transactions of the American Orthopaedic Association conference of hip replacement, pp 121–122
24. Cameron HU (1991) Ceramic head implantation failures (letter). J Arthroplasty 6:185–188
25. Sedel L, Nizard R, Kerboull L, et al (1994) Alumina-alumina hip replacement in patients younger than 50 years old. Clin Orthop 198:175–183
26. Kempf I, Semlitsch M (1990) Massive wear of a steel ball head by ceramic fragments in the polyethylene acetabular cup after revision of a total hip prosthesis with fractured ceramic ball. Arch Orthop Trauma Surg 109:284
27. Dorlot JM, Christel P, Meunier A (1989) Wear analysis of retrieved alumina heads and sockets of hip prostheses. J Biomed Mater Res Appl Biomater 23:299–310
28. Oonishi H, Igaki H, Takayama Y (1989) Comparisons of wear of UHMWPE sliding against metal and alumina in total hip prostheses. Bioceramics 1:272

29. McKellop H, Lu B, Benya B (1992) Friction, lubrication and wear of cobalt-chromium, alumina, and zirconia hip prostheses compared on a joint simulator. Trans Orthop Res Soc 17(2):402
30. Lancaster JG, Dowson D, Issac GH, et al (1997) The wear of ultra-high molecular weight polyethylene sliding on metallic and ceramic counterfaces representative of current femoral surfaces in joint replacement. J Eng Med 211(1):17–24
31. Walter IA (1992) On the material and the tribology of alumina-alumina couplings for hip joint prostheses. Clin Orthop 282:31–46
32. Bragdon CR, Jasty M, Kawate K, et al (1997) Wear of retrieved cemented polyethylene acetabula with alumina femoral heads. J Arthroplasty 12:119–125
33. Kummer FJ, Stuchin SA, Frankel VH (1990) Analysis of removed Autophor ceramic-on-ceramic components. J Arthroplasty 5:29–33
34. Wroblewski BM, Siney PD, Dowson D, et al (1996) Prospective clinical and joint simulator studies of a new total hip arthroplasty using alumina ceramic heads and cross-linked polyethylene cups. J Bone Joint Surg 78B:280–285
35. Dowson D (1994) A comparative study of the performance of metallic and ceramic femoral head components in total replacement hip joints. Wear 170:171–183
36. Jazrawi LM, Bogner E, Della Valle CJ (1999) Wear rate of ceramic-on-ceramic bearing surfaces in total hip implants. J Arthroplasty 14(7):781–787
37. Shih CH, Wu CC, Lee ZL, et al (1994) Localized femoral osteolysis in cementless ceramic total hip arthroplasty. Orthop Rev 23:325–328
38. Lerouge S, Huk O, Yahia LH, et al (1997) Ceramic-ceramic and metal-polyethylene total hip replacements. Comparison of pseudomembranes after loosening. J Bone Joint Surg 79B:135–139
39. Yoon TR, Rowe SM, Jung ST, et al (1998) Osteolysis in association with ceramic bearing surfaces. J Bone Joint Surg 80A:1459–1468
40. Mahoney OM, Dimon JH (1990) Unsatisfactory results with a ceramic total hip prosthesis. J Bone Joint Surg 72A:663–671
41. O'Leary JF, Mallory TH, Kraus TJ, et al (1988) Mittelmeier ceramic total hip arthroplasty. A retrospective study. J Arthroplasty 3:87–96
42. Garcia-Cimbrelo E, Martinex-Sayanes JM, Minuesa A, et al (1996) Mittelmeier ceramic-ceramic prostheses after 10 years. J Arthroplasty 11:773–781
43. Sedel L, Derboull L, Christel P, et al (1990) Alumina-on-alumina hip replacement. Results and survivorship in young patients. J Bone Joint Surg 72B:658–663

Medium-Term Results of a Modern Metal-on-Metal System in Total Hip Replacement

Michael Wagner

Summary. Since 1988, metal-on-metal articulation has been reintroduced into hip arthroplasty as an alternative to metal-on-polyethylene or ceramic-on-polyethylene components. Modular joint surfaces were developed for the second-generation metal-on-metal articulation using still introduced and proven prosthetic implants. Seventy-eight uncemented total hip replacements were followed up in a prospective study since 1990 with a mean follow-up time of 60 months. Three patients were lost to follow-up. The average age of the patient at the time of surgery was 48.8 years; 33 patients had been operated on previously. No early infections occurred; 1 late infection occurred after 3 years. Dislocation of the prosthesis occurred in 1 patient who was lost to follow-up. In 2 patients, ectopic ossifications were removed 17 and 27 months postoperatively, respectively. At the last follow-up examination, the Harris hip score was 96.8 points on average. There was no evidence that the metal-on-metal articulation gave rise to new problems or complications. Metal-on-metal articulation reduces wear considerably in the author's previous experience. It is hoped that foreign-body reactions are significantly reduced so that a hopeful alternative for total hip replacement in younger and active patients is now available.

Key words. Total hip arthroplasty, Hip, Metal-on-metal articulation, Wear, Aseptic loosening

Introduction

Aseptic loosening is a major problem of total hip arthroplasty that has not been solved satisfactorily [1–6]. The mechanism of particle-induced osteolysis was published as early as the 1970s [7]. Abraded particles are a logical result of motion. Most of the particles, therefore, are produced in the articulation [8–15]. However, particle abrasion also can arise because of impingement between implant and bone, from friction between prosthetic parts in the case of modular prostheses, and from micromotion between metallic implants, cement, and bone [16–22].

Orthopaedic Department, Zeisigwaldkliniken Bethanien, Zeisigwaldstraße 101, 09130 Chemnitz, Germany

Three-body wear represents a particular problem. Particle shedding outside the actual articulation can be avoided by choosing suitable implants and careful operative technique. The ultrahigh molecular weight polyethylene (UHMWPE) abrasion between a 32-mm CoCr metal ball and an UHMWPE cup is approximately 0.2 mm per year [23–26], which results in the urgent need to look for joint couples made of other materials that give rise to fewer abrasion particles and less volumetric wear. There is no doubt that the UHMWPE articulations in patients with a considerable life expectancy must be replaced by more effective systems [17,27].

Ceramic-on-ceramic articulation was introduced in the 1970s [28,29]. Mittelmeier and Heisel [30] reported an annual linear wear rate of 8 µm/year. Because of the hydrophilic molecular structure, ceramic materials can be wetted markedly better than metal, which favors lubrication of this articulation. Aluminium oxide ceramic is not a biomaterial, that is, cementless ceramic cups are not osseointegrated, which is an important cause of the frequent failure of these uncemented implants [31,32]. However, the particle chipping from the ceramic articulating surface when the cup is in a marked valgus position leads to considerable three-body wear with a steeply increasing rate of abrasion [33].

Examination of metal-on-metal McKee and Müller total hip prostheses using CoCr surfaces that were explanted more than 10 years postoperatively has shown an annual abrasion of 0.1–10 µm/year at the ball and 0.2–6 µm/year at the cups [34–43]. However, many of the prostheses inserted in the 1960s and 1970s failed after a short time. Problems in manufacturing are regarded as the main cause of failure. The surviving tribosystems showed a volumetric abrasion that was 250 times smaller compared with articulations with polyethylene cups and CoCrMo heads [41]. The metal particles are only 25 nm in size and the number of particles released per step corresponds to that of polyethylene articulations [37,44]. However, the extent of the tissue reaction to metal abrasion is markedly less compared with polyethylene abrasion.

The intracellular corrosion of the abraded particles is an important factor in ion release and activates the inflammatory reaction [45]. The friction of a metal-on-metal articulation is markedly greater than that of a metal-on-polyethylene articulation. In the Charnley pendulum testing frame, the in vitro oscillation figure of the metal-on-metal articulation with a ball diameter of 28 mm is equivalent to the metal-on-polyethylene articulation with a ball diameter of 32 mm [46]. Precise production technology has made it possible in recent years to manufacture metal-on-metal articulations from CoCrMo alloys with the necessary precision and with negligible dispersion [47,48] (Fig. 1).

Materials and Methods

Since 1990, the author has been using uncemented hip replacements with second-generation metal-on-metal articulation [49–51]. Modular joint surfaces were developed for this articulation of the hip replacement systems used by the author's group. The prosthetic stems and cups already had been introduced and proven. In this way, problems with this new technology could be recognized rapidly by immediate comparison with total hip replacements of the same design using UHMWPE and aluminium oxide ceramic ball heads. The modular prosthetic head for the metal-on-

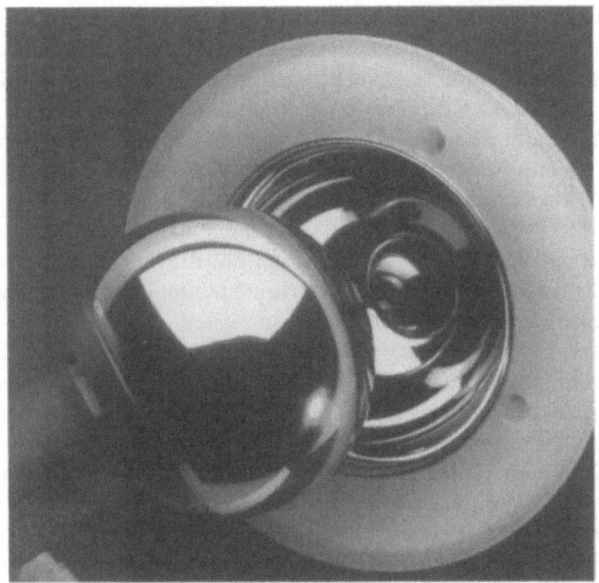

FIG. 1. Second-generation metal-on-metal articulation: a modular CoCr ball and a modular CoCr acetabular component. The articulating surface is mounted in a polyethylene liner

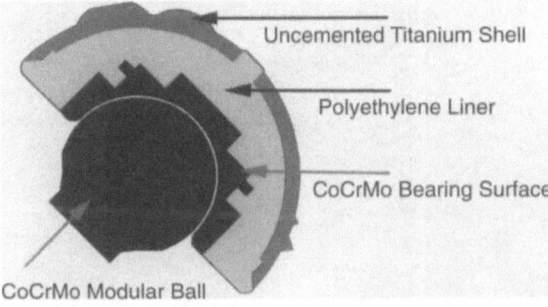

FIG. 2. Diagram of cross section through a metal-on-metal articulation with a modular acetabular component and a polyethylene liner with CoCrMo bearing surface

metal articulation is made from a forged CoCrMo alloy manufactured with particularly high precision [46].

For the acetabular component, a joint surface of CoCrMo alloy for the metal-on-metal articulation is pressed into polyethylene (Figs. 1, 2). By means of the manufacturing technology, the metal inlay is linked firmly with a polyethylene liner so that micromotion between the metal joint surface and the polyethylene will not occur (Fig. 2). The polyethylene inlay is inserted in the titanium acetabular component with a snap-fit coupling. The first metal-on-metal articulations were inserted with a conical threaded cup (manufacturer of all implants is Sulzer Orthopedics, Baar, Switzerland)

[52]. This implant is made of pure titanium with a conical outer thread and polar flattening. The outer thread serves to increase the surface and aids stable fixation in the acetabulum. In the case of bone defects, hip dysplasia, or hip prosthetic revisions, the cup can be reinforced with supplementary titanium cancellous screws. The implant is manufactured in outer diameters of 44–58 mm. An additional cup implant developed by the author's group is completely polyethylene free and nonmodular (primary cup) [50,51] (Fig. 3). The cementless press-fit cup is made of pure titanium with a factory-attached CoCrMo joint surface for metal-on-metal articulation. A shock absorption function by means of an intermediate layer of polyethylene does not seem necessary according to the results obtained with instrumented total hip arthroplasties [53]. This implant is available in diameters of 44–58 mm.

From January 1990 to January 1993, total hip prostheses with a metal-on-metal articulation were inserted in 78 patients in a prospective study. A conical threaded cup was used in 50 patients and a primary cup in 28 patients. All the stems were fixed without cement; there were 74 cone stems [49] and 4 cementless Spotorno stems [54] made of titanium alloy (Table 1). Modular heads for the metal-on-metal articulation of 28 mm diameter were put on the prosthetic taper.

All the patients were followed up according to the study protocol. Two patients did not return for follow-up, and 1 patient was not included because of late infection, so 75 hips were evaluated in 75 patients. The average follow-up was 60 months, the

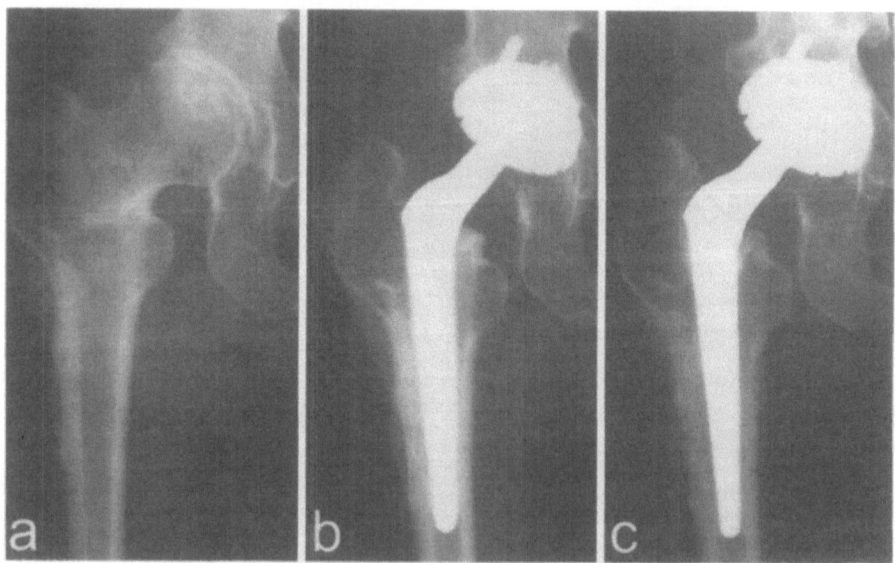

Fig. 3a–c. Radiographs of a 57-year-old woman with advanced osteoarthrosis of the right hip secondary to acetabular dysplasia 15 years after intertrochanteric osteotomy. a Radiograph obtained before total hip replacement. b Three weeks after total hip replacement using an uncemented cone stem, a press-fit nonmodular primary cup with metal-on-metal articulation. c At 5 years postoperatively, there are no radiolucencies, no ectopic ossification, and no implant migration. The Harris hip score is 100 points

TABLE 1. Implants of 75 evaluated metal-on-metal total hip arthroplasties

Components	Number
Cone stem	71
Cementless Spotorno stem	4
Conical threaded cup	42
Primary cup	33

TABLE 2. Functional results and diagnosis of metal-on-metal total hip arthroplasty

Diagnosis	Cases	Age (years)	Harris hip score Average preoperative	Average postoperative	Merle d'Aubigne score Average preoperative	Average postoperative
Osteoarthrosis	25	53.2	38.8	97.1	9.1	17.7
Dysplasiarthrosis	33	46.7	36.3	96.7	9.1	17.5
Aseptic loosening of resurfacing arthroplasty	10	50.1	36.7	94.9	10.0	17.7
Avascular necrosis	5	43.8	35.6	97.8	9.0	17.8
Slipped capital epihysis	1	45.4	42.6	100.0	10.0	18.0
Perthes disease	1	26.3	34.6	99.7	8.0	18.0

TABLE 3. Functional results of metal-on-metal articulations and previous surgery

Previous operations	Cases	Harris hip score Average preoperative	Average postoperative	Merle d'Aubigne score Average preoperative	Average postoperative
No operation	42	38.6	98.6	9.0	17.9
1 operation	8	37.8	97.2	8.6	17.6
2 operations	8	33.6	94.1	9.1	17.3
3 operations	8	35.0	94.5	9.3	17.5
4 operations	5	35.1	95.9	9.2	17.0
>4 operations	4	35.4	87.9	9.3	16.1

minimum follow-up was 44 months, and the maximum follow-up was 88 months. The average age of the patients at the time of surgery was 48.8 years; the youngest patient was 18 years of age and the oldest was 75 years of age; 15 patients were men and 60 were women. The indication for total hip replacement was osteoarthrosis in 25 patients, dysplasia arthrosis in 33, and avascular necrosis in 5 patients (Table 2).

In 10 patients, a cemented surface replacement using metal-to-polyethylene or ceramic-to-polyethylene articulation had to be converted into a stemmed total hip arthroplasty. Of 75 patients, 33 had undergone surgery previously (see Fig. 3; Table 3). A posterior approach to the hip was used in 49 patients and an anterior, modified Smith–Petersen approach in 26 patients. The Harris hip score [55] was 37.2 points on average preoperatively, with a minimum at 10 points and a maximum at 66 points.

The modified Merle d'Aubigne index [56] was 9.2 points on average preoperatively, with a minimum at 5 points and a maximum at 14 points (Table 2). All patients were followed up according to the same postoperative protocol. The patients were mobilized on the first postoperative day with partial weight-bearing of 25 kg on the leg that was surgically treated. This partial weight-bearing was maintained for 12 weeks. After the first follow-up examination 12 weeks after surgery, the load was increased to full weight-bearing.

To prevent ectopic ossification, all patients were treated with 100 mg of indomethacin for 3 weeks. As thrombosis prophylaxis, all patients received a subcutaneous injection of a low molecular weight heparine (Mono-Embolex NM; Novartis, Nuremberg, Germany) from the day before surgery until the day of discharge. On the day of surgery, patients received intravenous antibiotic prophylaxis with 2 g cefuroxime. After complete wound healing and rehabilitation, the patients were discharged on average 3 weeks after operation. Before the patient was discharged, radiographs of the hip that was surgically treated were obtained in two planes. Other imaging investigations were not included in the study protocol. At subsequent follow-ups, clinical examination and an anteroposterior radiograph were obtained. Follow-up examinations were scheduled 3, 6, and 12 months postoperatively and then annually.

Results

The early and medium-term clinical results were, as expected with modern joint replacements, very good. The function of the hip joints could be improved quickly. Major intraoperative problems such as fracture of the femoral shaft did not occur. In one patient who had a previous intertrochanteric osteotomy, a femoral fissure occured at the insertion of the femoral component. There was no instability of the femoral implant; therefore, no osteosynthesis was necessary. Peroneal palsy developed postoperatively in one patient in whom a posterior approach was used; this resolved completely during the first year postoperatively. No thrombosis or pulmonary embolism was observed. The Harris hip score was 96.8 points on average at the last follow-up examination, with a minimum of 64 points and a maximum of 100 points. The Merle d'Aubigne index at the last follow-up examination was 17.6 points on average, with a minimum of 14 points and a maximum of 18 points (see Table 2). No patient complained about thigh pain.

Compared with patients with the same implants using polyethylene and aluminium oxide ceramic joint surfaces, nothing abnormal was observed. No patient with a metal-on-metal articulation reported symptoms or signs that were different from the same implants with conventional ceramic-on-polyethylene articulating combinations. The best results were found in the group of patients with idiopathic osteoarthritis (see Tables 2, 3). Patients who underwent other surgeries before total hip replacement, such as intertrochanteric osteotomy, had somewhat poorer results than did the patients with severe hip dysplasia (Tables 2, 3).

On radiographic examination, no migration of the prosthetic cup or subsidence of the femoral component could be measured with the Müller template [57]. Osteolysis was not observed adjacent to the stem or adjacent to the cup. In seven prostheses, slight translucent lines less than 1 mm wide could be seen beside the femur and/or in

TABLE 4. Radiolucent lines around uncemented metal-on-metal components of hip arthroplasties

Acetabular component	Number of patients	Femoral component	Number of patients
Zone I	2	Zone 1	6
Zone II	1	Zone 2	2
Zone III	3	Zone 3	0
		Zone 4	0
		Zone 5	0
		Zone 6	4
		Zone 7	6

TABLE 5. Radiologic findings after 75 uncemented metal-on-metal total hip arthroplasties

Radiologic finding	Number of patients
Subsidence of the femoral component	0
Migration of the acetabular component	0
Osteolysis	0
Varus position of the femoral component	2
Femoral stress shielding	2

the acetabulum [58,59] (Table 4). No femoral prosthesis had radiolucent lines in more than three zones. Two femoral components were implanted in a slight varus position, and two other stems had some stress shielding (Table 5). These four patients were completely pain free and had an excellent functional result. Dislocation of the prosthesis occurred in one patient, and this patient did not return for additional follow-up examinations.

No early infection occurred; in one patient late infection appeared 3 years after surgery. The implants were removed 41 months after insertion because of a life-threatening infection with *Staphylococcus aureus* from an unknown source. No metallosis was apparent at the time of surgery, and the cementless implants were completely osseointegrated. Significant periarticular ossification occurred only in isolated cases. In nine patients who underwent previous surgery, major ectopic ossification existed before total hip replacement. Brooker grade III and IV ossification [60] were observed postoperatively in three patients (Table 6). In two patients periarticular ossifications were removed 17 and 27 months after implantation of the total joint replacement (Tables 6, 7). At revision surgery, no metallosis could be identified. Histological examination of the newly formed joint capsule and the ectopic bone did not show any signs of metal abrasion.

Discussion

There can be no doubt that every articulation of an arthroplasty causes abrasion [27,31,37,38]. The abraded particles lead to osteolysis caused by a foreign-body reaction that can lead to aseptic loosening of the prosthesis [7,31,61,62]. All types of wear

TABLE 6. Ectopic ossification after uncemented metal-on-metal arthroplasty

Ectopic ossification	Number of patients[a]
No ossification	52
Brooker 1	6
Brooker 2	3
Brooker 3	2
Brooker 4	1

Data of 64 patients without ectopic ossification before metal-on-metal total hip replacement

TABLE 7. Complications after uncemented metal-on-metal hip arthroplasty

Complications	Number of patients
Thigh pain	0
Early infection	0
Pulmonary embolism	0
Femoral fracture	0
Femoral fissure (no osteosynthesis necessary)	1
Transient peroneal palsy	1
Late infection	1
Dislocation	1
Revision of ectopic ossification	2

particles can create this reaction. Rapid wear of the polyethylene especially can be observed in young, physically active patients. The adjacent osteolysis often leads to aseptic prosthetic loosening after a few years. These associations have been shown in several studies [3,5]. Oxidation processes that are favored by gamma sterilization of the polyethylene further worsen the mechanical characteristics of the polyethylene [63–65]. There has been no proof hitherto that the hip replacements last longer with improved polymer materials [66].

For patients with limited life expectancy and/or limited physical activity, the ceramic-on-polyethylene or metal-on-polyethylene articulation is recommended. The ceramic-on-polyethylene articulation represents a proven joint replacement combination. Problems seldom are observed, and fracture of the ceramic head is a rare although serious event [67,68]. Revision surgery is undoubtedly difficult [69]. Because more and more young patients are being treated with hip arthroplasty, a solution of the problem of wear and osteolysis must be sought. [17,27,38]. There currently are two alternatives to this dilemma: metal-on-metal and ceramic-on-ceramic articulation. Against the ceramic, there is the risk of fracture of the brittle material and the possibility of particles chipping when the implant is in valgus position.

The metal-on-metal articulation was introduced in the 1960s [70–74]. Manufacturing problems led to this technology being largely abandoned [75,76]. Nonetheless, many of these prostheses are functioning after more than 20 years without significant signs of wear [34–36]. Obviously, optimal fit of the joint combination was achieved by chance because of individual variations in manufacturing with technology of the 1960s. The problem of the early prostheses was the inadequate size of the implants, so that the head and cup jammed because there was too little clearance between them and the cup loosened. If there was too much clearance, the contact surface of the pressure-transmitting surface was too small, resulting in considerable abrasion. The good results of the few well-functioning metal-on-metal prostheses in the past laid the foundation for a renaissance of this articulation. Already proven implant systems were provided with this articulating combination [51,77].

Meanwhile, 60 000 metal-on-metal articulations have been implanted since 1988 [43,48,49,51]. The short- and medium-term clinical results of the second-generation metal-on-metal articulation must be analyzed and interpreted very carefully [49–51,77] The superiority of a new joint combination will only become apparent in long-term clinical analysis because significant polyethylene wear can be anticipated in current polyethylene-on-aluminium oxide ceramic combinations only after 12–15 years. Whether hitherto unknown problems occur with the metal-on-metal articulation therefore must be investigated. The few revised arthroplasties with metal-on-metal articulation confirm the expectations of the metal-on-metal articulation: the measured abrasion corresponded to the low levels expected from laboratory tests [77]. Use of the metal-on-metal articulation undoubtedly demands a particularly careful operative technique. Incorrect positioning, dislocation, or an impingement of the prosthesis could lead to a considerable increase in abrasion [78].

Metal-on-metal articulation is also open to numerous criticisms and concerns [79,80]. The release of alloy constituents in particular is criticized frequently [45,81,82]. This kind of articulation has to be "broken in" first; that means that the resistance to friction and the abrasion of the articulation is clearly higher in the first months postoperatively than in subsequent years [83]. Metal-on-metal articulations undoubtedly produce abrasion, so the abrasion particles also must be detectable [44,62,84–86]. In a randomized prospective study of 27 patients with a modern metal-on-metal articulation, an average cobalt serum level of 1 µg/l could be detected, and markedly higher levels were detectable in individual cases [87]. A rise in the Co level also was observed after dislocation. The "breaking in" of a metal on metal articulation could be monitored by the serum cobalt levels. Co levels in the toxic range were not observed in this investigation. The authors postulated that the correct function of a metal-on-metal articulation can be monitored by the evaluation of the serum Co level. Black categorically rejects the metal-on-metal articulation because of increased biological risks [79]. In the current discussion, it should not be forgotten that every metallic implant releases alloy constituents [81,88–90] Loosened implants especially lead to considerably raised serum levels of the various elements. To date, there have been no clear indications of carcinogenicity. Visuri et al. [91] and Gillespie et al. [82] have published comprehensive articles concerning these questions. An estimated higher incidence of leukemia in patients with metal-on-metal implants must be analyzed very carefully in coming decades, but to date there are no statistical links [91].

Dislocation of a total hip arthroplasty using metal-on-metal articulation should always be avoided by positioning the implants correctly [24]. As a result of the dislocation, the CrCoMo prosthetic head can come in contact with the cup implant, and there may be a transfer of material from a titanium cup shell onto the prosthetic head.

After reducing the prosthesis, this titanium then is abraded again from the prosthetic head and metallosis probably develops. Tilting of the cup inlay of the acetabular component can lead to metal abrasion on the stem if the CrCoMo insert of the metal-on-metal articulation chafes on the neck of a prosthetic stem, with considerable damage of the femoral implant [78].

The metal-on-metal articulation should not be used in the case of allergies against individual alloy constituents. The great problem in assessing new articulations is the fact that only precise long-term observation permits a statement to be made. Problems of friction and wear can be expected after more than 10 years with the ceramic-on-polyethylene joint combination. Experiences with the metal-on-metal articulation give hope that these tribosystems represent a good alternative for the active patient. Furthermore, modern prostheses are different compared with the McKee or Müller metal-on-metal prostheses. The most important difference is the modularity of modern prostheses and the great precision of the articulating surfaces. The results of metal-on-metal articulations produced with modern technology have hitherto met the expectations of their users. New or unfamiliar problems were not observed. The described joint surfaces first were used in the modular implants that have been in use for years. These arthroplasties had proven themselves already in the past, so that a direct comparison between groups using polyethylene on ceramic and metal-on-metal joints is possible.

In the current study, 3 of 78 total hip arthroplasties were revised: in 2 patients, ectopic ossification was removed to improve the range of motion. One patient with a severe late infection required the removal of the implants. In all the three cases, the revison surgery was obviously not related to the metal-on-metal articulation. No metallosis could be detected in histological investigations. The most important provisional statement permitted by this study is that the hip joint prostheses using the metal-on-metal articulation give equally good results in clinical observation as modular prostheses of the same type with the polyethylene-on-ceramic articulation, and that the metal-on-metal articulation has not demonstrated any disadvantages or any new unexpected problems.

The longest experience with the the modular metal-on-metal articulation was that published by Weber [47,77]. There also have been no problems in this group of patients so far that could be attributed to the type of articulation used. It must be emphasized that only complete documentation of prospective series can give a final answer as to whether the metal-on-metal articulation represents a solution to the problem of aseptic loosening. Anecdotal individual results in active patients have shown that it is possible with these systems to avoid loosening attributable to osteolysis for more than 20 years [34].

References

1. Beckenbaugh RD, Ilstrup DM (1978) Total hip arthroplasty. A review of three hundred and thirty-three cases with long-term follow-up. J Bone Joint Surg 60A:306–313
2. Buckwalter JA, Lohmander S (1994) Current concepts review. Operative treatment of osteoarthrosis. Current practice and future development. J Bone Joint Surg 76A: 1405–1418

3. Chandler HP, Reineck FT, Wixon RL, et al (1981) Total hip replacement in patients younger than thirty years old. J Bone Joint Surg 63A:1426–1434
4. Collis DK (1984) Cemented total hip replacement in patients who are less than fifty years old. J Bone Joint Surg 66A:352–359
5. Cornell CN, Ranawat CS (1986) Survivorship analysis of total hip replacements. Results in a series of active patients who were less than fifty-five years old. J Bone Joint Surg 68A:1430–1434
6. Coventry MB (1981) Ten-year result of total hip arthroplasty. Orthop Trans 5:349–350
7. Willert HG, Semlitsch M, Buchhorn G, et al (1978) Materialverschleiß und Gewebereaktion bei künstlichen Gelenken. Orthopäde 7:62–83
8. Amis A (1996) Is polyethylene still the best prosthetic bearing surface? J Bone Joint Surg 78B:345–348
9. Jasty M, Bragdon C, Jiranek W, et al (1994) Etiology of osteolysis around porous-coated cementless total hip arthroplasies. Clin Orthop 308:111–126
10. Li S, Burstein AH (1994) Current concepts review. Ultra-high molecular weight polyethylene. The material and its use in total joint implants. J Bone Joint Surg 76A:1080–1090
11. McKellop HA, Campbell P, Park S-H, et al (1995) The origin of submicron polyethylene wear debris in total hip arthroplasty. Clin Orthop 311:3–20
12. Schmalzried TP, Jasty M, Harris WH (1992) Periprosthetic bone loss in total hip arthroplasty. J Bone Joint Surg 74A:849–863
13. Shanbhag AS, Rubash H (1993) Wear: the basis of particle disease in total hip arthroplasty. Adv Orthop 8:269–274
14. Tanzer M, Maloney WJ, Jasty M, et al (1992) The progression of femoral cortical osteolysis in association with total hip arthroplasty without cement. J Bone Joint Surg 74A:404–410
15. Willert HG, Bertram H, Buchhorn GH (1990) Osteolysis in alloarthroplasty of the hip. The role of ultrahigh molecular weight polyethylene wear particles. Clin Orthop 258:95–107
16. Agins HJ, Alcock NW, Bansal M, et al (1988) Metallic wear in failed titanium-alloy total hip replacements. A histological and quantitative analysis. J Bone Joint Surg 70A:347–356
17. Collier JP, Mayor MB, Surprenant VA (1990) The biomechanical problems of polyethylene as a bearing surface. Clin Orthop 261:107–113
18. Collier JP, Mayor MB, Williams IR, et al (1995) The tradeoffs associated with modular hip prostheses. Clin Orthop 311:91–101
19. Gilbert JL, Buckley CA, Jacobs JJ (1993) In vitro corrosion of modular hip prosthesis components in mixed and similar metal combinations. The effect of crevice, stress, motion and alloy coupling. J Biomed Mater Res 27:1533–1544
20. Horowitz SM, Doty SB, Lane JM, et al (1993) Studies of the mechanism by which the mechanical failure of polymethylmethacrylate leads to bone resorption. J Bone Joint Surg 75A:802–813
21. Nasser S, Campbell P, Kilgus DJ, et al (1990) Cementless total joint arthroplasty prostheses with titanium alloy articular surfaces: a human retrieval analysis. Clin Orthop 261:171–185
22. Urban RM, Jacobs JJ, Gilbert JL, et al (1994) Migration of corrosion products from modular hip prostheses. Particle microanalysis and histopathological findings. J Bone Joint Surg 76A:1345–1359
23. Streicher RM (1991) Examination of explanted hip joint cups made of UHMWPE. In: Willert HG, Buchhorn G, Eyerer P (eds) UHMWPE as a biomaterial in orthopaedic surgery. Hogrefe & Huber, Bern, pp 196–201
24. Streicher RM (1995) Tribology of artificial joints. In: Morscher E (ed) Endoprosthetics. Springer, Berlin, pp 34–48

60   M. Wagner

25. Zichner L, Lindenfeld T (1997) In vivo Verschleiß der Gleitpaarungen Keramik-Polyethylen gegen Metall-Polyethylen. Orthopäde 26:129–134
26. Zichner LP, Willert HG (1992) Comparison of alumina-polyethylene and metal-polyethylene in clinical trials. Clin Orthop 282:86–94
27. Harris WH (1995) The problem is osteolysis. Clin Orthop 311:46–53
28. Boutin P (1972) Arthroplastie totale de la hanche par prothèse en alumine fritée. Rev Chir Orthop 58:229–246
29. Sedel L, Kerboull, Christel P, et al (1990) Alumina-on-alumina hip replacement. Results and survivorship in young patients. J Bone Joint Surg 72B:658–663
30. Mittelmeier H, Heisel J (1990) Fifteen years of experience with ceramic hip prostheses. In: Aldinger G, Sell S, Beyer A (eds) Noncemented total hip replacement. Thieme, Stuttgart, pp 142–150
31. Böhler M, Knahr K, Salzer M, et al (1994) Long-term results of uncemented alumina acetabular implants. J Bone Joint Surg 76B:53–59
32. Mahoney OM, Dimon JH III (1990) Unsatisfactory results with a ceramic total hip prosthesis. J Bone Joint Surg 72A:663–671
33. Plitz W, Hoss HU (1980) Untersuchungen zum Verschleißmechanismus bei revidierten Hüftendoprothesen mit Gleitflächen aus Al_2O_3-Keramik. Biomed Tech 25:165–168
34. Amstutz HC, Grigoris P (1996) Metal on metal bearings in hip arthroplasty. Clin Orthop 329(suppl):S11–S34
35. Higuchi F, Inoue A, Semlitsch M (1997) Metal-on-metal CoCrMo McKee-Farrar total hip arthroplasty: characteristics from a long-term follow-up study. Arch Orthop Trauma Surg 116:121–124
36. Jantsch S, Schwägerl W, Zenz P, et al (1991) Long-term results after implantation of McKee–Farrar total hip prostheses. Arch Orthop Trauma Surg 110:230–237
37. McKellop H, Doorn P, Chiesa R, et al (1996) Twenty year retrieval analysis of metal-metal hip prosthesis. Trans Orthop Res Soc 21:456
38. Müller ME (1995) The benefits of metal-on-metal total hip replacement. Clin Orthop 311:54–59
39. Schmalzried TP, Szuszczewicz ES, Akizuki KH, et al (1996) Factors correlating with long term survival of McKee–Farrar total hip prostheses. Clin Orthop 329(suppl):S48–S59
40. Semlitsch M, Streicher RM, Weber H (1989) Verschleissverhalten von Pfannen und Kugeln aus CoCrMo-Gusslegierung bei langzeitig implantierten Ganzmetall-Hüftprothesen. Orthopäde 18:377–381
41. Semlitsch M, Willert HG (1995) Implant materials for hip endoprostheses: old proofs and new trends. Arch Orthop Trauma Surg 114:61–67
42. Täger G, Euler E, Plitz W (1997) Formveränderungen von McKee–Farrar-Hüftgelenkprothesen. Orthopäde 26:142–151
43. Weber BG, Fiechter T (1989) Polyethylen-Verschleiß und Spätlockerungen der Totalendoprothese des Hüftgelenkes. Neue Perspektiven für die Metall-Metall-Paarung für Pfanne und Kugel. Orthopäde 18:370–376
44. Soh EW, Blun GW, Wait ME, et al (1996) Size and shape of metal particles from metal-on-metal total hip replacements. Trans Orthop Res Soc 21:462
45. Doorn PF, Mirra JM, Campbell PA, et al (1996) Tissue reaction to metal on metal total hip prostheses. Clin Orthop 329(suppl):S187–S205
46. Schmidt M, Weber H, Schön R (1996) Cobalt chromium molybdenum metal com bination for modular hip prostheses. Clin Orthop 329(suppl):S35–S47
47. Weber BG (1992) Metall-Metall-Totalprothese des Hüftgelenkes: Zurück in die Zukunft. Z Orthop 130:306–309
48. Weber BG (1995) The reactivation of the metal-metal for the total hip prosthesis. In: Morscher E (ed) Endoprosthetics. Springer, Berlin, pp 49–59

49. Wagner H, Wagner M (1996) Metal/metal articulating interfaces. Orthopedics 19:749–752
50. Wagner M (1998) Indications, technical considerations, and early results with modern metal-on-metal couple in total hip arthroplasty. Semin Arthroplasty 9:143–156
51. Wagner M, Wagner H (1995) Preliminary results of uncemented metal on metal stemmed and resurfacing hip replacement arthroplasty. Clin Orthop 329(suppl):S78–S88
52. Wagner H (1987) Revisionsprothese für das Hüftgelenk bei schwerem Knochenverlust. Orthopäde 16:295–300
53. Bergmann G, Rohlmann A, Graichen F (1992) In Vivo Messungen der Belastung von Hüftendoprothesen—Konsequenzen für die Rehabilitation. In: Hipp E, Gradinger R, Ascherl R (eds) Die zementlose Hüftprothese. Demeter, Gräfelfing, pp 97–103
54. Spotorno L, Schenk RK, Dietschi C, Romagnoli S, Mumenthaler A (1987) Unsere Erfahrungen mit nicht-zementierten Prothesen. Orthopäde 16:225–238
55. Harris WH (1969) Traumatic arthritis of the hip after dislocation and acetabular fractures: treatment by mold arthroplasty. An end result study using a new method of result evaluation. J Bone Joint Surg 51A:737–755
56. Charnley J (1979) Numerical grading of clinical results. In: Charnley J (ed) Low arthroplasty of the hip. Theory and practice. Springer, New York, pp 23–24
57. Müller ME, Jaberg H (1982) Total hip reconstruction. In: McCollister EC (ed) Surgery of the musculoskeletal system, 2nd edn. Churchill Livingstone, New York, pp 2979–3017
58. DeLee J, Charnley J (1975) Radiological demarcation of cemented sockets in total hip replacement. Clin Orthop 121:20–32
59. Gruen TA, McNeice GM, Amstutz HC (1979) "Modes of failure" of cemented stem-type femoral components. A radiographic analysis of loosening. Clin Orthop 141:17–27
60. Brooker A, Bowerman JW, Robinson RA, et al (1973) Ectopic ossification following total hip replacement. J Bone Joint Surg 55A:1629–1632
61. Howie DW, Vernon-Roberts B, Oakeshott R, et al (1994) A rat model of resorption of bone at the cement-bone interface in the presence of polyethylene wear particles. J Bone Joint Surg 70A:257–263
62. Willert HG, Buchhorn GH, Göbel D, et al (1996) Wear behavior and histopathology of classic cemented metal on metal hip endoprostheses. Clin Orthop 329(suppl):S160–S186
63. Blunn GW, Bell CJ (1996) The effect of oxidation on the wear of untreated and stabilized UHMWPE. Trans Orthop Res Soc 21:482
64. Fisher J, Chan KL, Hailey JL, et al (1995) Preliminary study of the effect of aging following irradiation on the wear of ultra high molecular weight polyethylene. J Arthroplasty 10:689–692
65. Hamilton JV, Schmidt MB, Greer KW (1996) Improved wear of UHMWPE using a vacuum sterilization process. Trans Orthop Res Soc 21:20
66. Huber J, Plitz W, Walter A, et al (1997) Vergleichende Untersuchungen von Chirulen, Hylamer und Enduron gepaart mit AL_2O_3. Orthopäde 26:125–128
67. Holmer P, Nielsen PT (1993) Fracture of ceramic femoral heads in total hip arthroplasty. J Arthroplasty 8:567–571
68. Peiró A, Pardo J, Navarrete R, et al (1991) Fracture of the ceramic head in total hip arthroplasty. J Arthroplasty 6:371–374
69. Kempf I, Semlitsch M (1990) Massive wear of a steel ball head by ceramic fragments in the polyethylene acetabular cup after revision of a total hip prosthesis with fractured ceramic ball. Arch Orthop Trauma Surg 109:284–287
70. August AC, Aldam CH, Pynset PB (1986) The McKee-Farrar hip arthroplasty. J Bone Joint Surg 68B:520–527
71. Huggler AH (1968) Die Alloarthroplastik des Hüftgelenks mit Femurschaft- und Totalendoprothesen. Thieme, Stuttgart

72. McKee GK, Watson-Farrar J (1966) Replacement of the arthritic hips by McKee-Farrar prosthesis. J Bone Joint Surg 48B:245–259
73. McKee GK (1970) Development of total prosthetic replacement of the hip. Clin Orthop 72:85–103
74. Müller ME (1966) Protèses totales de hanches. In: Procedings Société Internationale de Chirurgie Ortopedique et de Traumatologie, Xth congress, Paris, pp 329–335
75. McKee GK (1982) Total hip replacement—past, present, and future. Biomaterials 3:130–135
76. Ungethüm M, Jäger M, Witt AN (1972) Sphärizitätsmessungen an Totalendoprothesen nach McKee-Farrar und Weber-Huggler. Arch Orthop Trauma Surg 73:1–6
77. Weber BG (1996) Experience with the Metasul total hip bearing system. Clin Orthop 329(suppl):S69–S77
78. Wagner M (1995) Beschädigung der Femur-Schaftprothese, eine vermeidbare Komplikation der Metall-Metall-Artikulation. Aktuel Traumatol 25:205–207
79. Black J (1996) Metal on metal bearings: a practical alternative to metal on polyethylene total joints? Clin Orthop 329(suppl):S244–S255
80. Howie DW, Rogers SD, McGee MA, et al (1996) Biologic effects of cobalt chrome in cell and animal models. Clin Orthop 329(suppl):S217–S232
81. Betts F, Wright T, Salvati EA, et al (1992) Cobalt-alloy metal debris in periarticular tissue from total hip revision arthroplasties. Clin Orthop 276:75–82
82. Gillespie WJ, Henry DA, O'Connell DL, et al (1996) Development of hematopoietic cancers after implantation of total joint replacement. Clin Orthop 329(suppl):S290–S296
83. Walker PS, Gold BL (1971) The tribology (friction, lubrication and wear) of all-metal artificial hip joints. Wear 17:285–299
84. Jacobs JJ, Skipor AK, Doorn PF, et al (1996) Cobalt and chromium concentrations in patients with metal on metal total hip replacements. Clin Orthop 329(suppl):S256–S263
85. Jin ZM, Dowson D, Fisher J (1996) Lubrication mechanisms in metal-on-metal hip joint replacements. Trans World Biomat Congr 5:787
86. Plitz W, Huber J, Refior HJ (1997) Experimentelle Untersuchungen an Metall-Metall-Gleitpaarungen und ihre Wertigkeit eines zu erwartenden in-vivo Verhaltens. Orthopäde 26:135–141
87. Brodner W, Bitzan P, Meisinger V, et al (1997) Elevated serum cobalt with metal-on-metal articulating surfaces. J Bone Joint Surg 79B:316–321
88. Case CP, Langkamer VG, James C, et al (1994) Widespread dissemination of metal debris from implants. J Bone Joint Surg 76B:701–712
89. Coleman RF, Herrington J, Scales JT (1973) Concentration of wear products in hair, blood and urine after total hip replacement. Br Med J 1:527–529
90. Kreibich DN, Moran CG, Delves HT, et al (1996) Systemic release of cobalt and chromium after uncemented total hip replacement. J Bone Joint Surg 78B:18–21
91. Visuri T, Pukkala E, Paavolainen P, et al (1996) Cancer risk after metal on metal and polyethylene on metal total hip arthroplasty. Clin Orthop 329(suppl):S280–S289

Part 3 Revision Total Hip Arthroplasty

Femoral Bone Remodeling in Hip Revision Surgery

Michael Wagner

Summary. The femoral revision stem bridges an extensive bone defect with an implant anchored in the diaphysis to restore the function of the limb. The transfemoral approach opens the medullary canal by creating a posterolateral bony lid that remains attached to the surrounding soft tissues. Then, the loosened component, the bone cement, and the granulation tissue are removed. After reaming of the intact femoral canal distal to the site of osteolysis, the noncemented revision prosthesis is inserted. Between 1969 and 1992, 69 revision procedures were performed using the transfemoral approach. The average follow-up period was 6.5 years (range, 5–9 years). All patients had an extensive loosening (Paprosky stage 2c and 3). In 4 patients, an infected component was exchanged. The transfemoral approach allows a radical debridement of infected implants. The Merle d'Aubigné score improved from a preoperative value of 6.9 points to 13.7 points at time of follow-up. At the time of the last follow-up, all patients were pain free. Without using bone grafts, bone remodeling of the osteolytic zones was observed in all patients. Careful attention to details is the key to the prevention of serious complications.

Key words. Total hip arthroplasty, Aseptic loosening, Uncemented femoral revision, Transfemoral approach, Preoperative planning

Introduction

Aseptic loosening in total hip replacement is associated with bone resorption. In advanced cases, the bone loss may be so severe that the firm fixation of a femoral prosthesis in the old implant bed will be difficult or even impossible (Fig. 1). Also, in periprosthetic fractures and in infected cases, implant fixation in the proximal femur very often is impossible. Cemented revisions have shown poor results in some studies [1–3].

The described uncemented femoral revision prosthesis (Sulzer Orthopedics, Baar Switzerland) bypasses the defective femoral segment like a medullary nail and is anchored in sound bone distal to the lesion. The revision prosthesis is designed

Orthopaedic Department, Zeisigwaldkliniken Bethanien, Zeisigwaldstraße 101, 09130 Chemnitz, Germany

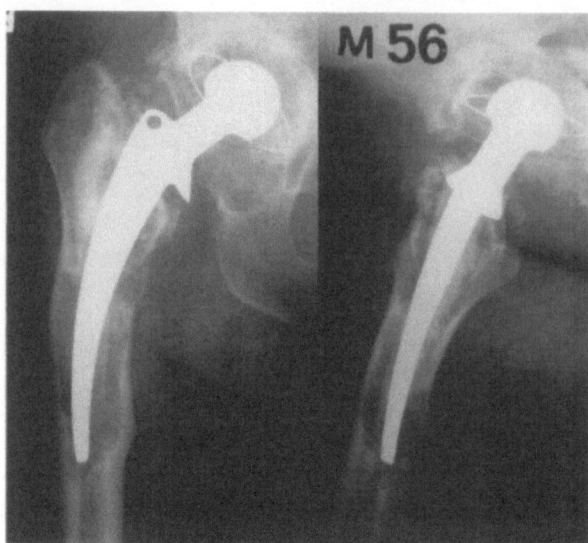

FIG. 1. This 56-year-old patient presented with severe femoral osteolysis at the aseptic loosening of a cemented total hip arthroplasty. The remaining proximal cortical bone does not allow the proximal fixation of an implant

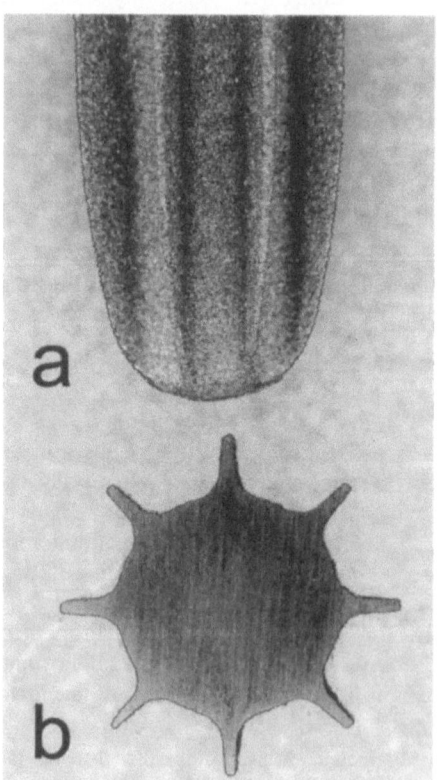

FIG. 2. **a** Rough blasted conical shaped tip of the revision stem. **b** Cross section of the revision stem demonstrating the eight longitudinal ribs of the implant

FIG. 3. Line drawing of revision stems in different lengths to accommodate the extent of the bony defect. Corresponding markings for the different prosthetic lengths are found on the reamer

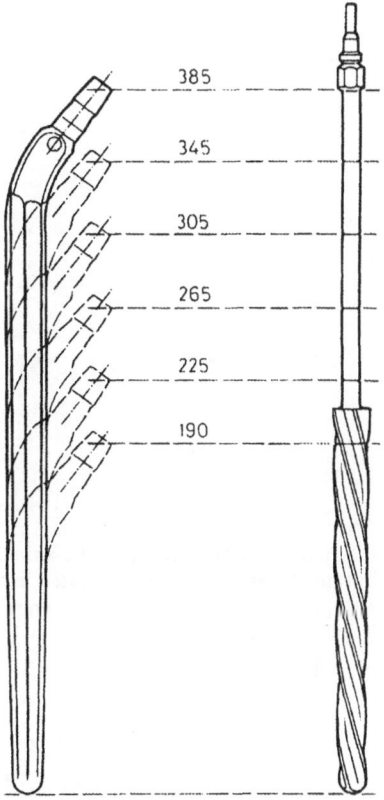

for cementless fixation with a cone junction, impacting a conical stem into the conically reamed femoral canal [4]. The implant is made from a titanium-aluminum-niobium alloy Protasul 100 (Ti6Al7Nb). The surface is blasted with corundum and the pore size of 20–200 μm thus obtained facilitates osteointegration of the femoral stem.

The femoral canal is opened through a posterolateral osteotomy and enlarged with conical reamers [5–7]. The starlike profile of the stem of the revision component is then fitted exactly into the femoral canal (Fig. 2). The length of the femoral component of 190, 225, 265, 305, 345, or 385 mm permits the bridging of defects of various sizes (Fig. 3). The reamers have the same shape as the femoral component. They are available in diameters varying from 14 to 25 mm with 1-mm increments. A rapid remodeling in the former osteolytic areas can be observed without using grafts [8].

In a sheep study, a very good remodeling of artificial defects was shown with this implant design [9]. A defect of 1-cm length was resected in the tibia of adult sheep. The defect was bridged with a conical implant with the starlike profile of the femoral revision stem. This rough blasted titanium implant was cemented in the proximal part of the tibia (Fig. 4). In the distal part, it was fixed uncemented.

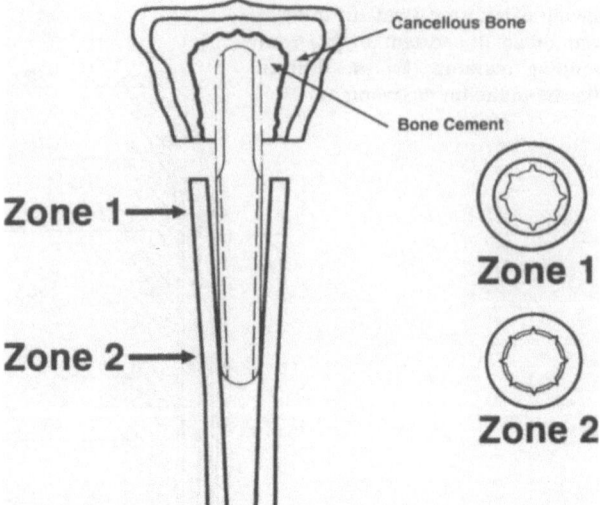

FIG. 4. Schematic drawing of the animal study. A gap is resected from the sheep tibia, and the intramedullary implant is anchored in the proximal part of the tibia with bone cement. In the distal part, the implant is fixed in *zone 2* in solid bone. No contact between implant and bone is achieved in *zone 1*

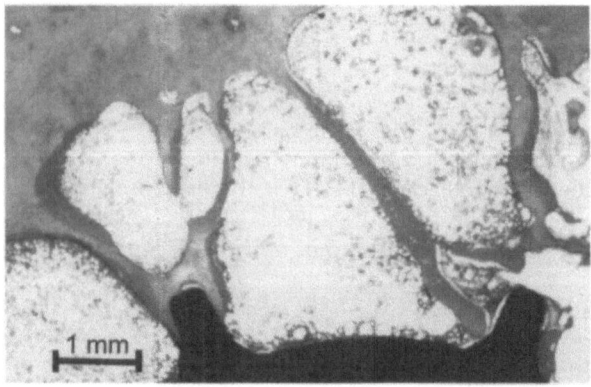

FIG. 5. Histological specimen from animal killed 3 months postoperative. The cross section in zone 1 shows newly formed bone growing on the ribs of the starlike profile of the stem

In zone 1, there was no contact to the endosteal bone; in zone 2, the implant was distally anchored in solid bone. In zone 1 a rapid bony ongrowth to the longitudinal ribs could be demonstrated. Gaps up to 4.5 mm were bridged by bone (Figs. 5,6). No proximal stress shielding combined with bone atrophy was observed in this animal study.

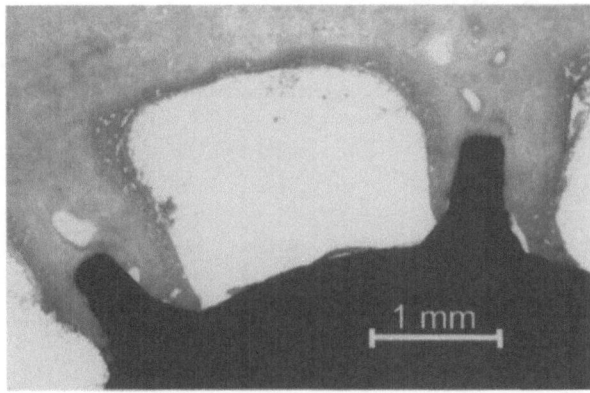

FIG. 6. Histological specimen at 6 months postoperative. Strong bony bridges have grown on the rough blasted titanium implant in zone 1

Preoperative Planning

Preoperative planning is indispensable for the determination of the sizes of the prosthetic components and the extent of the transfemoral approach. The proper length of the prosthesis and its required diameter are determined preoperatively. The most frequent error made during the planning and thus during insertion is the choice of a prosthetic stem that is too long and too narrow. If the diameter of the shaft has been properly selected, an anchorage over a distance of 10 cm is sufficient. The size of the prosthesis and the important length measurements are inscribed in the drawing: the depth of the tip of the loosened prosthesis, the depth of the old cement mantle, the depth of the planned revision component, and the site of the transverse osteotomy (Fig. 7).

Operative Technique

With the transfemoral approach, the femoral cavity is gently opened, facilitating the debridement and the preparation of the new implant seat distal to the bone defect (Fig. 8). The acetabular component can be revised through the same approach. It is essential for subsequent bone healing to protect the overlying muscles and not to release them from the bone surface. The patient is placed in a lateral position. After division of the subcutaneous tissues, the fascia lata and the glutaeus maximus are split. Exposure of the linea aspera of the femur is next. The semicircular, transverse osteotomy determines the distal border of the transfemoral approach. At the level of the transverse osteotomy, the femur is exposed anteriorly and posteriorly through a decortication. Only at this level will the muscles be detached from the femur. Splitting of the femur along the linea aspera up to the innominate tubercle. The osteotomy is continued to the tip of the trochanter. The tendon of the glutaeus medius may be split for a distance not exceeding 3 cm as a further split may injure the superior gluteal nerve. Then several stab osteotomies are made with a small flat chisel into the anterior border of the lid. The lid with the attached vastus lateralis can now be lifted and

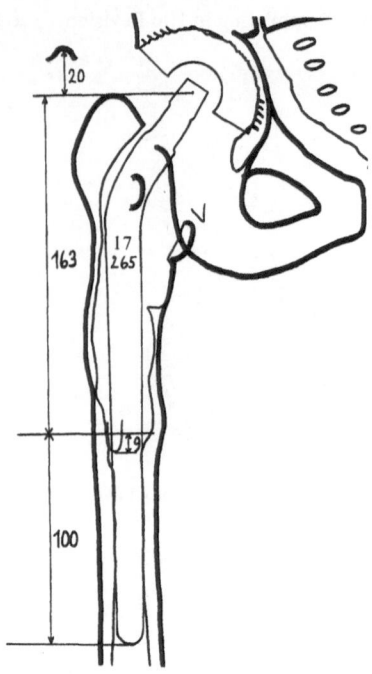

FIG. 7. Preoperative planning indicated a femoral revision stem of 265 mm length and 17 mm diameter in severe proximal osteolysis (see Fig. 1). The implant is anchored distally over 100 mm in solid bone. The transfemoral approach is made 163 mm distally to the greater trochanter

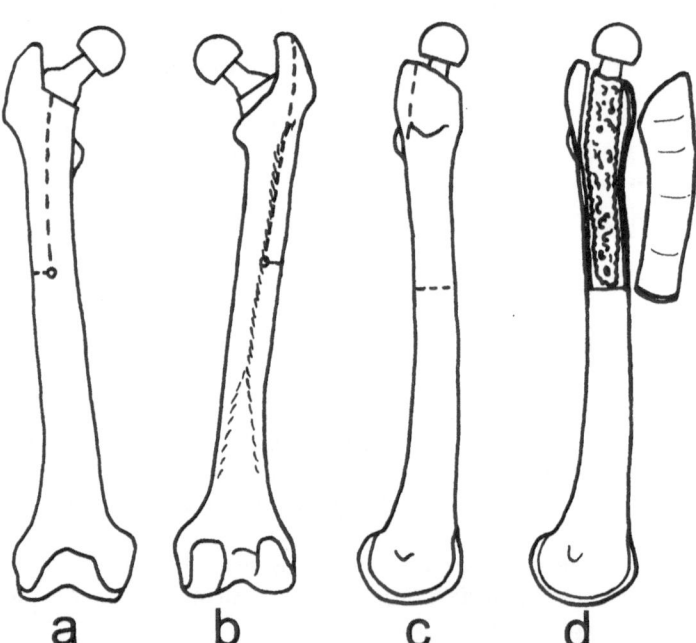

FIG. 8a–d. Schematic drawing of the transfemoral approach. The approach consists of a transverse osteotomy at the distal end, a longitudinal osteotomy along the linea aspera, and a number of puncture osteotomies along the anterior border of what is going to be the lid. a Anterior aspect. b Posterior aspect. c Lateral aspect. d The femur is opened like a door; the implant and the granulative tissue can be removed easily

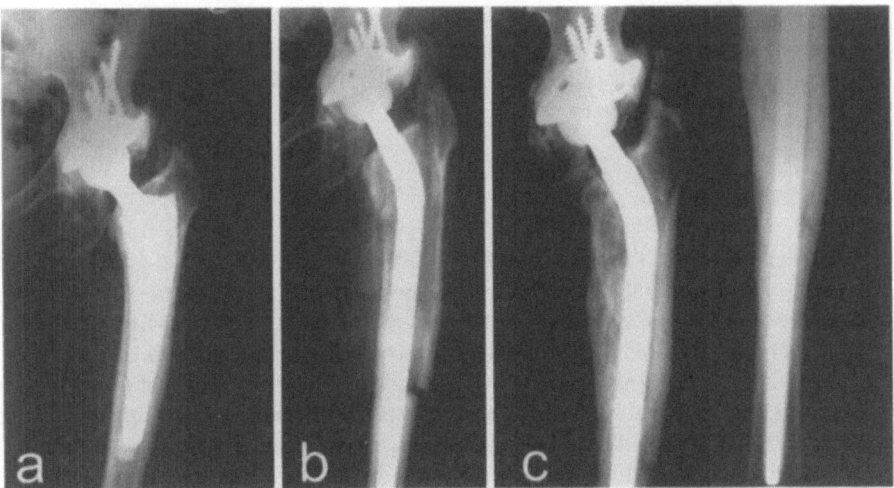

FIG. 9a–c. Bony reformation after transfemoral approach. **a** Loosening and subsidence of a cemented femoral component with cortical thinning in a 57-year-old woman 6 years after revision. **b** Three weeks after transfemoral approach with a femoral revision prosthesis. **c** Three years after transfemoral approach, previous bony defects are filled in

the femur opened like a door. At this point, tissue samples are removed for microbiological examination.

The femoral component can be extracted after resection of the reformed joint capsule. After removal of the granulation tissue, remnants of cement and perhaps the broken tip of the component, the femoral canal is widened with conical reamers until a firm resistance is felt. Distally to the transverse osteotomy, a double cerclage with 1.5-mm-diameter stainless steel wire may be applied if the bone is fragile. A depth of anchorage of the femoral revision stem of 7–10 cm is necessary. The implant is mounted on the inserter and introduced into the femoral canal. Autogenous bone particles, if present, as from heterotopic bone formation are apposed to the lateral surface of the lid. The postoperative neoosteogenesis is in general extensive enough to forego insertion of allogenic bone grafts (Fig. 9). Only in the presence of large lateral cortical defects bone grafting is recommended, because new bone formation on the lateral side of the thigh proceeds very slowly.

Once the physiological leg length has been reestablished, the tension of the gluteus medius muscle and vastus lateralis muscle will keep the posterolateral lid of the transfemoral approach in good position. The osteotomized greater trochanter is fixed with strong resorbable sutures. Should the soft tissues be flaccid, additional cerclage either with wire or strong resorbable sutures is recommended. Prevention of thrombophlebitis is accomplished with low molecular weight heparin until unassisted ambulation, in general for the duration of 6 weeks. For the prevention of heterotopic bone formation, 100 mg of indomethacine daily is prescribed for 3 weeks. Partial weight-bearing of 20–25 kg is permitted. The extent of partial weight-bearing depends mostly on the acetabular reconstruction. In general, the anchorage of the femoral revision component in solid cortical bone distal to the site of the first prosthesis allows full weight-bearing within the first 8 weeks. Radiographic controls are done before discharge and at 3, 6, and 12 months postoperatively. Patients are then checked clinically and radiologically every year.

Results

A consecutive series of 69 patients (31 men, 38 women) was operated between 1989 and 1992. All patients had a transfemoral approach, and the length of the femoral component varied between 265 and 305 mm. Stems with a diameter between 15 and 18 mm were mostly used. Of 69 patients, 41 were followed up according to the protocol using clinical examination and X-ray films. The average duration of follow-up was 6.5 years (5–9 years). Eleven patients died, 8 patients lived in a nursing home, precluding a clinical and radiological follow-up examination, and 9 patients could not be reached. All 69 patients, however, were examined postoperatively for at least 6 months, allowing assessment of early postoperative complications such as heterotopic bone formation or subsidence of the femoral component.

The average age at the time of surgery was 66 years (38–93 years). The extensive bone damage (Paprosky stages 2c and 3 [10]) necessitated a transfemoral approach. An infected prosthesis had to be changed in four patients, three times a broken femoral component had to be replaced, and in five patients periprosthetic fractures had to be treated. In most instances, the first revision was done for an aseptic loosening. The preoperative conditions of the patients were generally judged to be very poor and amounted to 6.9 points according to the Merle d'Aubigné scale [11] (minimum 0 points, maximum 10 points). The average value at the last follow-up examination of the 41 followed-up patients was 13.7 points (minimum 10, maximum 18 points). In spite of the relatively low score achieved by the patients, most of them were very satisfied with their result because of their freedom from pain. The average pain score was 5.1 points, (minimum 4, maximum 6 points). Three patients complained about pain at the thigh; in these cases, it was found that the stem had subsided by more than 1 cm. The other score parameters of Merle d'Aubigné, mobility and gait, had only improved partially.

Among those 69 operated patients, 54 had severe functional disturbances of the lower limbs and vertebral column preoperatively, which incapacitated their walking ability. In 16 of the 69 patients, 23 complications were observed (Table 1). Three times a revision was necessary due to subsidence of the stem of more than 1 cm. These patients complained of thigh pain. After a second revision, these complaints were eliminated. In 62 instances it was impossible to measure any subsidence with the template of Müller [12]. Seven patients presented with ossification of type 3 according to Brooker [13]. After revision and removal of heterotopic bone, an ossification recurred in 2 patients in spite of prophylactic treatment with indomethacine (Table 2). An ossification of type Brooker 4 was seen once. Two patients suffered from a postoperative dislocation. A delayed bony consolidation after the transfemoral approach was noted 4 times. In 57 patients, a rapid reformation of bone at the former site of the prosthesis was observed. In 8 patients, the bone defect filled very slowly. An atrophy of the newly formed bone was never observed. While trying to restore the original leg length

TABLE 1. Complications after transfemoral approach ($n = 69$)

Complication	No. of patients
Subsidence of prosthetic stem	7
Dislocation	2
Delayed consolidation	4
Transient paresis of peroneal nerve	2
Hematoma	7
Lung embolism	1
Thigh pain	0
Infection	0

TABLE 2. Heterotopic ossifications before and after revision with the transfemoral approach ($n = 69$)

Brooker type	Preoperative	Postoperative
0	17	29
1	30	20
2	14	17
3	7	2
4	1	1

a transient paralysis of the peroneal nerve occurred twice (Table 1). Aspiration of a hematoma was necessary in 7 patients, and 1 patient suffered from lung embolism. No infection or reinfection after the revision was seen.

Conclusion

The transfemoral approach in total hip revision arthroplasty provides ample and excellent exposure of the implants, the bone cement, and the granulomatous tissue, and thus facilitates the surgical procedure, saves operating time, and prevents excessive blood loss. The acetabular component can be revised through the same approach. Uncontrolled fractures and bone perforations in the defective femoral segment can be avoided, and bone repair is greatly stimulated. With a conventional nontransfemoral approach, the removal of the loose femoral prosthesis, the bone cement, and the granuloma is difficult and both time- and blood consuming, especially in the revision of long stems, and is fraught with the risk of uncontrolled fractures and perforations of the defective bone.

The use of the implant requires a precise preoperative planning; otherwise, malpositioning of the femoral component, subsidence of the femoral revision stem, dislocation of the total hip implant, and lengthening or shortening of operated limb may occur. A recurrent dislocation necessitates a revision. In this instance, the femoral component should be exchanged before osteointegration has taken place; once osteointegration has occurred, the femoral component can only be removed with great difficulties. During the first postoperative weeks some patients report a crepitation in the thigh, which is caused by the movement of the bony shell of the transfemoral approach. Experience indicates that this phenomenon disappears after a few weeks. The reports of the author's results compare favorably with those reported by others [14,15]. The most frequently reported complications were subsidence and dislocation of the prosthesis. The prompt restoration of the damaged bony structure and the absence of thigh pain are confirmed by their reports.

References

1. Callaghan JJ, Salvati EA, Pellicci PM, et al (1985) Results of revision for mechanical failure after cemented total hip replacement, 1979 to 1982: a two to five-year follow-up. J Bone Joint Surg 67A:1074–1085
2. Engelbrecht DJ, Weber FA, Sweet MB, et al (1990) Long-term results of revision total hip arthroplasty. J Bone Joint Surg 72B:41–45
3. Rorabeck CH, Bourne RB, Devane P, et al (1994) Cementless fixation of the femur: pros and cons. AAOS Inst Course Lect 43:329–338
4. Wagner H (1989) Revisionsprothese für das Hüftgelenk. Orthopäde 18:438–453
5. Wagner H, Wagner M (1997) Prothesenwechsel mit der Femur-Revisionsprothese. Med Orthop Tech 117:138–148
6. Wagner H, Wagner M (1998) L abord transfémoral dans les reprises de prothese totale de hanche. Maitrise Orthop 71:6–10
7. Wagner M, Wagner H (1999) Transfemoral approach for hip revision arthroplasty. Orthop Traumatol 7:260–276
8. Schenk RK, Wehrli U (1989) Zur Reaktion des Knochens auf eine zementfreie SL-Femur-Revisionsprothese. Histologische Befunde an einem fünfeinhalb Monate postoperationem gewonnenen Autopsiepräparat. Orthopäde 18:454–462
9. Wagner M (1996) Die konische Verankerung von Hüftendoprothesenschäften. Thesis, University Erlangen, Nuremberg
10. Paprosky WG (1990) Femoral defect classification: clinical application. Orthop Rev 14(suppl):9–15
11. Charnley J (1979) Numerical grading of clinical results. In: Charnley J (ed) Low friction arthroplasty of the hip. Theory and practice. Springer, New York, pp 23–24
12. Müller ME, Jaberg H (1982) Total hip reconstruction. In: McCollister EC (ed) Surgery of the musculoskeletal system, 2nd edn. Churchill Livingstone, New York, pp 2979–3017
13. Brooker A, Bowerman JW, Robinson RA, et al (1973) Ectopic ossification following total hip replacement. J Bone Joint Surg 55A:1629–1632
14. Hartwig CH, Böhm P, Czech U, et al (1996) The Wagner revision stem in alloarthroplasty of the hip. Arch Orthop Trauma Surg 115:5–9
15. Kolstad K, Adalbeth G, Mallmin H, et al (1996) The Wagner revision stem for severe osteolysis. Acta Orthop Scand 67:541–544

Uncemented Femoral Revision

Seiya Jingushi, Yasuo Noguchi, Toshihide Shuto,
Yasuharu Nakashima, and Yukihide Iwamoto

Summary. Loss of bone stock is the most difficult problem in femoral revision surgery. Even when the bone defect is moderate or severe, immediate fixation of the femoral component should be mainly supported by native bone. Additionally, in the remaining bone loss, bone tissue is grafted as much as possible. According to these principles, we prefer uncemented femoral revisions rather than cemented revisions. This chapter shows short-term clinical results of femoral revisions in our department mainly using an uncemented femoral component. From 1993 until 1999, 55 femoral revisions have been performed. We reviewed 50 hips. Mean age at operation was 64 (range, 41–82) years. All revisions were due to aseptic loosening. Twenty-one patients were followed for at least 2 years (range, 2–6 years; mean, 3.8 years) for clinical evaluation. Intraoperative complications occurred in 9 hips (18%); 7 hips had perforation, and 2 hips had fracture. All the complications occurred in revision of failed cemented components. Using the scoring system of Merle d'Aubigne and Postel as modified by Charnley, average pain and gait scores at the latest evaluation were 5.1 and 4.0, respectively. No rerevision was undergone. Six hips (29%) were radiographically loosened. The advantages of uncemented femoral revisions are to enable restoration of bone stock and biological fixation by native bone. Furthermore, an uncemented component could be removed relatively easily if it failed in the future. The survival rate of revision arthroplasty is low compared with that of primary THA. In addition to the present revision, a possible next operation in the future should be considered when we plan revision surgery.

Key words. Revision, Hip, Uncemented, Bone loss, Femur

Introduction

The goals of femoral revision arthroplasty are to achieve stability of the femoral component, to restore biomechanical function of the hip joint, and to restore the femoral bone stock. To accomplish such an ideal revision arthroplasty, several points

Department of Orthopaedic Surgery, Graduate School of Medical Sciences, Kyushu University, 3-1-1 Maidashi, Higashi-ku, Fukuoka 812-8582, Japan

should be remembered before and during the revision arthroplasty, such as exposure, removal of the failed component, restoration of bone loss, placement of the new component, and hip stability. Appropriate options of femoral components for revision depend on the degree of femoral bone loss. When the bone loss is minimal, a standard length component can be used as in primary total hip arthroplasty (THA). When it is moderate or severe, special components and techniques are necessary.

Loss of bone stock is the most difficult problem in femoral revision surgery. It causes complications during the operation such as fracture or perforation, and also results in difficulty in achieving stability of the component. Even when the bone defect is moderate or severe, immediate fixation of the femoral component should be mainly supported by native bone. Additionally, in the remaining bone loss, bone tissue is grafted as much as possible.

In accord with these principles, we prefer uncemented femoral revisions rather than cemented revisions. This article shows the short-term clinical results of femoral revisions in our department mainly using an uncemented femoral component.

Patients and Methods

From 1993 until 1999, 53 femoral revisions have been performed. We reviewed 50 hips. Mean age at operation was 64 (range, 41–82) years. All revisions were due to aseptic loosening. Seven hips were post hemiarthroplasty, and 43 hips were after THA. Revised femoral components were standard length cemented type (32 hips, 64%); standard length uncemented type (17 hips, 34%); or cemented long length type (1 hip, 2%).

Femoral bone loss was evaluated according to the American Association of Orthopedic Surgeons (AAOS) criteria [1]. One hip was segmental, 19 were cavitary, 29 were combined, and 1 hip was of malalignment type. Most hips were cavitary or combined type. The level of the bone loss in 3 hips was type I, in 4 hips, type II, and in 43 hips, type III. The grade in 6 hips was type I, in 38 hips, type II, and in 6 hips, type III. Allogenic bone was grafted in 42 hips (84%). All the grafted bone was chipped or morselized. A standard length uncemented stem was used for 23 revisions (46%), a standard length cemented stem for 2 revisions (4%), a midsized, fully coated uncemented stem for 5 revisions (10%), and a long-curved, proximally coated uncemented stem for 20 revisions (40%).

Twenty-one patients were followed for at least 2 years (range, 2–6 years; mean, 3.8 years) for clinical evaluation. Three patients were excluded because 2 patients had neurological disease and 1 had died. Pain and walking ability were classified using the scoring system of Merle d'Aubigne and Postel as modified by Charnley [2]. Restoration of bone loss was reviewed in 12 femoral revisions using a long-curved, proximally coated uncemented component in which cases were followed for at least 1 year. The type of bone loss was cavitary in 4 cases or combined type in 8 cases. The level was all type III. Restoration of bone stock in the latest radiographs was assessed by comparing with the postoperative radiographs.

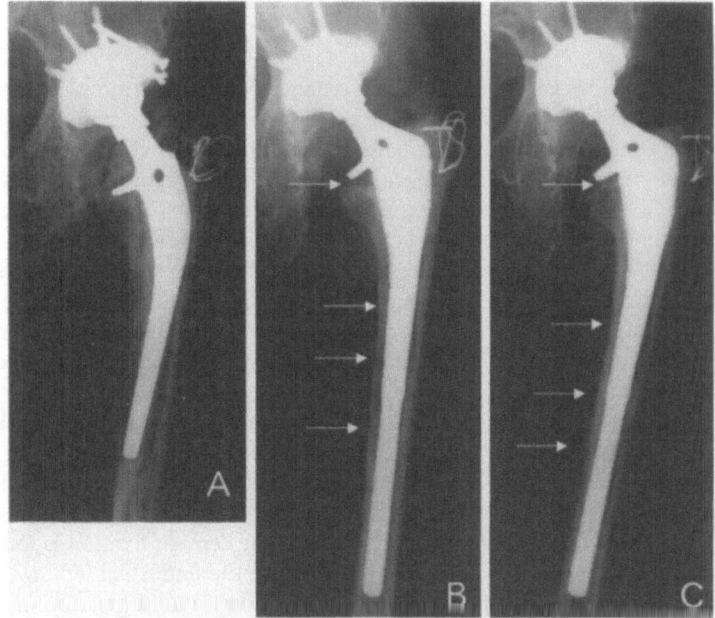

FIG. 1A–C. Restoration of bone stock in a representative femoral revision case using a long-curved, proximally coated uncemented component. **A** Before revision. **B** Just after revision. **C** One year after operation. Restoration of bone stock is observed in the proximal calcar segmental defect (*single arrow*) and in the diaphyseal cavitary defect (*triple arrows*)

Results

Intraoperative complications occurred in nine hips (18%). Seven hips had perforation and two hips had fracture. All the complications occurred in revision of failed cemented components. After revisions, two femoral fractures occurred at the cortical window for cement removal and at the perforated lesion. Both the femoral cortical window and the femoral perforation had occurred during removal of the cemented component. In three hips, dislocations were repeated more than three times.

Average of pain and gait scores at the latest evaluation were 5.1 and 4.0, respectively. No rerevision was undergone. Six hips (29%) were radiographically loosened. Four revisions were undergone with a standard length uncemented stem, and the level of the bone loss was type III. Cement remained in the femoral canal of the two revisions. In all the reviewed cases using a long-curved, proximally coated uncemented component, bone stock of the femur was restored where the bone was grafted and also where not grafted (Fig. 1).

Discussion

Cemented femoral revision has the disadvantage of difficult removal of the prosthesis when it has failed. Removal of a cemented component has a high possibility of complications, including perforation and fracture. During revision arthroplasty of a cemented femoral component using a modern cement technique, removal of the cement mantle is difficult, time-consuming, and hazardous. The cement mass distal to the tip of the femoral component is the most difficult to remove because it is often well fixed [3]. The removal procedure has a high risk of causing femoral perforation or fracture. Furthermore, in rerevision, the cement fixation is often beyond the isthmus and into the distal bone defect, and revised cemented femoral components would be more difficult to remove. On the contrary, loosened uncemented components can be removed relatively easily.

The uncemented stem has the advantage of bone stock restoration. Simultaneous bone graft induces restoration of bone stock. Restored bone tissue will support the component, and this improvement of the bone stock would be beneficial when it has failed again in the future. Cemented revision has the disadvantage of placement of the implant compared with primary cemented THA. The cement fixation is less effective in revision than in primary cemented THA because the endosteal femoral surface is smooth and sclerotic. Furthermore, if it is a long stem, second-generation technique is difficult beyond the isthmus.

We prefer uncemented components that will enable rotational stability in the proximal femur and axial stability in both the proximal and the distal femur. In the remaining defect, usually in the proximal posterior portion of the femoral canal, bone chips are packed. A long uncemented nonmodular or modular implant is chosen for the case in which bone loss is moderate or severe. Severe bone loss of the proximal femur results in variability of three-dimensional geometry in revision surgery. It is a problem to gain rotational stability for uncemented components. The modular type of uncemented component has quite a variability, and it could fit such a variable geometry to gain the stability. A midsized uncemented fully coated implant is also used when bone loss is moderate.

Femoral-impacting bone graft is an interesting technique [4]. Its use is suggested to gain an immediate fixation of the implant by cement and simultaneously to restore bone loss using packed morselized bone tissues. However, it is reported to cause several problems [5]. For packing bone tissue, a large amount of bone tissue is necessary. Especially when the bone loss is severe, there is a high possibility of fracture during packing. Many reports have shown the high incidence of subsidence, and this may be technically demanding.

The advantages of an uncemented femoral revision is to enable restoration of bone stock and biological fixation by native bone. Furthermore, it could be removed relatively easily if it failed in the future. The survival rate of revision arthroplasty is low compared with that of primary THA [6]. In addition to the present revision, a possible subsequent operation in the future should be considered when we plan revision surgery.

References

1. D'Antonio J, McCarthy JC, Bargar WL, Borden LS, Cappelo WN, Collis DK, Steinberg ME, Wedge JH (1993) Classification of femoral abnormalities in total hip arthroplasty. Clin Orthop 296:133–139
2. Charnley J (1972) The long-term results of low-friction arthroplasty of the hip performed as a primary intervention. J Bone Joint Surg 54B(1):61–76
3. Jingushi S, Noguchi Y, Shuto T, Nakashima Y, Iwamoto Y (2000) A device for removal of femoral distal cement plug during hip revision arthroplasty: a high-powered drill equipped with a centralizer. J Arthoplasty 15(1):231–233
4. Gie GA, Linder L, Ling RS, Simon J-P, Slooff TJJH, Timperley AJ (1993) Impacted cancellous allografts and cement for revision total hip arthroplasty. J Bone Joint Surg 75B(1):14–21
5. Leopold MSS, Rosenberg AG (1999) Current status of impaction allografting for revision of a femoral component. J Bone Joint Surg 81A(9):1337–1345
6. Malchau H, Herberts P (1998) Prognosis of total hip replacement. Revision and re-revision rate in THR: a revision-risk study of 148 359 primary operations. Presented at the scientific exhibition, 65th AAOS meeting, February 19–23, New Orleans, LA, USA

Radiographic Results of Cemented Stem Revision in THA

Hirotsugu Ohashi, Akira Matsumura, Yuki Imai, and
Yoshiki Yamano

Summary. Radiographic and clinical results of revision and rerevision total hip arthroplasties (THA) with cemented stem were reviewed over 2-year follow-up. Revision THA was performed in 57 hips at an average age of 61.4 years. The average follow-up duration was 8.5 years. The average JOA (Japanese Orthopaedic Association) score at final follow-up was 77.6 points. Eight stems were revised because of aseptic loosening, and 1 stem was explanted because of infection. Radiographically, 6 hips showed loosening whereas 42 stems remained intact. Compared to the standard stem, the revision rate was lower when using the long stem. Proximal bone atrophy was observed in both standard and long stems. Rerevision THA was performed in 8 hips at an average age of 65.0 years. The average follow-up duration was 5.4 years. The average JOA score at final follow-up was 72.0 points. One stem was revised because of aseptic loosening and 1 stem was revised because of infection. Radiographically, 1 hip showed loosening and 5 stems remained intact. These results indicated that revision THA with a cemented stem expressed good radiographic results. Although rerevision after cemented stem loosening seems to be difficult, the results of rerevision cases in our series were satisfactory.

Key words. Revision THA, Rerevision THA, Cemented stem, Radiographic results, Bone loss

Introduction

As total hip arthroplasties (THA) are widely performed, the number of revision surgery is increasing. The most common etiology of failure is aseptic loosening, especially as the result of osteolysis. Thus, the strategy of revision THA focuses on the restoration of bone stock and the stable fixation of new implant. For fixing a femoral stem, diminished cancellous structure weakens the interlocking with bone cement and decreases the biological fixation with a cementless stem. Thin cortical bone and structural bone defects affect implant stability for both cemented and cementless stems.

Department of Orthopaedic Surgery, Osaka City University Medical School, 1-4-3 Asahi-machi, Abeno-ku, Osaka 545-8585, Japan

These factors may deteriorate the implant fixation. The question is how to stabilize a new implant to bone. We can select a cemented stem and a cementless stem for revision surgery.

In our department, revision total hip arthroplasties have been performed using the cemented stem. In this study, radiographic and clinical results of revision and rerevision THA with the cemented stem were reviewed over 2-year follow-up.

Materials and Methods

Revision THA

Up to 1997, 78 revision THAs in 72 patients were performed in our department using the cemented stem. Of these, 57 hips in 52 cases could be reviewed over 2 years. The average age at primary surgery was 50.9 ± 9.1 years (range, 26–68 years) and that at revision surgery was 61.4 ± 10.0 years (range, 31–81 years). The diagnosis at the time of the primary arthroplasty was osteoarthritis in 48 hips, avascular necrosis in 3 hips, and femoral neck fracture in 6 hips. Primary surgery was performed with monopolar endoprostheses in 6 hips, bipolar endoprostheses in 8 hips, and total hip arthroplasties in 43 hips; 46 stems were cemented and 11 stems were uncemented. The etiology of failure was aseptic loosening in all cases.

Bone loss before revision surgery was classified according to the American Academy of Orthopaedic Surgeons (AAOS) classification [1]. Seven hips were categorized in segmental deficiencies, 39 hips in cavitary deficiencies, 6 hips in combined deficiencies, 4 hips in malalignment, and 1 hip in stenosis. Three bipolar endoprostheses and 54 total hip arthroplasties were performed for revision surgery. All stems were cemented. In 25 hips, a long stem was used. All sockets were cemented, with or without bone graft. The average follow-up duration was 8.5 ± 5.1 years (range, 0–18 years).

Clinical results were assessed using the Japanese Orthopaedic Association hip score (JOA hip score; full mark = 100 points). Radiographically, a femoral stem was considered loose when the radiolucent lines greater than 2 mm were present all around the stem or the subsidence of stem was more than 2 mm.

Rerevision THA

In this series, rerevision THA was performed in eight hips. The average age at primary surgery was 46.4 ± 15.5 years (range, 26–64 years), that at revision surgery was 53.4 ± 13.9 years (range, 31–68 years), and that at rerevision surgery was 65.0 ± 13.7 years (range, 40–82 years). In revision surgery, the standard stem was used in seven hips and the long stem in one hip. The cause of failure was aseptic loosening in all cases.

According to the AAOS classification, two hips were categorized as segmental deficiencies, three hips as cavitary deficiencies, and three hips as combined deficiencies. Bone loss before revision surgery and that before rerevision surgery is shown in Table 1. For rerevision surgery, total hip arthroplasties with a cemented stem were performed in all cases. The standard stem was used in two hips and the long stem in four hips. In two hips, morselized allografts were impacted in the femoral canal and the

TABLE 1. Progress of bone loss after revision surgery

	Before revision	Before Rerevision
Type I (segmental)	2 hips ⟶	2 hips
Type II (cavitary)	5	3
Type III (combined)	0	3
Type IV (malalignment)	1	0

CPT stem (Zimmer, Warsaw, IN, USA) was fixed with bone cement. All sockets were cemented with or without bone graft. The average follow-up duration was 5.4 ± 4.2 years (range, 1–11 years).

Results

Revision THA

The average JOA hip score was 77.6 ± 10.7 points (range, 51–95 points) at final follow-up. Eight stems were revised because of aseptic loosening. One stem was explanted due to MRSA infection, and hip disarticulation was finally performed to treat the infection. Radiological loosening was observed in 6 hips; the other 42 stems remained intact.

Comparing the standard stem to the long stem, eight standard stems (25.0%) were revised or explanted, whereas a long stem (4.0%) was revised. Radiological loosening was observed in three hips (9.4%) after standard stem revision and in three hips (12.0%) after long stem revision. Proximal bone atrophy was observed in four hips; two with a standard stem and two with a long stem.

Rerevision THA

Bone loss before rerevision THA progressed to be classified as combined deficiencies in three hips (see Table 1). The average JOA hip score was 72.0 ± 13.7 points (range, 50–82 points) at final follow-up. One long stem was revised due to aseptic loosening. One standard stem was revised because of infection, and single-stage exchange arthroplasty was performed using antibiotics-loaded bone cement. Radiological loosening was observed in one long stem, and the other five stems remained intact. No radiological loosening was observed in CPT stem with impaction allografting. The overall results are summarized in Table 2.

Case Presentations

Case 1

A 52-year-old woman underwent THA using a Müller prosthesis. Thirteen years postoperatively, subsidence of the stem and focal osteolysis were observed (Fig. 1a). Revision THA was performed using a standard cemented stem (Fig. 1b), and no loosening was observed at 11 years after the revision (Fig. 1c).

TABLE 2. Results of revision and rerevision surgery

Revision	Results	Rerevision	Results
Standard stem 32 hips	L(−) 21 hips L(+) 3 Rev 7	Standard stem 2 hips	L(−) 1 hip Rev 1 (infection)
		Long stem 4	L(−) 2 L(+) 1 Rev 1
	Exp 1 (infection)	CPT 1	L(−) 1
Long stem 25	L(−) 21 L(+) 3 Rev 1	CPT 1	L(−) 1

L(−), no loosening; L(+), loosening; Rev, revision; Exp, explanted

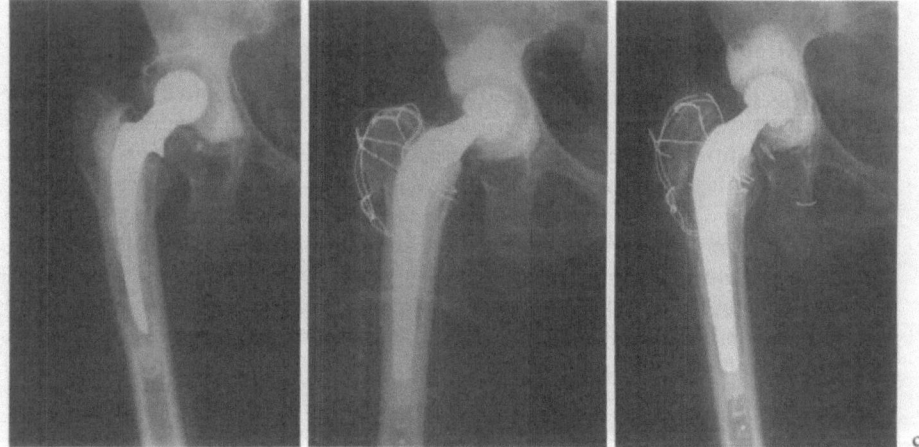

a,b   c

FIG. 1a–c. Case 1. **a** Before revision. **b** Immediately after revision. **c** Eleven years after revision

Case 2

A 39-year-old woman underwent THA using a Weber–Huggler prosthesis. Fourteen years postoperatively, extensive osteolysis was observed (Fig. 2a), and revision THA was performed using a long stem (Fig. 2b). Proximal bone atrophy was observed at 13 years after the revision (Fig. 2c).

Case 3

A 30-year-old woman underwent THA using a Müller prosthesis. Eleven years later, the prosthesis became loose (Fig. 3a), and revision THA was performed using a long stem (Fig. 3b). Fifteen years after the revision, loosening of the prosthesis was again observed (Fig. 3c). Rerevision THA was performed using impaction techniques (Fig. 3d).

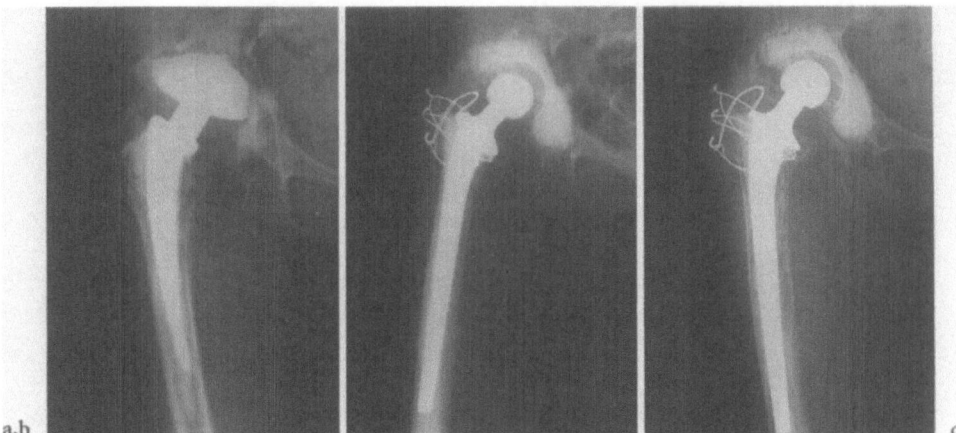

a,b

c

FIG. 2a–c. Case 2. **a** Before revision. **b** Revision using a long stem. **c** Proximal bone atrophy observed (13 years after revision)

Discussion

Revision total hip arthroplasty is a challenging procedure because the patients often have bone loss, soft tissue deficiencies, and leg length discrepancy. Selection of the prosthesis depends mainly on the bone loss. It should be decided whether an implant is fixed with bone cement or not; however, it is still controversial which method of fixation is superior for revision THA.

When using a cementless stem, the design of the stem, as well as the operative techniques, affects the results. Proximally porous coated stems and distally fixed stems brought good results [2,3]. One of the benefits of the cementless stem is to be able to expect the spontaneous healing of osteolytic lesions and bone defects, whereas the results are unreliable when the fixation with bone is poor.

In our department, revision total hip arthroplasties have been performed with the cemented stem. Recently, the cemented femoral revision was reported to be a durable option when improved cementing techniques are used [4]. In our series, bone cement was inserted by fingers or was injected with a cement gun. There was no difference for the results between these cementing techniques. Raut et al. reported good results of cemented Charnley revision arthroplasty [5]. Their results suggested that the cemented stem revision arthroplasty was promising in the presence of extensive femoral osteolysis, even without the use of bone grafts.

However, a roentgen stereophotogrammetric study reported that the fixation of the femoral components after cemented revision was less secure than after primary arthroplasty [6]. The reason was presumed to be femoral canal enlargement and inadequate cement filling. Potential limitations of cemented stem revision are considered to be poor interlock with bone cement in the sclerotic, smooth, deficient proximal femur and that it mandates use of a longer stem to obtain fixation in normal bone and fails to address bone stock, making subsequent revision more difficult.

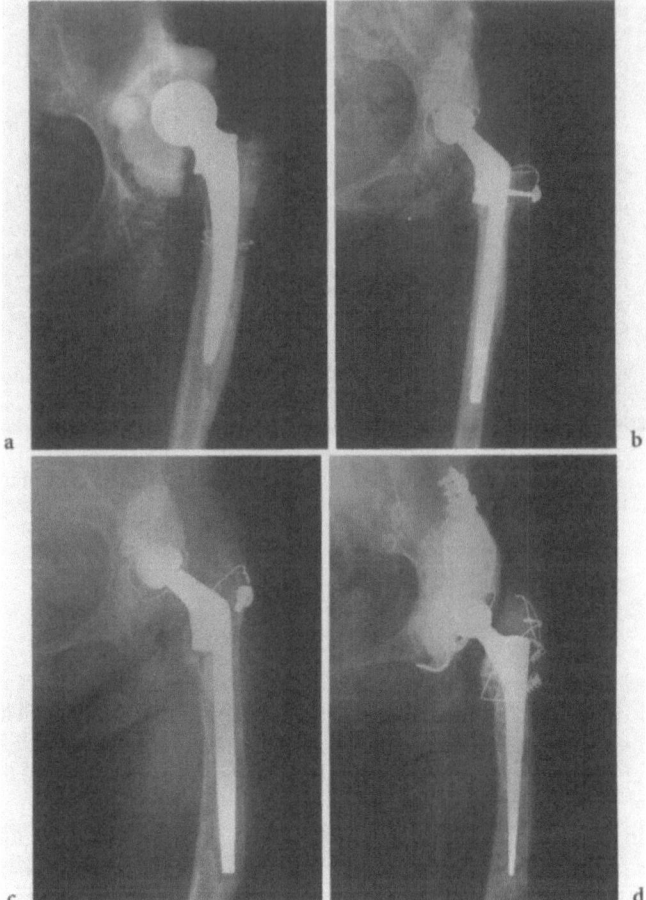

Fig. 3a–d. Case 3. **a** Before revision. **b** Revision using long stem. **c** Before rerevision. **d** Rerevision using impaction techniques

The use of the long stem is controversial. A long stem has advantages in being able to fix bone cement in the intact femoral canal, while proximal bone atrophy may be brought about by distal fixation. In our series, a long stem was used in 25 hips (44%). Fortunately, proximal bone atrophy was observed in 4 hips (2 standard stems, 2 long stems). Radiographic results showed that 11 (34%) standard stems were loose or revised whereas there were 4 (16%) using the long stem. Thus, the use of a long stem was considered to be profitable unless facing the revision after stem loosening.

These results indicated that the results of cemented stem revision in THA were satisfactory and that the results of rerevision were also good. Except for infection, all hips are functioning well, including two hips that have undergone a third revision. The results of the long stem were better; however, it is suggested that the use of a long stem is not strongly recommended.

References

1. D'Antonio J, McCarthy JC, Barger WL, et al (1993) Classification of femoral abnormalities in total hip arthroplasty. Clin Orthop 296:133–139
2. Moreland JR, Bernstein ML (1995) Femoral revision hip arthroplasty with uncemented, porous-coated stems. Clin Orthop 319:141–150
3. Chandler HP, Ayres DK, Tan RC, et al (1995) Revision total hip replacement using the S-ROM femoral component. Clin Orthop 319:130–140
4. Mulroy WF, Harris WH (1996) Revision total hip arthroplasty with use of so-called second-generation cementing techniques for aseptic loosening of the femoral component. J Bone Joint Surg 78A:325–330
5. Raut VV, Siney PD, Wroblewski BM (1995) Cemented Charnley revision arthroplasty for severe femoral osteolysis. J Bone Joint Surg 77B:362–365
6. Franzén H, Mjöberg B, Önnerfält R (1992) Early loosening of femoral components after cemented revision. A roentgen stereophotogrammetric study. J Bone Joint Surg 74B:721–724

Part 4 Custom-Made Hip Prostheses

Preoperative Simulation System for the ZCHW Custom Hip Prosthesis and Its Usage Through the Internet

Hirotaka Iguchi[1], Nobuhiko Tanaka[2], Yukio Yoshida[2],
Toshiyuki Kawanishi[2], Yoichi Taneda[2], Nobuo Matsui[2], Jia Hua[3],
and Yoshiro Hattori[4]

Summary. The ZCHW custom hip prosthesis has been developed at the Department of Biomedical Engineering, University College of London, by Peter S. Walker and colleagues since 1988. About 3000 cases have been performed under the name of CAD-CAM Hip in the U.K., with very good results. We have been joining in the project since 1990, and 19 cases have been done since 1995 when the Japanese Ministry of Health and Welfare issued permission for it usage. A 3-D preoperative simulation system was developed to determine if there were problems, and the system was refined so as to be able to use it over the Internet. In this article, the results of these cases and the utility of the preoperative simulation system are presented.

Key words. Preoperative simulation, Custom hip, 3-D, Computer-aided surgery, CAD-CAM

Introduction

To make an off-the-shelf (OTS) press-fit stem that will function longer without pain, many trials have been done. Most of the trials were related to the stem design. To get better fit and fill at the proximal part of the stem, canal geometries were assembled and many optimal designs were tried. Another approach uses the surface structures.

However well an OTS pressfit stem is well, it is still made for the majority. In press-fit stem cases, distal migration was often seen in the early period, which is not often seen among cemented cases. It is considered that the following two reasons could apply:

1. An OTS press-fit stem is designed to fit the majority. Each case has its own canal geometry, and OTS stems cannot fit all.

[1] Nagoya Midori Municipal Hospital, 1-77 Shiomigaoka, Midori-ku, Nagoya 458-0037, Japan
[2] Nagoya City University Medical School, 1 Kawasumi, Mizuho-cho, Mizuho-ku, Nagoya 467-8601, Japan
[3] Department of Biomedical Engineering, University College of London, Brockley Hill, Stanmore, Middlesex, UK
[4] Central Hospital, Instute of Tokai Health Services, 1 Nishimarune, Arao-cho, Tokai, Aichi 476-8511, Japan

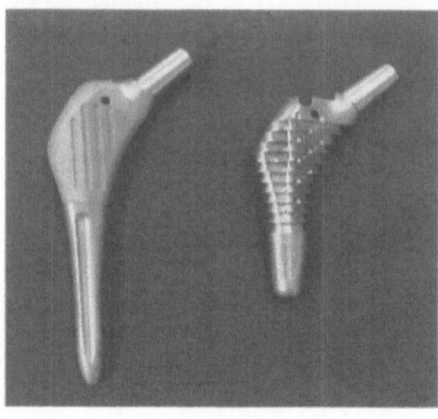

Fig. 1. ZCHW and its custom rasp are manufactured

2. During insertion, when a part of the stem is attached to the cortical bone, the operators are apt to consider that it is inserted to the optimal position. However, over several months the stem moves down until it is settled.

If the stem is designed optimally for each canal, the fit can be maximized, and these problems could be resolved.

Resent computer technology made many impossible things possible. CAD-CAM technology [1] made it possible to manufacture a custom stem. To achieve this technology, the following three steps must be done for each case:

1. Analyze the three-dimensional (3-D) geometry for each proximal canal.
2. Design an optimized stem for the 3-D geometry.
3. Manufacture a stem for the design.

To achieve these three aims, a workstation was developed that is called an orthopedic workstation. Using this workstation, ZCHW was designed and manufactured (Fig. 1).

Materials and Methods

Nineteen hips on which ZCHW was performed with or without the preoperative simulation system are reviewed; 13 cases were handled without preoperative simulation and 6 were with simulation. Among the 6 simulation cases, 3 were simulated via the Internet.

Concept of ZCHW

ZCHW uses plain AP and ML X-rays for its designation whereas most custom stems use CT. ZCHW is not designed to have the same geometry as the proximal canal but to have an optimized smooth surface for each canal. In other words, ZCHW uses the method of designing an OTS stem for each case. CT can give the 3-D geometry of the canal, but its definition is about 0.5 mm, and while extracting the 3-D geometry more error can occur. Thus, CT is not considered sufficiently accurate for designing custom stems. On the contrary, plain X-rays can give much higher definition. Using this method, a smooth surface is designed to avoid stress concentration. It is considered that if a custom stem were given irregular geometry, stress concentration could occur. The ZCHW is an OTS stem system that has infinite sizes and curves.

Designing the ZCHW

First, very accurate AP and ML plain X-rays were taken with a scale. Then, the medial, lateral, anterior, and posterior curves of the canal were digitized. Those curves were used to transform the average proximal canal geometry database, and design canal geometry was constructed. The design canal can be said to be smoothed and optimized canal geometry to be used to design a stem for the case. The accuracy of the design canal was examined, using eight retrieved proximal femurs. In the proximal part the difference was 0.30 mm, in lesser trochanter part, 0.30 mm, and 0.14 mm in the distal part [2,3] (Fig. 2). Thus, obtaining the geometry from plain X-rays can give better geometry than from a CAT scan. Second, an algorithm was used to design a stem for the design canal. The most proximal one-third was designed to obtain a very tight fit, the middle third was designed to have a less tight fit to reduce stress shielding, and the distal third was designed to lead the stem to the appropriate position. All the surface was designed to be very smooth, so-called mathematically smooth; this is essential for this concept. Finally, a tool path for the designed stem was created for the CNC machine, and the stem was then manufactured.

Hua and Walker [4] have reported the comparison of micromotion between the optimal size of OTS stem and ZCHW using retrieved proximal femurs. In the study, ZCHW showed better stability (Fig. 3). Hua et al. also reported proximal stress shielding compared among custom stems, OTS stems, and cemented stems. ZCHW showed the least stress shielding among the three [5] (Fig. 4).

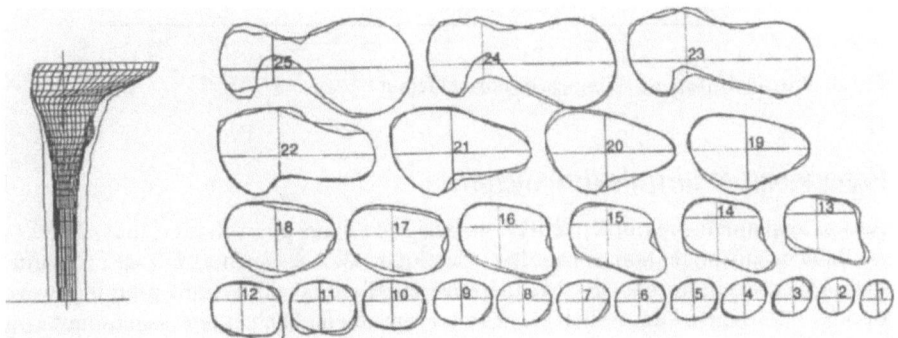

FIG. 2. Accuracy of reconstructed design canal

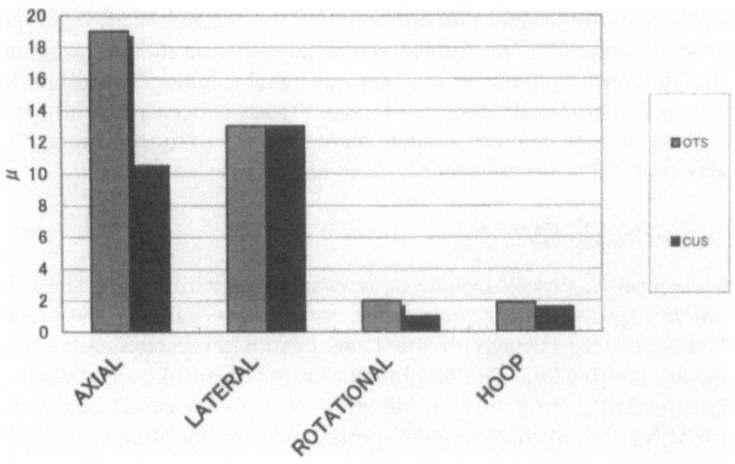

FIG. 3. MicroMotion

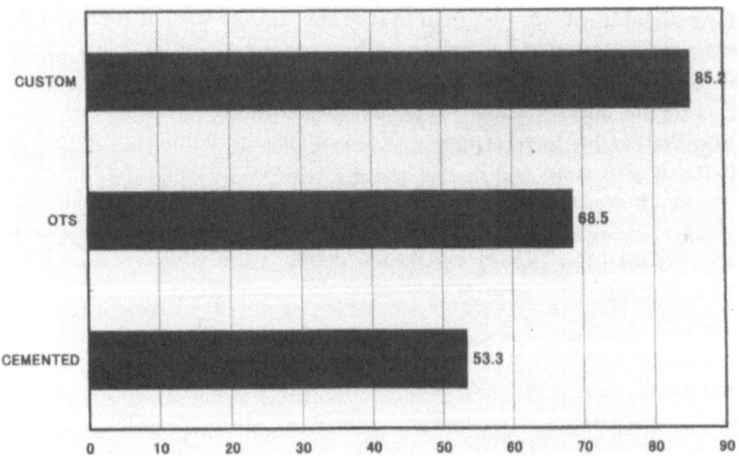

FIG. 4. Proximal stress shielding (% of normal femur)

Preoperative Simulation System

As was explained previously, ZCHW is designed from plain X-rays; thus, ZCHW is available at hospitals that do not have particular devices such as DICOM CT, and it has proved accurate enough. Preoperative simulation will be still useful, however, because there can be unpredictable geometric problems such as after osteotomy. Thus, a preoperative simulation system was developed on a Sun workstation.

The 3-D geometry of the proximal canal is obtained from DICOM files of a CAT scan. Recent CAT scans store data as DICOM files, and these files are sent to the Sun workstation. On the workstation, the slice data are processed and the 3-D geometry of the proximal canal can be extracted. Two ways to extract the canal geometries were prepared in our preoperative simulation system: one uses the threshold of the Hounsfield unit, and another uses neural network technology [6]. The first method is an easy and fast way to extract the geometry, but in some cases it is difficult to get smooth geometry. In those cases, the latter method was used. Neural network technology is a simulation of the human brain to find out the border of the cortical bone and canal. The 3-D geometry of the stem is provided from the ZCHW maker, then transferred to an available format.

Those two geometries are displayed using 3-D data display software, then observed from many directions. When proximal canal geometry is displayed transparently, the stem settlement can be observed, and when a section is displayed, the bone–prosthetic interface can be well observed.

Preoperative Simulation System Usage Through the Internet

Although the preoperative simulation system is very useful, it can be used only at a hospital where the workstation is located. Because the workstation costs are very high, it is impossible to prepare this simulation system at every hospital, and thus the same resource was expected to be used by many hospitals. As the workstation at Nagoya City University (NCU) is connected to the Internet by a 1.5 M-bps digital line, and the computer system at Midori Municipal Hospital (MMH) is also connected by a 128 K-bps digital line, we attempted to use the system through the Internet. Patient CT data were transferred to NCU by Internet, the staff at NCU ran the workstation, and the 3-D geometry was extracted. Then, using the browsing software the canal geometry and designed stem geometry were overlapped and checked. Preferable views were preset. After all the preparations were done, the browsing software was started from MMH through Internet using Window System X (so-called X window).

Results

Figure 5a shows a typical preoperative simulation (Internet case.) A very accurate fit could be seen from many directions, and no design modification was required in this case. The next case (Fig. 5b) was a postosteotomy case. By the proximal distortion, it is obvious that insertion requires partial resection. Figure 5c is a revision case. Bipolar arthroplasty was performed for a femoral neck fracture 8 years ago. Because of a problem with the ultrahigh molecular weight polyethylene (UHMWPE), severe loosening had occurred around the stem. One could see how the space should be filled by preoperative simulation.

Discussion

Using the preoperative simulation system made the ZCHW operation more accurate and easier. ZCHW is not intended to have the same geometry as the canal. It is designed to have global fit to the optimized canal geometry, which means very small

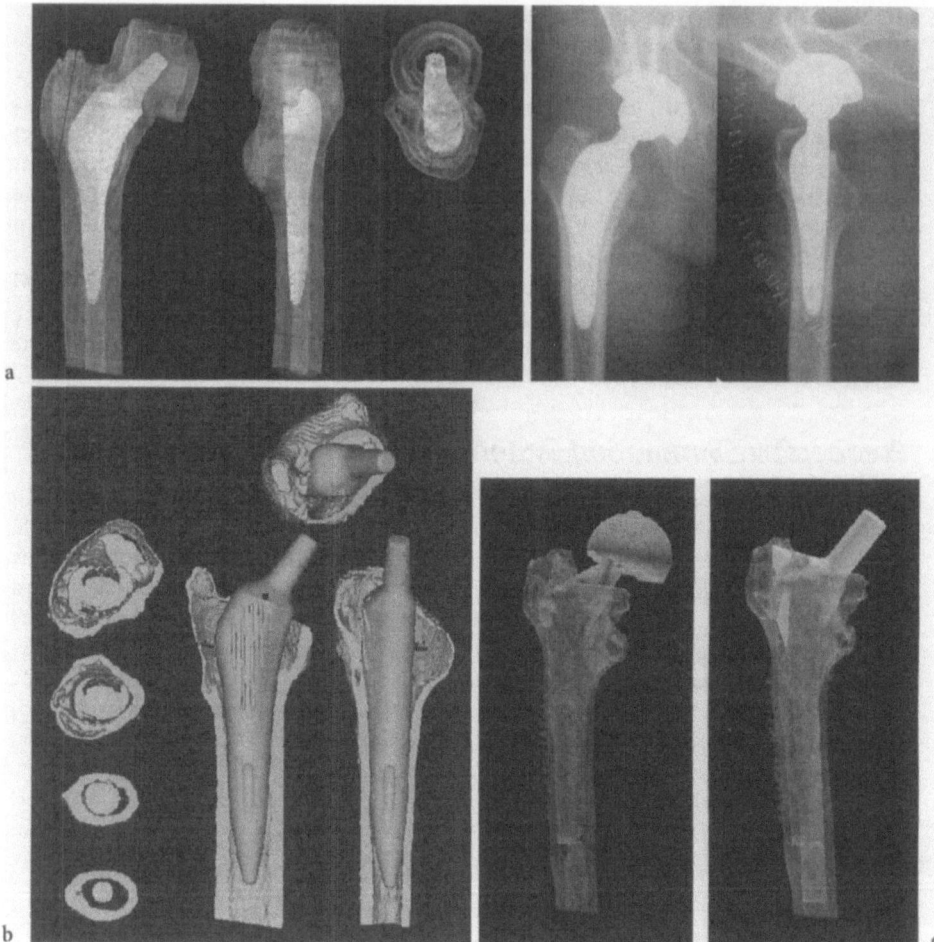

FIG. 5a–c. Preoperative simulation images. **a** Primary case. **b** Post osteotomy case. **c** Revision case

differences of the canal are ignored. To reduce such problems, 3-D preoperative simulation was very useful.

Use of the preoperative simulation system was limited to a hospital where the system was located, but using the system through the Internet made remote usage possible. As free software is available to run the browsing software on a workstation at NCU on a remote personal computers, the cost for a remote user is not so high. Using the window system through Internet is a little too difficult, but when the preferable views were preset, the load was minimized and the remote user could get better utility.

Thus, sharing workstations and the preoperative simulation system provided a great advantage.

References

1. Walker PS, Hua J, Culligan S, et al (1998) Analysis and 6-year clinical experience with a CAD-CAM custom hip in primary cases. J Bone Joint Surg [B] 80:41
2. Iguchi H, Hua J, Walker PS (1992) Fit-and-fill analysis of custom hips and its prediction. J Bone Joint Surg Orthop Proc 74B:166–167
3. Iguchi H, Hua J, Walker PS (1996) Accuracy of using radiographs for custom hip stem design. J Arthroplasty 11:312–321
4. Hua J, Walker PS (1994) Relative motion of hip stems under load: an in vitro study of symmetrical, asymmetrical and custom asymmetrical designs. J Bone Joint Surg 76A(1):95–103
5. Hua J, Walker PS, Muirhead-Allwood W, et al (1995) The rationale for CAD-CAM uncemented custom hips: an interim assessment. Hip Int 5:52–62
6. Iguchi H, Yoshida Y, Kawanishi T, et al (1996) Determination of 3-D coordinates of the skeletal system using neural-network technology. J Jpn Soc Clin Biomech Relat Res 17:1–4

Results with a Custom-Made Stem

Kenji Kawate[1], Tetsuji Ohmura[1], Susumu Tamai[1], and
Yumiko Natsume[2]

Summary. Ninety-one cementless custom-made stems manufactured according to CT
(computed tomography) data were investigated. Patients average age at surgery was
59 years (range, 44–79) with a mean follow-up of 5 years and 4 months (range, 4–7
years). The JOA (Japanese Orthopaedic Association) score was improved from a preoperative mean of 45 points (range, 12–74) to a postoperative mean of 88 points
(range, 49–98). Four patients (4.4%) complained of thigh pain. To date, no patients
have undergone revision of the stem. Radiographically, according to Engh's classification system, there was bone-ingrown fixation in 86 hips (94.5%), stable fibrous
fixation in 2 (2.2%), and unstable fixation in 3 (3.3%). Cortical bone width ratio was
smaller and stem diameter was greater in the 5 stress-shielding hips than in the
remaining 86 hips. Cortical bone width ratio was smaller in 4 hips with a complaint
of thigh pain than in the remaining 87 hips. Careful indication is needed for patients
with thin cortical bone width. Although further follow-up is needed, the results
obtained with this custom-made stem system over a mean follow-up period of 5 years
and 4 months were excellent.

Key words. Custom-made stem, CT data, Fixation, Stress shielding, Cortical bone
width ratio

Introduction

In Japan, the majority of patients with coxarthrosis for whom total hip arthroplasty
is indicated are those with secondary coxarthrosis associated with dysplasia. The characteristics observed in a number of patients include not only the presence of acetabular dysplasia but morphology of the femur that is not suitable for ready-made
components. We have therefore had produced custom-made stems based on CT (computed tomography) data and have used them since 1992 [1]. We report here the results
of more than 4 years of follow-up of these custom-made stems.

---

[1] Department of Orthopaedic Surgery, Nara Medical University, 840 Shijo-cho, Kashihara, Nara
634-8522, Japan
[2] Department of Orthopaedic Surgery, National Nara Hospital, 1-50-1 Higashikidera-cho, Nara
630-8305, Japan

Materials and Methods

A total of 91 hips in 79 patients consisting of 6 hips in 5 men and 85 hips in 74 women were investigated. The average age at surgery was 59 years (range, 44–79 years). Mean follow-up period was 5 years and 4 months (range, 4–7 years), and the follow-up rate was 88%.

Underlying diseases were secondary coxarthrosis in 75 hips, primary coxarthrosis in 1, dislocation coxarthrosis in 5, rheumatoid arthritis in 4, necrosis of the femoral head in 3, and rapidly destructive coxarthrosis in 3. Surgical treatments performed before total hip arthroplasty include valgus osteotomy in 4 hips, rotational acetabular osteotomy in 3, varus osteotomy in 1, and rotational osteotomy of the femoral head in 1.

CT studies were performed with 5-mm slice intervals and 2-mm slice widths. Thirty-nine slices from the top of the head to the diaphysis of the femur and 1 slice at the femoral condyle of the knee joint were taken, and data were input into a personal computer. Two circles were drawn along the internal margin of the mediolateral cortical bone. A line was drawn between these two circles. A tapered stem was produced with this line as the side (Fig. 1). Measurements of anteversion of the femoral neck were performed with the slice of the femoral condyle of the knee joint as the base. Adjustment of derotation at the femoral neck was made at stem preparation for patients with excessive anteversion.

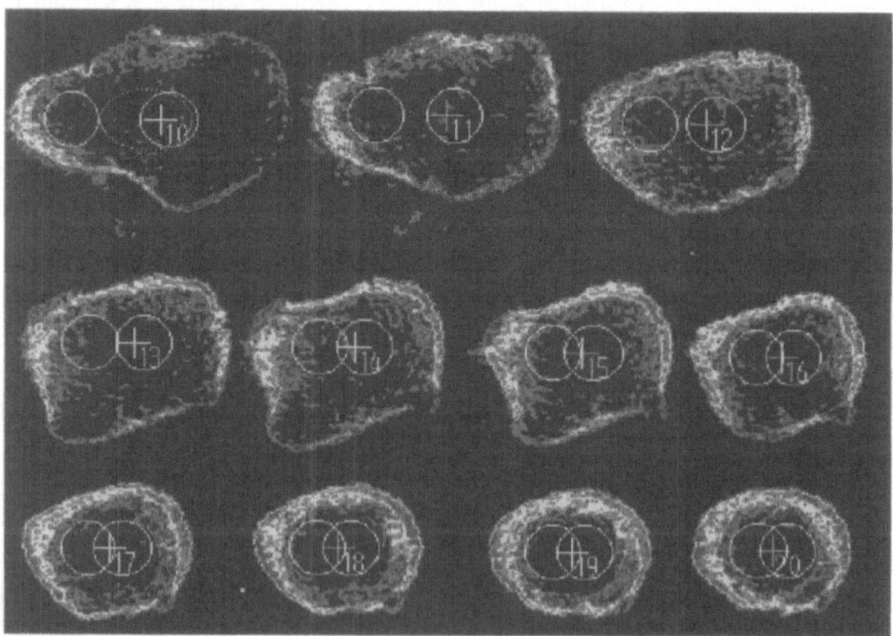

FIG. 1. Design of a custom-made stem

FIG. 2. Cortical bone width ratio (CR): CR = $(b + c)/a \times 100$

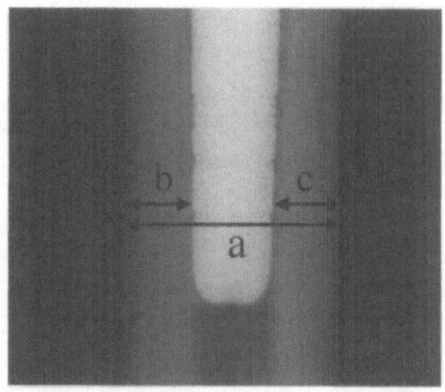

Utilizing a stem (Expert System Ver. 1.0; Kyocera, Kyoto, Japan) made of Ti-6Al-4V, we produced stems with between two-thirds of the proximal surface treated with sandblasting and the entire surface treated with sandblasting. Characteristics of the procedure used for this custom-made stem system include direct insertion of stem following confirmation of the direction with use of a elevatorium without a reamer or rasp.

In the present study, the JOA score (Japanese Orthopaedic Association score) and thigh pain along with radiographical Engh's classification [2], reactive line, sinking, atrophy, stress shielding, cortical bone width ratio at 1 cm above stem tip (Fig. 2), canal filling ratio of the stem at 1 cm above stem tip, and other parameters were examined. Statistical analysis on stress shielding and thigh pain was performed using Mann–Whitney's U-test.

Results

The JOA score was improved from a preoperative mean of 45 points (range, 12–74 points) to a postoperative mean of 88 points (range, 49–98 points). Four patients (4.4%) complained of thigh pain.

Dislocation occurred in 1 hip, fracture in 2, infection in 1, and nonunion of the greater trochanter in two. To date, no patients have undergone revision of the stem. Radiographically, according to Engh's classification system, bone-ingrown fixation occurred in 86 hips (94.5%) (Fig. 3), stable fibrous fixation in 2 (2.2%), and unstable fixation in 3 (3.3%). In addition, distal densification was seen in 65 hips (71.4%), spot welds in 18 (19.8%), calcar resorption in 42 (46.2%), cortical hypertrophy in 5 (5.5%), canal widening in 3 (3.3%), pedestal in 17 (18.7%), varus of the stem in 3 (3.3%), and reactive line in 28 joints (30.8%). A reactive line was found in 15.4% through 30.8% of zones 3, 4, and 5 on both anteroposterior and lateral views. Sinking greater than 2 mm was found in 7 patients (7.7%). Atrophy was observed in 33% to 73.6% of the proximal site of zones 1, 2, 6, and 7 on anteroposterior view, while severe stress shielding was found in 5 hips (Fig. 4). The rate of canal filling ratio of the stem was 91% at 1 cm distal on the lesser trochanter, 90.1% at 1 cm proximal from the stem tip, and 90.8% in between.

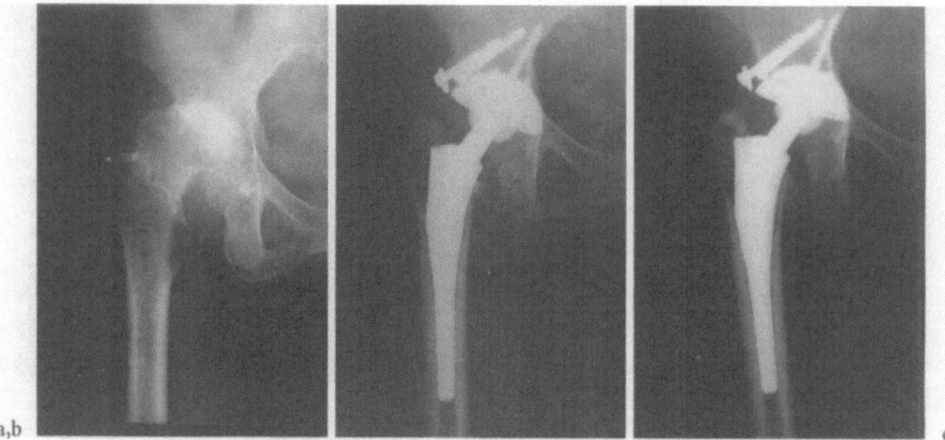

a,b   c

FIG. 3a–c. Radiographs of a 60-year-old woman with congenital dysplasia. a Before operation.
b Immediately after total hip arthroplasty (THA). c Seven years after operation, showing good
fixation

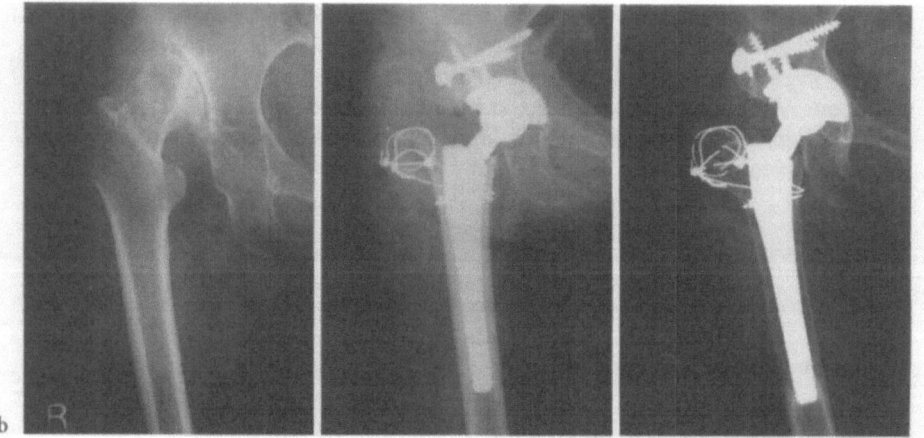

a,b   c

FIG. 4a–c. Radiographs of a 52-year-old woman with a dislocated hip. a Before operation.
b Immediately after THA. c Seven years after operation, showing severe stress shielding

   The relationships between cortical bone width ratio, canal filling ratio of the stem,
and stem diameter at 1 cm proximal from the stem tip and 5 hips exhibiting severe
stress shielding were examined and compared with those for the remaining 86 hips.
A statistically significant difference was observed in cortical bone width ratio and
stem diameter. Cortical bone width ratio was smaller and stem diameter was greater
in the stress-shielding patients than in the remaining patients (Table 1). Concerning
the relationships among cortical bone width ratio, canal filling ratio of the stem, and

TABLE 1. Results of cortical bone width ratio, canal filling ratio of the stem, and stem diameter at 1 cm proximal from the stem tip in 5 hips exhibiting severe stress shielding and the remaining 86 hips

	SSS ($n = 5$)	Other ($n = 86$)
Cortical bone width ratio (%)	37.2 ± 10.6*	52.5 ± 6.3
Canal filling ratio (%)	90.9 ± 4.4	90.0 ± 7.7
Stem diameter (mm)	12.3 ± 0.99*	10.1 ± 1.7

SSS, severe stress shielding
* $P < 0.01$

TABLE 2. Results of cortical bone width ratio, canal filling ratio of the stem, and stem diameter at 1 cm proximal from the stem tip in 4 patients with thigh pain and the remaining 87 hips

	Thigh pain ($n = 4$)	Other ($n = 87$)
Cortical bone width ratio (%)	36.7 ± 14.6*	52.1 ± 6.6
Canal filling ratio (%)	82.7 ± 9.4	90.3 ± 7.3
Stem diameter (mm)	10.5 ± 1.7	10.2 ± 1.7

* $P < 0.01$

stem diameter at 1 cm proximal to the stem tip and in 4 hips with a complaint of thigh pain, a statistically significant difference was observed in cortical bone width ratio, which was small in patients with thigh pain (Table 2).

Discussion

For fixation of a cementless stem, Matsumoto et al. [3] described new endosteal bone formation and a distal radiolucent line as characteristics of proximal fixation and proximal bone atrophy as characteristic of distal fixation. Approximately two-thirds of the present patients could undergo distal fixation.

Engh and Bobyn [4] noted that AML stem (Anatomic Medullary Locking stem; Depuy, Warsaw, IN, USA) patients who had stress shielding were those who had a thick stem with a diameter greater than 13.5 mm. In our patients, five hips that had severe stress shielding had a mean diameter larger than the other hips but had smaller cortical bone width ratios. Four hips that had thigh pain had smaller cortical bone width ratio than the other hips. Thus, careful indication is needed for patients with thin cortical bone width.

Yu et al. [5] reported that the procedure used for this custom-made stem system, with direct insertion of the stem without using a reamer or rasp, provided excellent initial fixation compared with conventional procedures in experimental studies. Goldberg et al. [6] noted that surface condition is excellent with grit-blasting.

Although further follow-up is needed, the results obtained with this custom-made stem system over a mean follow-up period of 5 years and 4 months were excellent.

References

1. Ohneda Y, Kakihana T, Kawate K, et al (1993) CT assisted femoral canal measurement and computer simulation of uncemented THA (in Japanese). Hip Joint 19:168–171
2. Engh CA, Glassman AH, Suthers KE (1990) The case for porous-coated hip implants. The femoral side. Clin Orthop 261:63–81
3. Matsumoto K, Okumura H, Ishimaru K, et al (1998) Radiographic assessment of femoral component of A-W glass ceramic coated cementless THA (in Japanese). Hip Joint 24:533–537
4. Engh CA, Bobyn (1987) The influence of stem size and extent of porous coating on femoral bone resorption after primary cementless hip arthroplasty. Clin Orthop 231:7–28
5. Yu L, Clark JG, Dai QG, et al (1999) Improving initial mechanical fixation of a porous coated femoral stem by a cancellous bone compaction method. Trans ORS 45:863
6. Goldberg VM, Stevenson S, Feighan J, et al (1995) Biology of grit-blasted titanium alloy implants. Clin Orthop 319:122–129

Custom-Made Cementless Total Hip Arthroplasty (Kyocera Expert 2)

Yutaka Oneda and Yumiko Natsume

Summary. This article describes a method for designing our custom cementless stem (Expert 2). The three-dimensional shape of the femoral canal is described by using CT data of a femoral axial scan. Our computer program decides the shape of an optimal-fit custom stem that can be inserted into the femoral canal. We have performed total hip replacements using this custom stem since 1997. Eighty-seven of the hips have reached 1 year or more after operation. The mean JOA score has been improved from 42 points preoperatively to 88 points the time of last follow-up. Short-term clinical results are considered to be successful.

Key words. Custom-made, Cementless, Total hip arthroplasty, Computed tomography, Design

Introduction

We had formerly developed a custom-made cementless total hip arthroplasty (THA) [1] (Kyocera, Kyoto, Japan; Expert 1) and had used it since 1992. However, it lacked flexibility in design of the stem and it was also difficul to fit optimally because the cross section of stem of Expert 1 consisted of two circles and tangents. Therefore, we changed the computer-aided software to design the cross section of the stem in any shape or form (Fig. 1). The new custom stem designed by the new software, named Expert 2, is able to be inserted into the femoral canal. We report here the method of designing the stem and preliminary results of this custom cementless stem.

Method of Stem Design

First, we obtain CT scans of the patient's proximal femur and femoral condyle. Axial scans, 2 mm thick, are taken every 5 mm, starting from the top of the femoral head to 20 cm distal. Moreover, one CT scan of the femoral condyle is taken to measure the

---

Department of Orthopaedic Surgery, National Nara Hospital, 1-50-1 Higashikidera-cho, Nara 630-8305, Japan

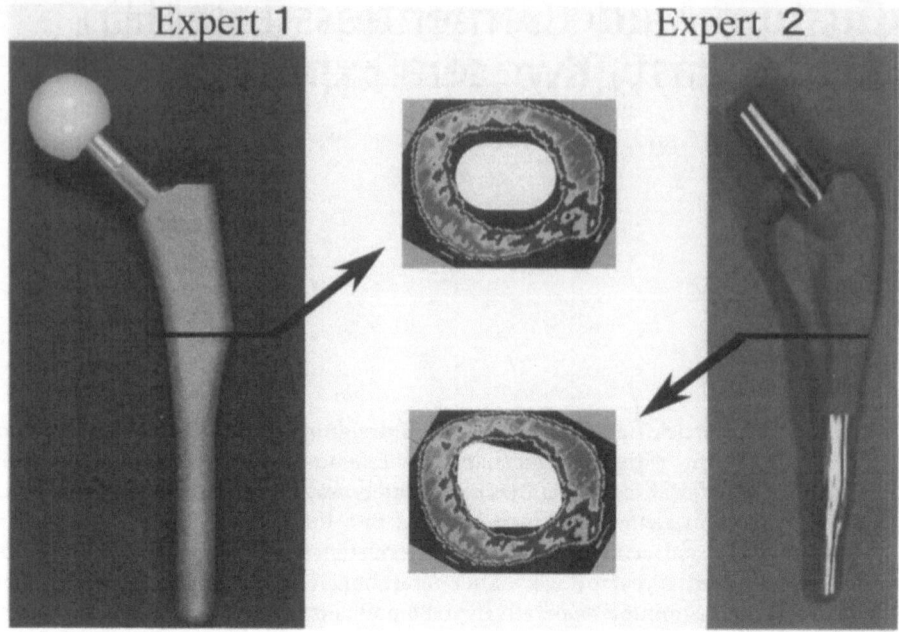

FIG. 1. The cross-section of Expert 2 is designed for any shape or form

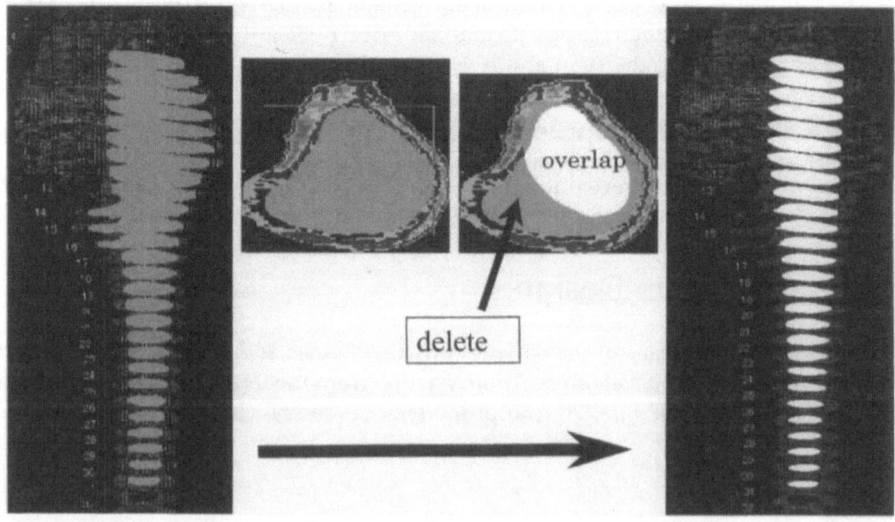

FIG. 2. Each cross section of stem uses only the part overlapping with the upper part of another cross section

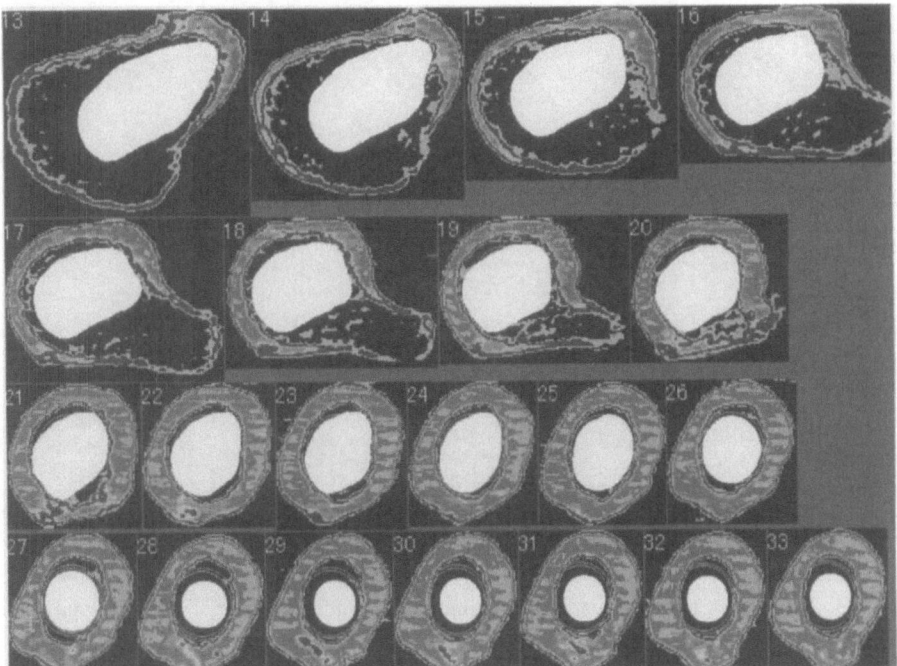

FIG. 3. Cross sections of femur and stem

rotation of the patient's lower limbs at the CT scan. These images of the CT scan are preserved on a magnetoptical disc. In our CAD sytem, the computer directly reads these CT images and processes them in three dimensions.

The design of the custom stem begins with the decision on the axis of inserted stem. The axis depends on drawing inscribed circles on two CT images of the femoral shaft. Next, we draw manually the inner cortical contours of the cross sections of the femur on the computer display. Then, the fundamental shape of stem is fixed. Nevertheless, it is impossible to insert this fundamental shape of the stem itself into the femoral canal. Thus, each cross section of the stem uses only the part overlapping with the upper part of each cross section (Fig. 2). After these procedures, the optimal-fit custom stem that can be inserted into the femoral canal is designed (Figs. 3, 4).

Material and Results

We have performed total hip replacements by using Expert 2 since 1997. Among them, 87 of the hips have reached more than 1 year after operation; for instance, the average period is about 14 months (range, 12–24 months). The average age of the patients at the operation is about 60 years (range, 42–76 years). The mean JOA (Japanese Orthopedic Association) score has been improved from 42 points at preoperatively to 88 points at the time of last follow-up. Short-term clinical results are considered to be successful, because these results do not indicate that the patient has the thigh pain that occasionally occurs after conventional uncemented THA (Fig. 5).

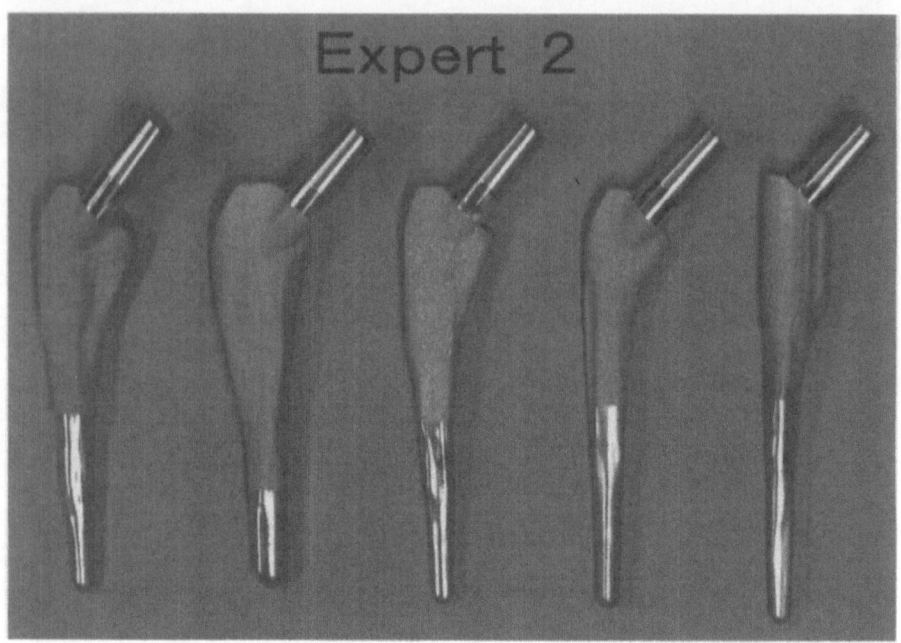

FIG. 4. The Expert 2 stem is made with titanium alloy and the proximal part of its surface is sandblasted

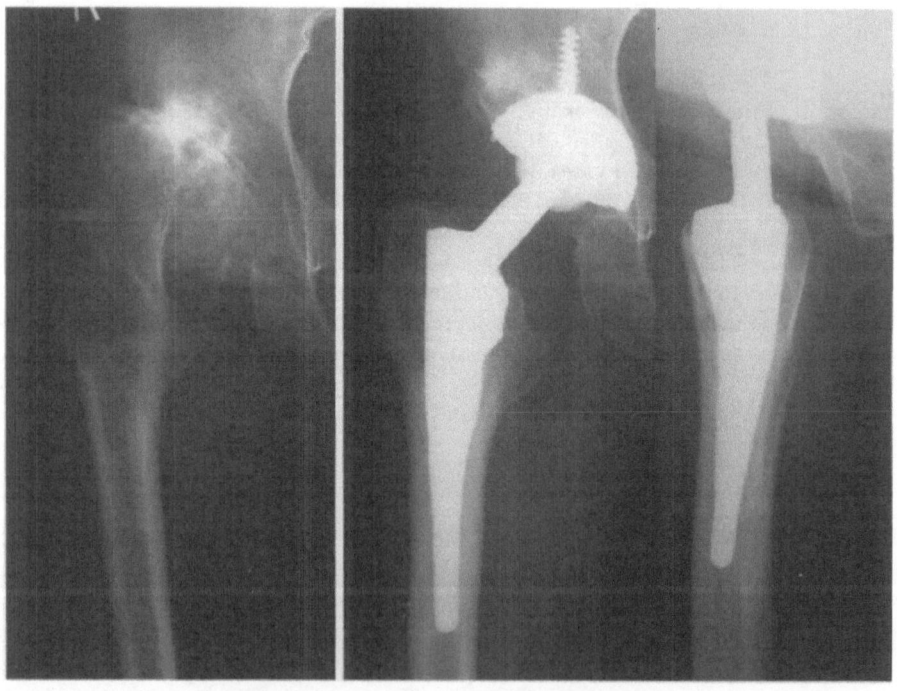

FIG. 5. This 42-year-old woman received a Pauwels valgus osteotomy 15 years ago; she has no pain and walks without a crutch 1 year and 6 months after custom THA

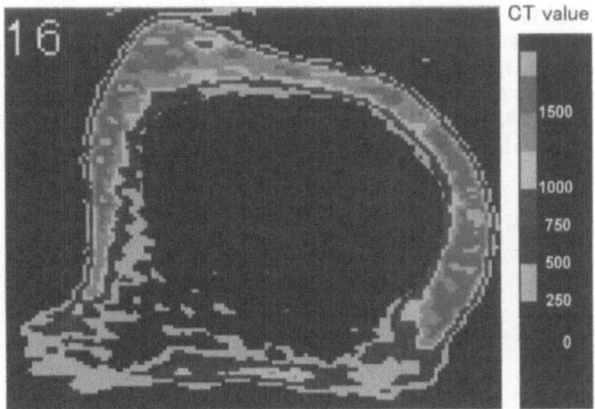

FIG. 6. This photograph is black and white. In our real software, cross sections of femur are displayed in color according to the CT value so that it is easy for the designer to recognize the boundary of the inner cortex

In addition, the studies provide the good canal filling rate that we expected before the operation. Canal filling rate on the anteroposterior radiographs was 94% ± 4% below the lesser trochanter, 92% ± 6% at the midpoint of the lesser trochanter and stem tip, and 79% ± 8% at the stem tip.

Discussion

There have been some reports of custom THA since 1988 [2–5]. Logically, the best way for the cementless stem is to design an optimal form for each patient by using CT scans and the computer. However, some authors have stated that the clinical results obtained with custom THA are inferior to those of conventional THA. There are several unresolved problems in the design of the custom THA, and especially the performance of CAD may have effects on the clinical results of a custom THA. At least, the cross sections of the femur should be displayed in color, which can assist the judgement of the CT value; the designer of a custom stem may not be able to judge the boundary between a hard bone and a soft bone if cross sections of the femur are displayed in black and white. In our CAD software, cross sections of the femur are displayed in color according to the CT value (Fig. 6), so that the designer can recognize the boundary of the inner cortex. That step is why successful clinical results have been obtained in our custom THA.

References

1. Yutaka O (1995) Development of custom-made cementless THA and clinical results (in Japanese). East Jpn J Clin Orthop 7:458–463
2. Garg A, Deland JT, Walker PS (1985) Design of intramedullary femoral stems using computer graphics. Eng Med 14:89–93

3. Robertson DD, et al (1987) Design of custom hip stem prosthesis using 3-D CT modeling. J Comput Assist Tomogr 11:804–809
4. Stulberg SD, Stulberg BN, Wixson RL (1989) The rationale, design characteristics, and preliminary results of a primary custom total hip prosthesis. Clin Orthop 249:79–96
5. Bargar WL (1989) Shape the implant to the patient: a rationale for the use of custom-fit cementless total hip implants. Clin Orthop 249:73–78

Cementless Total Hip Arthroplasty Using a Custom-Made Femoral Component with Sand-Blasted Surface

Takashi Sakai[1], Nobuhiko Sugano[1], Minoru Matsui[2], Seung-Bak Lee[2], Takashi Nishii[1], Keiji Haraguchi[1], Katsuya Nakata[3], Takahiro Ochi[1], Hideki Yoshikawa[1], and Kenji Ohzono[1]

Summary. This study reviews the clinical and radiographical results of 98 cementless total hip arthroplasties (THAs) using custom-made, 125-mm-long femoral components with a sand-blasted surface at a mean of 52 months follow-up. All 76 patients were diagnosed as having secondary osteoarthritis of the hip, and their mean age at operation was 54 years. With the Japan Orthopaedic Association's scoring system for osteoarthritis of the hip (JOA hip score), 93 hips (95%) were clinically evaluated as excellent, 4 (4%) as good, and 1 (1%) as poor. Radiographically, 86 hips (87%) were assessed as bone-ongrown fixation, 8 (9%) as stable fibrous fixation, and 4 (4%) as unstable. Both clinical and radiographical results were better than those reported elsewhere for cementless custom-made femoral components with surface finish insufficient for bone ongrowth. The four unstable hips had intraoperative cracks or varus positioning of the components. Such technical errors were thought to be due to the length of the stems, which was designed to obtain the maximum fill of implant in the medullary canal. We therefore reduced the stem length of the custom-made femoral components to 100 mm.

Key words. Custom-made femoral component, Cementless total hip arthroplasty (THA), Surface finish, Stem length, Canal filling

Introduction

To achieve optimal fit and canal filling for patients with variable femoral geometry, we have been using cementless custom-made total hip arthroplasty (THA) since 1994 for patients with secondary osteoarthritis of the hip [1]. A curved stem was designed to obtain not only maximum fill of implant in the medullary canal, but also to make implantation possible based on computer simulation of the insertion. To investigate the clinical and radiographical results for cementless custom-made THA, we reviewed

[1] Department of Orthopedic Surgery, Osaka University Medical School, 2-2 Yamadaoka, Suita, Osaka 565-0871, Japan
[2] Department of Orthopaedic Surgery, Osaka National Hospital, Osaka, Japan
[3] Department of Orthopaedic Surgery, Kansai Rousai Hospital, Amagasaki, Hyogo, Japan

the results of 98 hips using custom-made, 125-mm-long femoral components with sand-blasted surface.

Patients and Methods

Between January 1994 and July 1997, 76 patients had 98 custom-made total hip femoral components implanted primarily, for acetabular dysplasia or congenital dislocation of the hip with resultant degenerative arthritis. There were 69 women and 7 men, with mean age at operation of 54 years (range, 40–73 years). The mean postoperative follow-up period was 52 months (range, 30–72 months).

Custom-made femoral components (Cremascoli, Milano, Italy) were produced with the aid of computerized tomography (CT). The inner and outer contours of the femur were digitized on serial 3- to 5-mm pitch axial CT images, after which the maximum implantable femoral component with a stem length of 125 mm was designed. The femoral component was made from titanium alloy (Ti-6Al-4V) with a sand-blasted surface.

The operations were performed under general anesthesia through the posterolateral approach. The hip then was dislocated posteriorly during surgery. No trochanteric osteotomies were performed. The femoral canal was opened with a custom-made broach that precisely duplicates the shape of the custom-made prosthesis so as to provide a close and exact fit. After insertion of the femoral components, modular neck and head systems were used. The modular head system consisted of three increments of alumina ceramic head. On the acetabular side, in 82 hips a spongy metal socket and polyethylene cup insert (ESKA, Lubeck, Germany) was inserted and in the remaining 16 hips an ANCA-fit socket and alumina ceramic cup insert (Cremascoli).

All patients received prophylactic intravenous antibiotics (2 g second-generation cephalosporins at the time of anesthesia and then 2 g every 12 h for 72 h). Anticoagulants were not administered. Elastic stockings were used to prevent thromboembolic disease for the first 2 postoperative weeks. In cases without complications, partial weight-bearing was started at 1 week, and full weight-bearing was allowed at 3 weeks after surgery. The treatment of any intraoperatively incurred cracks or fractures consisted of 6 weeks of partial weight-bearing with crutches.

Clinical results were evaluated before surgery and at the latest follow-up using the Japan Orthopaedic Association scoring system for osteoarthritis of the hip (JOA hip score). Presence of thigh pain was also checked at the latest follow-up. Radiologically, the mode of femoral component fixation at 2 years postoperatively was evaluated according to the criteria of Engh et al. [2]: bone-ongrown, stable fibrous, and unstable fixation. Migration of femoral components was determined on the basis of measurements of the following values: the vertical distance from the shoulder of the stem to the midpoint of the lesser trochanter, and the varus angle of the stem formed by the axis of the stem and the the axis of the proximal femur. More than 2 mm of subsidence in the vertical distance or changes of more than 2° in the varus angle was considered to indicate stem migration. The canal filling on the AP and lateral radiographs 3 weeks after surgery was measured at 1 cm below the lesser trochanter level and at 1 cm above the stem tip level. Presence of stress shielding [2] and osteolysis of the femur were also assessed at the latest follow-up.

Results

Clinical Evaluation

Clinical results are shown in Table 1. The respective mean pain and total scores were 16 and 45 before THA and 39 and 96 at the latest follow-up. Ninly-three hips (95%) were evaluated as excellent (a score of 90 or more), 4 (4%) as good (a score of 80 or more), and 1 (1%) as poor (less than 80). Thigh pain was detected in 2 hips (2%) at the latest follow-up.

Radiological Evaluation

Examination of the mode of femoral component fixation at 2 years postoperatively resulted in 86 hips (87%) being assessed as bone-ongrown fixation, 8 (9%) as stable fibrous fixation, and 4 hips (4%) as unstable fixation. Bone densification and bridging were detected from the middle to the distal part of the stem (Fig. 1).

Of the four unstable hips, two had intraoperative cracks of the proximal femur and two had varus positioning of the stem. One hip showed more than 10 mm subsidence and one 2 mm subsidence, while the other two hips showed varus migration of the femoral components.

Canal filling is shown in Table 2. At 1 cm below the lesser trochanter level, the mean filling on the anteroposterior (AP) view was 91.9% and the mean filling on the lateral view was 90.6%. At 1 cm above the stem tip level, the corresponding values were 77.6% and 74.6%.

Stress shielding of the proximal femur was detected in 78 hips (80%) at the latest follow-up, with 58 hips (60%) showing first-degree and 20 hips (20%) second-degree shielding. No osteolysis was observed in any hips at the latest follow-up.

TABLE 1. Japan Orthopaedic Association scoring system (JOA score) for osteoarthritis of the hip

Factor	Before THA	At the latest follow-up
Total	45 ± 11 (17–70)	96 ± 5 (60–100)
Pain	15 ± 8 (0–35)	39 ± 2 (20–40)
Range of motion (ROM)	10 ± 4 (1–19)	17 ± 1 (12–20)
Gait	9 ± 3 (5–15)	20 ± 1 (10–20)
Activity of daily life (ADL)	11 ± 3 (4–20)	20 ± 1 (14–20)

THA, total hip arthroplasty

TABLE 2. Canal filling of the custom-made femoral component (%)

Position	Anteroposterior (AP) view	Lateral view
1 cm below the lesser trochanter level	91.9 ± 4.7 (78.2–100)	90.6 ± 4.3 (79.8–98.3)
1 cm above the stem tip level	77.6 ± 7.6 (61.5–93.8)	74.6 ± 7.1 (60.3–91.1)

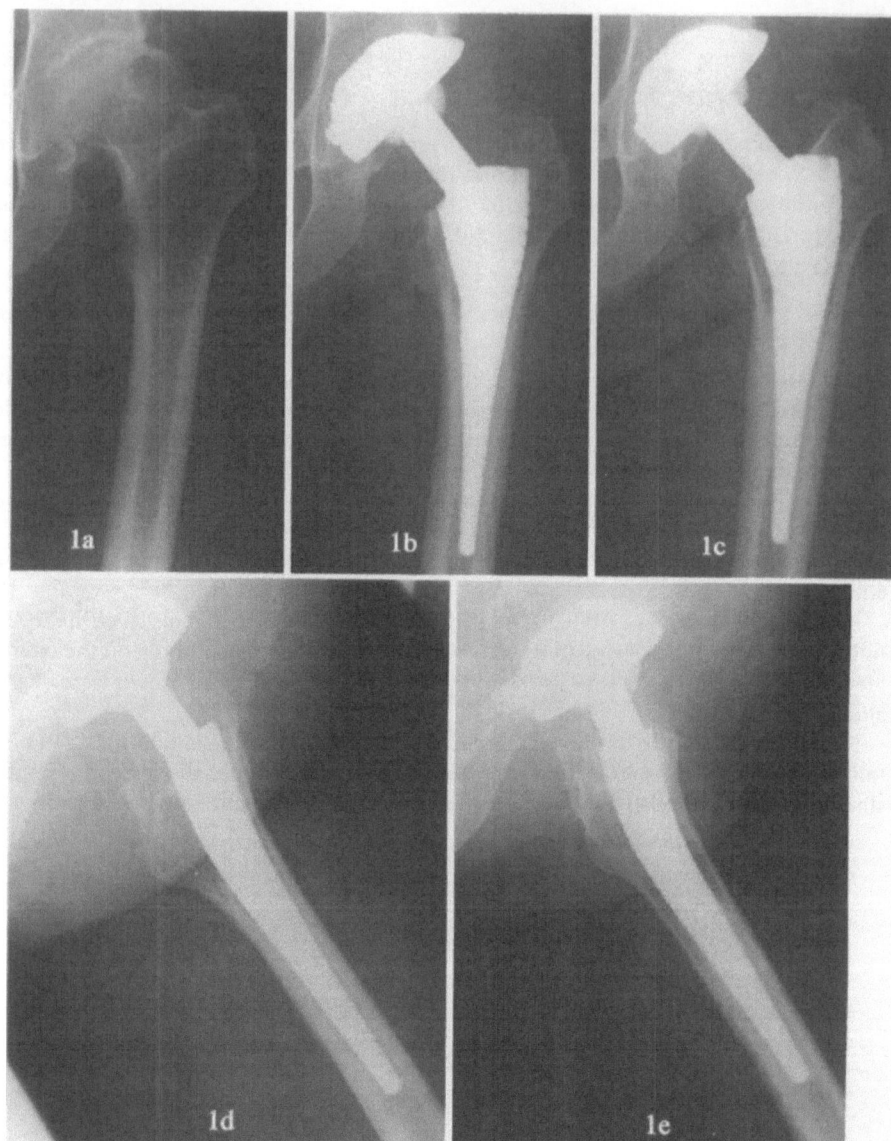

FIG. 1a–e. Secondary osteoarthritis in a 45-year-old woman caused by developmental dislocation of the hip. **a** Anteroposterior (AP) view before surgery. **b** AP view at 6 months postoperatively. **c** AP view at 5 years postoperatively. **d** Lateral view at 6 months postoperatively. **e** Lateral view at 5 years postoperatively

Discussion

Optimal fit and canal filling [2,3] as well as surface finish [3–5] are important for stable fixation in cementless total hip arthroplasty (THA). To achieve the optimal fit and fill in patients with variable femoral geometry, especially in cases of osteoarthritis secondary to hip dysplasia, custom-made femoral prostheses [6–13] or modular prostheses [14] are more effective than off-the-shelf components.

However, some clinical studies have failed to show any significant improvement in clinical success or implant longevity for custom-made prostheses because their surface finish, either smooth or proximal titanium mesh pads, was not optimal for cementless THA [7,8,11]. In this study, the custom-made femoral components have a blasted surface, and the efficacy of this surface has been reported [4]. Clinically, 97 hips (99%) showed excellent or good results, and radiographically 94 (96%) achieved stable fixation. Both clinical and radiographical results were better than those reported elsewhere for cementless custom-made femoral components with surface finish unsuitable for bone ongrowth [7,8,11].

Four unstable hips showed intraoperative cracks of the proximal femur or varus positioning of the components. Such technical errors were thought to be due to the length of the stems (125 mm), which was designed to result in maximum fill of implant in the medullary canal. We therefore, discontinued the use of the 125-mm-long custom-made femoral components and reduced the stem length of the custom-made femoral components to 100 mm. This improvement of the stem design concept is expected to produce better results.

References

1. Sakai T, Sugano N, Nishii T, et al (1999) Stem length and canal filling in uncemented custom-made total hip arthroplasty. Int Orthop 23:219–223
2. Engh CA, Glassman AH, Suthers KE (1990) The case for porous-coated hip implants. The femoral side. Clin Orthop 261:63–81
3. Bourne RB, Rorabeck CH, Burkart BC, et al (1994) Ingrowth surfaces. Plasma spray coating to titanium alloy hip replacements. Clin Orthop 298:37–46
4. Feighan JE, Goldberg VM, Davy D, et al (1995) The influence of surface-blasting on the incorporation of titanium-alloy implants in a rabbit intramedullary model. J Bone Joint Surg 77A:1380–1395
5. Geesink RGT, Hoefnagels NHM (1995) Six-year results of hydroxyapatite-coated total hip replacement. J Bone Joint Surg 77B:534–547
6. Barger WL (1989) Shape the implant to the patient. A rationale for the use of custom-fit cementless total hip implants. Clin Orthop 249:73–78
7. Bert JM (1996) Custom total hip arthroplasty. J Arthroplasty 11:905–915
8. Lombardi AV, Mallory TH, Eberle RW, et al (1995) Failure of intraoperatively customized non-porous femoral components inserted without cement in total hip arthroplasty. J Bone Joint Surg 77A:1836–1844
9. McCarthy JC, Bono JV, O'Donnell PJ (1997) Custom and modular components in primary total hip replacement. Clin Orthop 344:162–171
10. Mulier JC, Mulier M, Brady LP, et al (1989) A new system to produce intraoperatively custom femoral prosthesis from measurements taken during the surgical procedure. Clin Orthop 249:97–112

11. Robinson RP, Clark JE (1996) Uncemented press-fit total hip arthroplasty using the Identifit custom-molding technique. A prospective minimum 2-year follow-up study. J Arthroplasty 11:247–254
12. Stulberg SD, Stulberg BN, Wixson RL (1989) The rationale, design characteristics, and preliminary results of a primary custom total hip prosthesis. Clin Orthop 249:79–96
13. Xenaklis TA, Gelalis ID, Koukoubis TD, et al (1996) Neglected congenital dislocation of the hip. Role of computed tomography and computer-aided design for total hip arthroplasty. J Arthroplasty 11:893–898
14. Gorski JM (1988) Modular noncemented total hip arthroplasty for congenital dislocation of the hip. Clin Orthop 228:111–116

Part 5 Computer Assisted Surgery

Computer-Assisted Procedures in Orthopedic Surgery

MARTIN BOERNER, ULRICH WIESEL, and ARMIN LAHMER

Summary. The first successful robot-assisted total hip replacement (THR) was performed at BGU (Berufsgenossenschaftliche Unfallklinik) Frankfurt in 1994 and has become a standard procedure at BGU. Operating room time decreased to an average of 90 min, and it was possible to change the system from three to two pins. The robot guarantees precise transformation of the preoperative plan during surgery. Femur fractures, a common complication in THR, can be avoided. In January 2000, the 2500th operation using Robodoc was performed successfully at BGU Frankfurt. The results were supported by a dog study at the Small Animal Clinic in Auburn, Alabama, in 1995 comparing a robot group to a hand-broached group of male greyhounds. The next important step was the introduction of the Robodoc Pinless System at BGU Frankfurt in mid-1998. The system also contains a revision software. Now, the pinless procedure has become everyday routine at BGU just like the pin-based procedure.

Key words. Robodoc, THR, Revision THR, CAOS, Hip

Introduction

Each year, hundreds of thousands of patients undergo total hip arthroplasty. Indications for total hip arthroplasty are severe pain and disability resulting from osteo-, rheumatoid, or posttraumatic arthritis of the hip joint, or avascular necrosis of the femoral head.

The modern era of total hip replacement started in the late 1960s with the Charnley cemented total hip replacement system. The disadvantage of cemented hip replacements is that the cement can crack, loosen, or give rise to osteolysis, causing failure of the implant. Implant design has advanced since the Charnley era, and probably the greatest advance occurred with the development of cementless implant systems. Cementless implant systems rely on "natural" fixation from bone growing into the porous metal surfaces of the implant [1]. Clinical and basic science research has shown that for ingrowth to occur, the cavity of the femur must be very exact, such that any gap between bone and porous surface is less than 0.25 mm.

Berufsgenossenschaftliche Unfallklinik Frankfurt am Main, Friedberger Landstrasse 430, D-60389 Frankfurt am Main, Germany

In the traditional method of preparing the femur for a cementless implant a series of handheld reamers and broaches is used to create the general size and shape of the cavity in bone. Although implant components are manufactured to a high level of precision, the method of creating the bone cavity has been much less precise. The reamers and broaches follow the canal of the bone, and precise alignment is not always possible. In addition the tools tend to bounce off hard cortical bone and tear away softer trabecular bone, leaving large gaps that may result in improper ingrowth and early loosening of the implant. An additional complication of the traditional approach is intraoperative fractures of the femur, which can occur if the implant is placed in a misshaped cavity [2].

Developments

In 1991, Paul Hap, a veterinarian in Sacramento, California, convinced scientists at the University of Davis in California in cooperation with engineers from IBM to start a research project with the goal to be able to implant a prosthesis into canine femora by using a computer-controlled milling device to prepare the cavity.

IBM engineers had started in 1986 to develop an automated machine language that was applied successfully to tasking an industrial robot to mill simplified shapes in synthetic bone. Later on, an imaging system was developed based upon 3-D registered data that retains pixel size accuracy for registration. Also, a computer workstation was developed to preplan prosthesis selection and positioning. Human and canine cadaver bones were milled in vitro using a modified industrial robot to reach accuracies equal to or better than implant tolerances.

As a next step, specifications were developed for a surgical robot designed to operate in the sterile OR environment. A canine study using 26 dogs with a dysplasia of the hip was performed successfully. The use of the system did not cause any major problems, and the subject dogs that had received robot-assisted total hip replacement showed faster recovery than those dogs whose prosthesis was implanted in the traditional way. The improved precision was verified. No untoward risks were identified. Given the results of the canine study, a ten-patient feasibility study was completed in California. No unforseen risks were identified. All surgeries were successfully completed [3–5].

In 1993, a 300-patient randomized multicenter trial was started in the United States. Patients to be included in this study had to be candidates for cementless total hip replacement. Specific inclusion and exclusion criteria were utilized. Patients had to be at least 21 years of age but no older than 80 years of age. Excluded were patients with an active systemic or local infection, patients requiring revision surgery, patients with metallic implants in the operative hemipelvis or femur, and patients with pathological skeletal conditions. Some other exclusion criteria were applied. The patients were randomized into either the control group or the Robodoc group. The average age for the Robodoc group was 52 years and for the control group it was 55 years. Osteoarthritis dominated in both groups. Two different implants were used: the Osteolock (Howmedica) and the AML (Depuy). Patients were reviewed separately according to implant-specific criteria.

The average surgery time was longer for the Robodoc group (266 versus 125 min). The average length of hospital stay was not significantly different. There were *no* intraoperative femoral fractures in the Robodoc group compared to two fractures in the control group. Radiographic review by Dr. Charles Engh (Anderson Clinic, Arlington, VA) and Dr. William Bargar (Sutter General, Sacramento, CA) of the AMLs showed significant differences when comparing Robodoc to control: correct size, 100% versus 78%; correct position, 97% versus 61%; and reaming defects, 3% versus 14%. These factors have been shown to be surrogate indicators for long-term outcome and suggest an improvement for long-term clinical results using this technique. The clinical trial is still under consideration by the FDA for approval of Robodoc [2,6].

Designing a system for use in human operating rooms imposes strict performance, safety, and user interface requirements. The feasibility of using a robot to prepare a femoral cavity for total hip replacement (THR) was shown by operating with a prototype on canine patients. The prototype functioned as intended, but all the canine surgeries required extensive engineering assistance. Many changes were necessary to prepare the second-generation system for unsupervised use by trained but technically unskilled personnel in human clinical trials. Changes were applied to both the presurgical planning component of the system and the surgical robot [7].

System Setup

The Robodoc Surgical Assistant System consists of three major components: the preoperative planning workstation called Orthodoc, the surgical robot, and the robot control unit that receives the preoperative planning data and controls the Robodoc. At the beginning of the procedure three titanium pins had to be implanted, one in the greater trochanter and two in the medial and lateral femoral condyle. The number of pins was later reduced to two and the pin in the lateral condyle was omitted. Cannulated pins are being used to ensure the implantation can be performed with as little as possible soft tissue damage. These pins are the landmarks for the following procedures.

A CT scan is made of the proximal femur and the distal pin(s). A rod is laid on the patient's leg to detect the motion during CT scan. About 75 CT slices are taken; the thickness of the CT slices is 1 mm. The CT data are transferred to the Orthodoc workstation on an optical disk. The Orthodoc is a very powerful graphic workstation based on a PC. One patient's CT data averages 20–30 megabytes. The system automatically computes the distances between the pins and the axes of the pins. Orthodoc also checks the CT data to determine whether the patient moved during the CT scan. For this, the center of the rod is computed for each CT scan. The program checks if all the points are on a line. The planning system has the capability of building a 3-D model of the femur.

The Orthodoc displays three orthogonal cross sections of the femur (AP, lateral, and cross section) on a high-resolution screen. A manipulation on one of the cross sections is shown in nearly real time on the other two cross sections. The first step of the planning procedure is to adjust the axis of proximal femur in the AP and lateral views by rotating and translating the images. The surgeon can zoom in and zoom out to facilitate this procedure. The second step is to mark the rotation center of the femur head in three dimensions relative to the CT coordinates. This step is necessary for an exact reconstruction of the leg length and the anteversion. After finishing this, the surgeon selects an implant model from an implant library. At present, it is possible to choose from five different implants.

The surgeon interactively adjusts the position of the implant in the proximal femur by using the computer mouse. The system provides a resolution of 1 mm for shifting the implant. It is possible to use any type of implant with the Robodoc system provided that the implant dimensional data are loaded into the Orthodoc system. For optimizing the fit of the prosthesis in the proximal femur, it is possible to rotate the implant with a resolution of 0.1° in each direction. For optimizing the planning, the systems allow the surgeon to show the density of the bone with different colors on the screen and also to zoom in to the important areas of bone–implant contact. The implant can also be displayed as opaque, transparent, or an outline. Thus, the surgeon has the possibility to select the best implant for his patient. After finishing the planning, a transfer tape that can be loaded into the Robodoc is created.

The robot first runs a diagnostic program. A sterile ball probe is attached to a tool interface below the force sensor, and the robot is covered with a sterile drape. The patient data tape is loaded into the robot controller and the robot is placed into standby mode. The patient is prepared and draped in the normal manner. Surgery proceeds normally until the acetabular component of the implant is implanted and the head of the femur is removed. The robot is brought up to the OR table and the femur is rigidly attached to the robot base using a specially designed fixator. The two (three) titanium pins are exposed manually. The robot's bone motion monitor is attached to the bone. The top center of each pin is then located by the ball probe on the tip of the robot arm. The controller of the robot compares the distances and angles measured by the preoperative planning system with the data measured intraoperatively. Now the ball probe is removed and a sterile cutting tool is attached to the robot. The robot will start cutting only if all distance differences are less than 3 mm.

This provision is only one of the safety features of the system. Robodoc reams out the cavity with an accuracy better than 0.5 mm. If the bone motion monitor detects any sign of bone motion (i.e., the patient moving on the OR table) that goes beyond a certain tolerance, the process is stopped and the pin-finding process has to be restarted. The reaming takes between 15 and 30 min; this means that the implant is placed in the position the surgeon planned on the Orthodoc during surgery. The contact between the implant and bone is optimized for good stability, which should result in an optimized ingrowth of the bone to the surface of the implant [8–12].

Clinical Introduction

In 1991, first contacts between the Berufsgenossenschaftliche Unfallklinik (BGU) Frankfurt am Main and Integrated Surgical Systems (ISS) in Sacramento, the developers of Robodoc, were established. Since that time, parallel to the ongoing studies in the United States, transition of this technology to the European market was discussed and planned. There were several prerequisites for the Robodoc transfer to Germany. Apart from the FDA approval, German regulations required the TÜV testing of the system, which, contrary to the FDA procedure, did not challenge the efficacy of the system but put emphasis on its technical safety. Regarding the system as a tool in the surgeon's control, its use and the evaluation of its benefits were left to the surgeon's jugdement.

The major issue in the transfer of Robodoc to Germany was the different surgical approach. Although many American surgeons operate on total hips through a posterior approach, with the patient in a lateral decubitus position, most German and European surgeons prefer the anterolateral approach in which the patient is positioned supine on the OR table. Extensive testing led to modifications of the fixator arm of the robot, the bone motion monitor, and the lower leg holder. Pins were placed and found in a different orientation, so software had to be adapted.

After obtaining TÜV certification, the system was installed at BGU in Frankfurt in July 1994. The first two cases, performed in the same week, had to be aborted because of inaccurate CT data. These cases nevertheless proved the safety of the system. The computer detected an error in table motion of the "somewhat dated" CT scanner during pin finding. Lacking accuracy in pin data, the computer refused to complete the procedure. The first successful surgery with a hand-corrected CT was performed in August 1994. In November 1994, a new CT scanner was installed. Subsequently, between November 1994 and November 1995 150 cases were attempted; 142 patients were successfully operated on with the Robodoc, and 8 procedures had to be aborted. In 2 cases there was a CT error, 2 cases had to be aborted due to pin loosening, 1 case due to a software error, another case due to mechanical error, and in 2 cases there was a user error.

All these cases could be completed by hand, although the preoperatively planned implant sizes could not be manually executed by the surgeon. The first 150 cases proved that robotic surgery can be performed on patients without exposing them to uncertain risks. While OR time in the first 15 cases averaged 180 min, the succeeding patients were operated on in an average time of 120 min, and the fastest cases required 69 min. The overall complication rate was lower than in a comparable cementless series previously published. No fractures occurred, a rather common complication in cementless hip replacement. In all robot cases, the preoperatively chosen implant could be implanted, and postoperative X-rays showed that positioning of the implant was performed with a high degree of exactness when related to the preoperative plan. Consequently, immediate full weight-bearing was recommended to the patients [9,10,12].

Dog Study

To support these results, a dog study was started at the Small Animal Clinic at Auburn University in Auburn, Alabama, in 1995. The goals of the study were clinical performance (fractures), gait analysis, and histological evaluation (healing implant–bone); 20 male greyhounds with a weight of 60–70 pounds were used in the study. Preoperatively all the dogs received vaccination, and clinical examination, gait analysis, and X-rays were performed.

The robot group received pin implantation in general anesthesia and a subsequent CT scan. Surgery was planned on the Orthodoc, and robot-assisted hemiarthroplasty was performed in general anesthesia. In the hand-broached group, surgery was planned with templates that were put over X-rays, and the dogs received conventional hemiarthroplasty. Postoperatively, both groups received polychrome sequence labeling. A gait analysis was performed after 6 weeks. Necropsy was performed in three intervals, after 35, 84, and 365 days.

The results showed that surgery time in the Robodoc group was 30 min longer compared to the hand-broached group. In the hand-broached group, there were two fractures and none in the Robodoc group; two persistent nerve palsies were found in the hand-broached group and none in the Robodoc group. Gait analysis was superior in the Robodoc group. Histology showed that in the Robodoc group there were signs of primary healing. Also, there was closer alignment of the prosthesis to strong cortical bone. The hand-broached group showed signs of major repairs and more disturbances, as well as less cortical contact of the prosthesis.

The conclusions of the study were that in the Robodoc group there were no fractures, an exact transformation of the preoperative plan, superior gait analysis, and histological signs of primary healing [13].

Clinical Experience

In January 2000, the 2500th operation with Robodoc was performed successfully at BGU Frankfurt; 58.8% were male patients and 41.2% were female. The indication for the operation was osteoarthrosis in 69.9%, posttraumatic osteoarthrosis in 13.9%, dysplasia in 12.7%, and 3.5% were revision cases. Complications were nerve palsy (3.5%), dislocation of the hip (2.9%), deep vein thrombosis (2.5%), pulmonary embolism (0.9%), and infection (0.2%).

The OR time decreased from an average of 209 min for the first 10 operations to an average of 90 min after the 500th case. Due to the milling process, which takes an average of 20–30 min, OR time cannot be reduced much further at present. Most patients we operated on were in the age group from 46 to 65 years. Of these patients, 4.7% have received bilateral THR with the Robodoc. The most common complication of cementless THR, the fracure or fissure of the femur, was reduced to 0.0% in the group of the 2500 Robodoc patients. The disadavantages of using Robodoc are the increased radiation of the CT scan compared to conventional X-rays, the second operation for the pin implantation when using the pin-based system, the increased OR time, and the postoperative knee pain caused by the distal pin.

There are costs for additional material used, additional staff costs, and costs for the additional operation for the pin implantation. Absolute contraindications for using Robodoc are morbid obesity, poor bone quality, parkinsonism, and an uncooperative patient. Relative contraindications are patients above the age of 70 years.

The increased OR time could be lowered substantially by changing from the three-pin to the two-pin system. The next important step in using Robodoc at BGU Frankfurt was the introduction of the pinless system in mid-1998 [9,10,14,15].

In 12 patients who had both hips replaced with the Robodoc system, we compared the actual position of the shaft 300 days after robot-assisted total hip replacement to the original planning on the Orthodoc. This comparison was possible by reconstructing the opposite hip in the CT scan when the CT scan for the second surgery was performed, and this did not cause any additional radiation exposure. Eight patients were male, four were female. We found a dislocation of no more than 0.6 mm in the proximal area vertical to the axes of the shaft. The variation along the axes of the shaft was 1.5 mm in the mean, and the differences in the axes were 0.6°. In our study we measured all the inaccuracies of the system and of the CT scan. We also registered all the changes of the implant position between the first and the second surgery. Our results showed an excellent correspondence between the planning and the actual position of the prosthesis [16].

Robot-Assisted Revision THR

The Orthodoc also contains a revision software that enables us to plan and execute total hip revision surgery with Robodoc. The program uses a special technique to enhance the CT images so that all the existing bone cement in the cavity and around the old prosthesis is clearly visible and can be distinguished from bone structures. Also, metal artifacts caused by the existing prosthesis are minimized. A cutting path can be planned to remove all the existing bone cement.

The next step is the planning of the new prosthesis. Any prosthesis available in the Orthodoc's software library can be used. The new prosthesis is planned above the old prosthesis. Just as in the program for primary THR, the prosthesis can be adjusted in any direction until a satisfactory position is reached. The data again are transferred onto a tape and loaded into the Robodoc. Intraoperatively, after the normal pin-finding procedure, the robot mills out the existing bone cement and creates a new cavity for the planned implant.

As mentioned before, this procedure cannot be performed with the pinless system. The advantages of using Robodoc for revision surgery are obvious. Optimized preoperative planning of the procedure is possible, the anteversion can be corrected, and the fibrous membrane and sclerosis in the cavity are removed by the cutter. The duration of the operation is greatly reduced compared to the traditional method of removing the bone cement manually. There is no risk of intraoperative fractures. There are several options for revision surgery. A loose uncemented prosthesis can be replaced by a new uncemented implant. A loose cemented prothesis can be replaced by either a cemented or an uncemented implant. If a cemented implant is used as the new implant, only the removal of the bone cement can be planned on the Orthodoc, not the prosthesis itself [17,18].

Conclusions

Robot-assisted surgery in total hip replacement using the Robodoc system can be performed without exposing the patient to uncertain risks. Working with Orthodoc is a revolution in presurgical planning. The robot guarantees precise transformation of the preoperative plan during surgery. Femur fractures, a common complication in cementless total hip replacement, can be avoided. Surgery times are longer but within a reasonable range. Robodoc proved to be a reliable and safe technology that can be handled by a trained surgeon without permanent on-site support. The rather short follow-up (5 years) and the results of the dog study give us reason to hope that long-term results will be favorable. The long-term outcome measure for total hip replacement requires more than 10-year follow-up.

Certain short-term variables can be shown to correlate with outcome, hence, "surrogate variables." Outcomes of new techniques and devices can be implied by measuring surrogate variables. We believe that proper implant selection, position, and fit are "surrogate variables" for long-term outcomes of cementless total hip arthroplasty.

Future applications of Robodoc will be computer-assisted planning and positioning of the acetabular cup in total hip replacement, total knee replacement, and osteotomies. Clinical trials on the implantation of the acetabular component have already started at BGU. Total knee replacement and osteotomies are planned to go to the clinical trial stage later this year, and software development for total knee replacement is well underway [19–21]. By January 2000, 2500 patients had undergone total hip replacement successfully using Robodoc.

References

1. Noble PC, Alexander JW: Robotic vs. manual preparation of the femur: the stability of the cementless femoral implant interface
2. Bargar WL, Blumenfeld T, Parise C: Stress shielding in cementless THA: a DEXA study comparing Robodoc vs. conventional surgical techniques
3. Kazanzides P, Mittelstadt B, Musits B, et al (1995) An integrated system for cementless hip replacement: robotics and medical imaging technology enhance precision surgery. IEEE Eng Med Biol, pp 307–313
4. Mittelstadt B, Paul H, Kazanzides P, et al (1993) Development of a surgical robot for cementless total hip replacement. Robotica 11:553–560
5. Mittelstadt BD, Kazanzides P, Zuhars J, et al (1994) The evolution of a surgical robot from prototype to human clinical use. In: Proceedings, first international symposium on medical robotics and computer assisted surgery, vol 1. Pittsburgh, PA, pp 36–41
6. Bargar WL, Bauer A, DiGioia A, et al (1999) Robodoc clinical trial status. Center for Orthopaedic Research, http://www.cor.ssh.edu/projects /robodoc/status.html
7. Cain P, Kazanzides P, Zuhars J, et al (1993) Safety considerations in a surgical robot. ISA, paper #93-035, pp 291–294
8. Integrated Surgical Systems (1998) Robodoc kurz gefaßt. Integrated Surgical Systems B.V., Nieuwegein, Germany
9. Börner M, Bauer A, Lahmer A (1997) Computerunterstützter Robotereinsatz in der Hüftendoprothetik. Unfallchirurg 100:640–645
10. Börner M, Bauer A, Lahmer A (1997) Rechnerunterstützter Robotereinsatz in der Hüftendoprothetik. Orthopäde 26:251–257
11. Di Gioia AM, Colgan BD (1997) Robotics, image guidance, and computer assisted orthopaedic surgery. In: Proceedings, second annual North American program on computer assisted orthopaedic surgery (CAOS/USA), pp 35–49
12. Lahmer A, Boerner M, Bauer A (1997) Experiences with an image directed workstation (Orthodoc) for cementless hip replacement. In: Proceedings, 11th international symposium and exhibition on computer assisted radiology and surgery (CAR '97), pp 939–943
13. Bauer A, Boerner M, Lahmer A (1997) Tierstudie: Roboterassistierte vs. Handgeraspelte Endoprothese. Langenbecks Arch Chir I (Forumband 1997):465–469
14. Wiesel U, Lahmer A, Boerner M, Skibbe H (1999) Robodoc® at Berufsgenossenschaftliche Unfallklinik Frankfurt (BGU): experiences with the pinless system. CAS 4(6):342
15. Wiesel U, Lahmer A, Börner M, Skibbe H (1999) Robodoc at Berufsgenossenschaftliche Unfallklinik Frankfurt (BGU): experiences with the pinless system. In: CAOS/USA '99,

third annual program on computer assisted orthopaedic surgery, Pittsburgh, PA, pp 113–117

16. Lahmer A, Bauer A, Hollmann G, Börner M (1998) Is there a difference between the planning and the real position of the shaft 300 days after a robot assisted total hip replacement? In: Proceedings, 12th international symposium and exhibition on computer assisted radiology and surgery (CAR '98), pp 694–698

17. Bargar W, Bauer A, Boerner M (1998) Primary and revision total hip replacement using the Robodoc system. Clin Orthop 354:82–91

18. Skibbe H, Börner M, Wiesel U, Lahmer A (1999) Revision THR using the Robodoc system. In: CAOS/USA '99, third annual program on computer assisted orthopaedic surgery, Pittsburgh, PA, pp 110–111

19. Boerner M, Wiesel U (1999) Einsatz computerunterstützter Verfahren in der Unfallchirurgie. Trauma Berufskrank 1:85–90

20. Di Gioia AM (1998) What is computer assisted and image guided orthopaedic surgery? Clin Orthop 354:2–4

21. Jerosch J, v Hasselbach C, Filler T, et al (1998) Qualitätssteigerung in der präoperativen Planung und intraoperativen Umsetzung durch die Verwendung von computerassistierten Systemen und Operationsrobotern—eine experimentelle Untersuchung. Chirurg 69:973–976

A Novel Combined Acetabular and Femoral Computer Navigation System

Nobuhiko Sugano[1], Takashi Nishii[1], Takashi Sakai[1],
Shunsaku Nishihara[1], Kenji Ohzono[1], Kazuo Yonenobu[1],
Yoshinobu Sato[2], Toshihiko Sasama[2], Kei Nakahodo[2],
Shinichi Tamura[2], and Takahiro Ochi[3]

Summary. A combined acetabular and femoral navigation system for total hip arthroplasty (THA) using infrared light-emitting diode markers and an optical camera (OPTOTRAK) was developed. We utilized this navigation system for 18 patients who underwent THA for osteoarthritis secondary to hip dysplasia. The efficacy of the system for precise placement of the acetabular cup was confirmed in this study, as for the previously reported benefits of using the HipNav. The expanded application of navigation on the femoral side was advantageous when deciding the femoral neck osteotomy level, aligning the stem with the medullary axis, and modifying femoral anteversion. Moreover, the use of this novel navigation system revealed the relative movement of the components during the intraoperative check of the safe range of motion. This information is useful to provide postoperative explanation of the functional range of motion for individual patients.

Key words. Total hip arthroplasty, Navigation, Optical sensor, Computer-assisted surgery, Simulation

Introduction

Total hip arthroplasty (THA) is one of the most reliable reconstruction methods for a hip joint disabled because of rheumatoid arthritis, osteoarthritis, or osteonecrosis. Improvements in THA implant materials, implant designs, and instruments have reduced the incidence of complications and have improved durability. However, surgeons, or more precisely their surgical skills, are still the most significant factor affecting patient outcomes. Success in THA depends on precise planning and accurate placement of total hip components.

Recently, to assist surgeons in overcoming their limitations, computer-assisted surgery (CAS) utilizing robotic- or image-guided technologies has been introduced

[1] Department of Orthopaedic Surgery, [2] Division of Functional Diagnostic Imaging, [3] Department of Computer Assisted Orthopaedic Surgery, Osaka University Medical School, 2-2 Yamadaoka, Suita, Osaka 565-0871, Japan

in various orthopedic fields [1]. The CAS systems for THA include ROBODOC and HipNav. ROBODOC is a robotic system designed to prepare the optimal surgical treatment plan for femoral components and facilitate precise femoral canal preparation for the implants [2,3]. HipNav is a navigation system to guide acetabular component placement [4,5]. However, to understand the complete motion and stability of total hip joints, surgeons require information about both the acetabular and femoral sides. Therefore, we developed a combined acetabular and femoral navigation system using infrared light-emitting diode (LED) markers and an optical camera [6]. We report herein our navigation system and the preliminary results of its clinical use.

Materials and Methods

Our navigation system consists of the following three steps: (1) making a computer model of the object to be used in the operation from the preoperative medical image data; (2) registration of the computer model and the real object; and (3) tracking and measurement of the object and operative tools during operation. Preoperatively, transverse images from the level of the superior anterior iliac spines to the level of the femoral canal isthmus were obtained using a helical CT scanner. Slice thickness was 3 mm and slice pitch was 3 mm, with the exception of a portion between 2 cm below the lesser trochanter and the femoral canal isthmus where the slice pitch was 10 mm (Fig. 1). Several reference images of the femoral condyles were also taken to measure femoral anteversion. Image data were stored on an optical disk and then transferred to a workstation. Three-dimensional (3-D) acetabular and femoral bone surface models were reconstructed from the CT data.

Two coordinates systems were defined for preoperative planning: one was the standard anatomic pelvic coordinates that referred to the plane through the superior anterior iliac spines and the pubic tubercles (Fig. 2), and the other was the femoral coordinates that referred to the proximal medullary axis and the table plane through the posterior prominent of the greater trochanter and the posterior femoral condyles (Fig. 3) [7,8]. The cup size was determined from the AP diameter of the acetabulum, and placement of the cup was planned to be at 40° of abduction and 20° of anteversion. A cementless total hip system with a changeable modular neck and head components (ANCA-FIT, Cremascoli, Milan, Italy) was used (Fig. 4). A ceramic-on-ceramic bearing couple was selected. Eighteen patients who underwent THA for osteoarthritis secondary to hip dysplasia are the subjects of this study.

In the operating room, the optical three-dimensional position sensor (OPTOTRAK 3020, Northern Digital, Waterloo, Canada) was placed at the wall caudal to the patient. The operating table was placed so that the surgical area was within 2.5 m from the position sensor. Patients were placed in a lateral decubitus position, and a posterolateral approach was used. A flat plate with 6 LED markers with a rod was fixed to the iliac crest using an extraskeletal fixation system (Hoffmann, Howmedica, Rutherford, NJ, USA). A triangular plate with a socket was fixed to the lateral aspect of the greater trochanter so that the socket connected a rod that was used to attach a 25-LED-marker OPTOTRAK pen probe employing the Hoffmann system. The pen probe can then be removed and reattached at the same place during the procedure without disturbing the procedure.

Fig. 1. Protocol for taking CT scan images of the hip

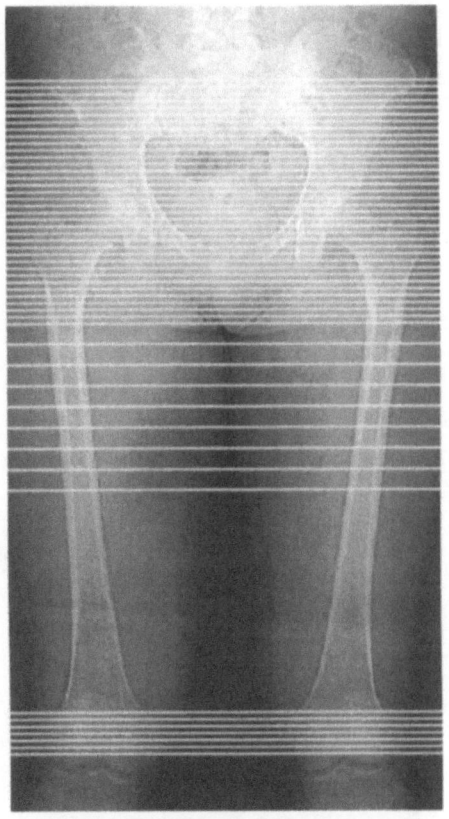

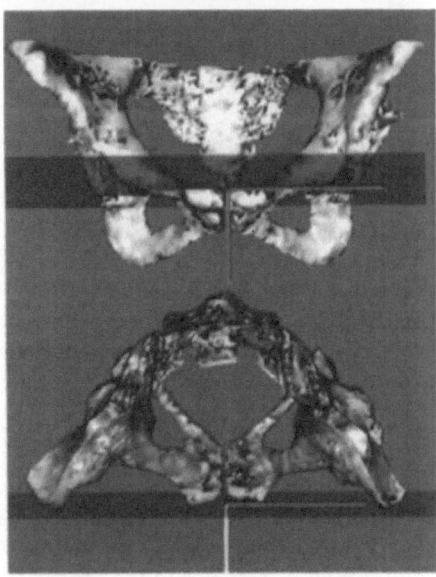

Fig. 2. Coordinates of the pelvis

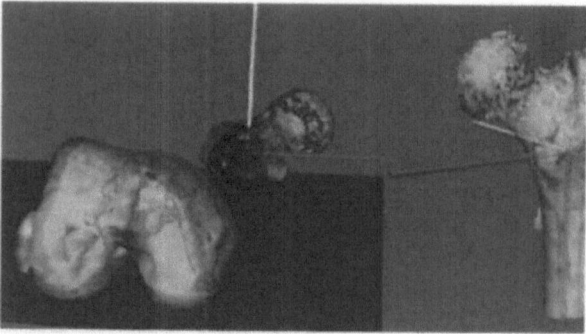

FIG. 3. Coordinates of the femur

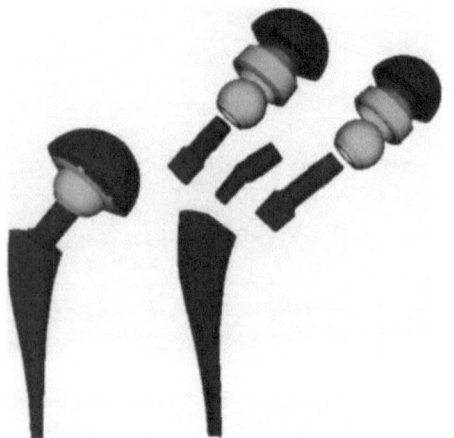

FIG. 4. Cementless cup, alumina ceramic insert (Biolox), alumina head (Biolox), modular femoral neck components, and cementless femoral stem used for surgical treatment of total hip arthroplasty (THA)

Shape-based surface registration of the previously constructed bone models to the real objects was performed in two steps. First, the surgeon digitized 4 surface points to provide the starting position for matching, and then 30 surface points were digitized for the final registration (Fig. 5). After shape-based surface registration, the following indices were measured: femoral neck osteotomy level, position of the cup center, cup angle, femoral anteversion, femoral offset, and limb length discrepancy. The relative movement of the pelvis and the femur was also recorded when the final range of motion was tested intraoperatively.

Results

The navigation tool effectively indicated the femoral neck osteotomy level planned preoperatively (Fig. 6). To avoid malalignment of the stem, it was also useful for femoral broaching because the proximal medullary axis was visible on the computer monitor with reference to the broach (Fig. 7).

FIG. 5. Shape-based registration

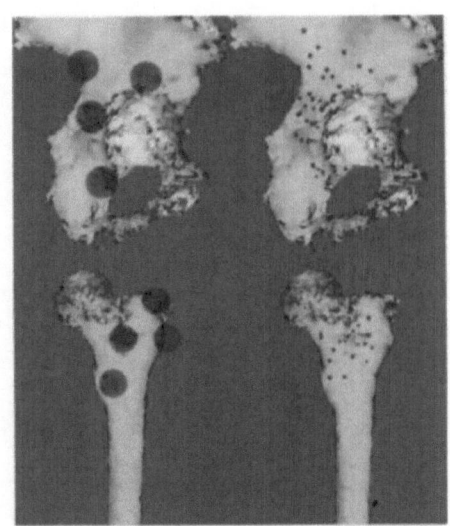

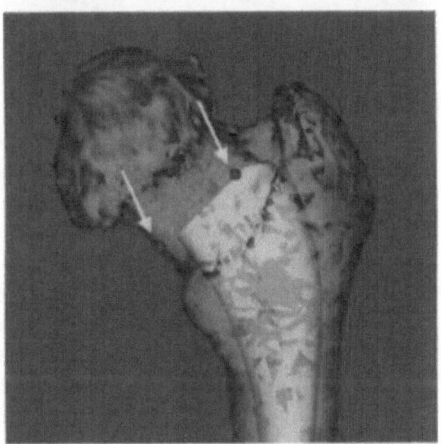

FIG. 6. Indication of the femoral neck osteotomy level

Inclination of the anatomic plane of the pelvis on the operation table as measured by the navigation system revealed a mean 10° of flexion (SD, 6.8°; range, 1°–25°), 0° of abduction (SD, 4°; range, 12°–9°), and 3° of external rotation (SD, 8°; range, 15°–16°). The acetabular cup angle showed a mean 42° of abduction (SD, 3°; range, 37°–48°) and 23° of anteversion (SD, 7°; range, 10°–35°). After implantation of the cup and femoral stem, the limb length discrepancy, femoral neck anteversion, and offset were optimized choosing the best combination of version and length of the modular neck and head system according to the simulation. The limb length discrepancy was achieved within 5 mm in all cases without X-ray control. The range of motion was monitored after reduction of the hip joint. For maximum flexion, the relative flexion of the femur to the pelvis in each patient ranged from 79° to 92°, and no impingement of the implants was observed.

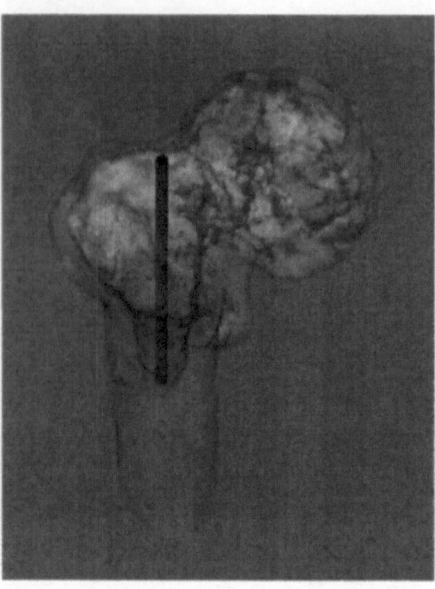

FIG. 7. Visualization of the femoral proximal medullary axis

Discussion

The efficacy of computer navigation systems employing an optical camera and LED markers for the acetabular cup placement was confirmed in this study, thus showing similar results to those previously reported for the HipNav [4,5]. The expanded application of navigation on the femoral side was advantageous when deciding the femoral neck osteotomy level, aligning the stem with the medullary axis, and modifying femoral anteversion, particularly in cases of hip dysplasia in which femoral anteversion is highly variable [8]. Femoral navigation can also provide information about limb length. In the present study, limb length discrepancy was adjusted without intraoperative X-ray. Limb length discrepancy measured on the postoperative X-ray revealed that the maximum error of the intraoperative estimate of the limb length discrepancy using the novel navigation system was 5 mm. Moreover, the navigation revealed the relative movement of the components during the intraoperative check of the safe range of motion. The data acquired intraoperatively can be used in the individual postoperative education of a safe range of motion (ROM).

   In conclusion, our combined acetabular and femoral navigation system using Optotrak enables surgeons to control acetabular orientation, femoral anteversion, and limb length. It provides ROM simulation of each hip and aids our understanding of the safe ROM in individualized cases.

References

1. DiGioia AM (1998) Symposium: computer assisted orthopaedic surgery: medical robotics and image guided surgery. Editorial comment. Clin Orthop 354:2–4

2. Paul HA, Bargar WL, Mittlestadt B, et al (1992) Development of a surgical robot for cementless total hip arthroplasty. Clin Orthop 285:57–66
3. Bargar WL, Bauer A, Borner M (1998) Primary and revision total hip replacement using the Robodoc system. Clin Orthop 354:82–91
4. Jaramaz B, DiGioia AM III, Blackwell M (1998) Computer assisted measurement of cup placement in total hip replacement. Clin Orthop 354:70–81
5. DiGioia AM, Jaramaz B, Blackwell M (1998) The Otto Aufranc Award. Image-guided navigation system to measure intraoperatively acetabular implant alignment. Clin Orthop 355:8–22
6. Sugano N, Sato Y, Sasama T, et al (1999) Control of limb length and femoral anteversion in total hip arthroplasty using Optotrak. Comput Aided Surg 4:343
7. Sugano N, Noble PC, Kamaric E (1998) A comparison of alternative methods of measuring femoral anteversion. J Comput Assist Tomogr 22:610–614
8. Sugano N, Noble PC, Kamaric E, et al (1998) The morphology of the femur in developmental dysplasia of the hip. J Bone Joint Surg 80B:711–719

Robodoc at Berufsgenossenschaftliche Unfallklinik (BGU) Frankfurt: Experiences with the Pinless System

ULRICH WIESEL, MARTIN BOERNER, and ARMIN LAHMER

Summary. The Robodoc Pinless System was introduced at BGU Frankfurt in mid-1998. In the preoperative planning phase, using the 3-D CT data, the surgeon places a model of the implant into position and the Orthodoc determines the cut path for Robodoc. The surgeon then creates a 3-D surface model that is used intraoperatively for pinless registration. In the operating room, the points are compared to the surface model created on the Orthodoc to register the robot to the femur position. Using the pinless system, 95%–98% of all patients can be operated on. Exclusion criteria are severely disfigured posttraumatic cases, revision cases, and cases with a nontitanium implant in the opposite leg, because there are too many metal artifacts in the CT scan. The number of pinless procedures has risen steadily since its introduction. The major advantages of the pinless procedure are that only one operation is needed. Postoperative knee pain is eliminated in most cases, and costs per surgery are reduced. Surgical time and radiation exposure are the same as in the pin-based system, and system accuracy and reliability are equal to the pin-based system.

Key words. Robodoc, THR, Pinless system, Arthroplasty, CAOS

Introduction

This article discusses the development and progress of robotic total hip replacement (THR) at Berufsgenossenschaftliche Unfallklinik (BGU) Frankfurt with a special emphasis on the introduction and clinical use of the pinless system.

Background

In 1991, Berufsgenossenschaftliche Unfallklinik Frankfurt am Main, Germany, and Integrated Surgical Systems (ISS) in Sacramento, California (USA) the developers of Robodoc, first established contact [1–3]. Since that time, while studies in the United States were still going on, the transition of Robodoc to Germany was initialized [4].

Berufsgenossenschaftliche Unfallklinik Frankfurt am Main, Friedberger Landstrasse 430, D-60389 Frankfurt am Main, Germany

Although there was still no FDA approval for the system in the United States, the first successful robot-assisted total hip replacement using a three-pin-based system was performed at BGU Frankfurt [5].

The use of Robodoc for total hip surgery has become a standard procedure at BGU. Operating room time decreased to an average of 90 min per case, and it was also possible to change the system from three to two pins, which not only helped to save a considerable amount of time during surgery but also reduced the postoperative knee pain in our patients.

The advantages of the Robodoc system are well known nowadays. The robot guarantees precise transformation of the preoperative plan during surgery. Femur fractures, a common complication in cementless total hip replacement, can be avoided. Robodoc proved to be a reliable and safe technology that can be handled by a trained surgeon without permanent on-site support [6–9].

In January 2000, the 2500th operation using Robodoc was performed succesfully at BGU Frankfurt. The results we have found in those 2500 patients were supported by a dog study at the Small Animal Clinic in Auburn, Alabama (USA) that was performed in 1995 comparing a Robot group to a Hand-broached group of male greyhounds. No fractures were found in the Robodoc group and no nerve palsies; gait analysis was superior, and there was closer alignment of the prosthesis to strong cortical bone [10].

Design and Methods

The next important step was the introduction of the Robodoc Pinless System at BGU Frankfurt in mid-1998. Extensive clinical trials had been run at our hospital before introducing the system into everyday practice. The system was officially released to all Robodoc users by ISS in October 1998. The system is based on the current Robodoc surgical system but does not require the preoperative insertion of registration markers (pins). The pinless system consists of a modified Orthodoc and Robodoc.

The pinless procedure consists of three phases. The first is a preoperative planning phase in which the surgeon downloads the CT data into the Orthodoc system. Using the three-dimensional (3-D) CT data, the surgeon places a model of the implant into position and the Orthodoc determines the cut path for Robodoc. The surgeon then creates a 3-D surface model from the CT data using a surface model generation program, which is also running in the Orthodoc. The bone surface model is a geometric representation of the bone. This surface model is used intraoperatively for pinless registration.

The planning of the prosthesis on the Orthodoc is performed in the same way as it is for the pin-based system. The planning software has not been changed, and it can be used for pinless and pin-based planning on the same Orthodoc at the same time.

In the operating room, after the head of the femur has been surgically removed in the normal manner, the Robodoc is moved into position and a digitizer is used to collect points both proximally and distally on the femur. The distal femur is not exposed during surgery, and the distal data are collected percutaneously using a long, thin probe. A graphic indicator on the computer display assists the surgeon in collecting the data over the distal region of interest. The proximal femur is exposed in the conventional manner during surgery, providing adequate access to the proximal region of bone where surface data must be collected. During the surface data collection, the computer display shows pictorial images of a proximal femur with the desired point collection sites indicated. Once the bone surface data are collected, the registration process is started. These points are compared to the surface model created on the Orthodoc to register the robot to the femur position. This registration allows the robot to accurately position the cutter relative to the bone in the operating room as the surgeon has planned in the Orthodoc.

The registration is verified by viewing independently digitized points superimposed on cross-sectional CT images; this is a visual check of the registration correctness using independently collected data. The system prompts the surgeon to digitize additional bone surface points at specific locations. The locations are selected to identify translational or rotational errors in any of the six possible degrees of freedom. As each point is digitized, it is displayed superimposed on the bone CT image. Because the digitized point is on the actual bone surface, the displayed point should appear on the surface edge of the CT bone image. By viewing the prescribed sequence of points the surgeon can verify that those points lie on or very close to the bone surface.

Once all the data have been collected, Robodoc starts cutting the implant cavity, which is the same procedure that is used for the pin-based system. Because of the high neck cut required by the pinless procedure, a small amount of additional bone needs to be removed after the milling of the cavity. Two "recovery markers" are installed into the bone before the surface point collection process. These markers are installed proximally and distally. Once the registration has been determined, the markers are measured with the digitizing arm. The distal marker is measured twice: once directly, and the second time with an "extender sleeve" that provides directional as well as positional information. If bone motion occurs during the milling of the cavity, the markers are remeasured in the same manner. It is possible to calculate an updated registration that takes the bone motion into account. Compared to the pin-based system, once bone motion occurs, it takes about 30 s to relocate those markers to be able to resume the operation. This also is a great advantage compared to the pin-based system in which the pin-finding process, which requires about 6 min, must be repeated once bone motion occurs [11–13].

Results and Conclusions

The major advantages of the pinless procedure are that only one operation is needed, providing greater scheduling flexibility for the patient and the surgeon. Postoperative knee pain is eliminated in most cases. The costs per surgery are reduced. The surgical time and radiation exposure are the same as in the pin-based system, and system accuracy and reliability are equal to the pin-based system. After using the pinless system for almost a year, we believe that 95%–98% of all patients can be operated on using the pinless system. Exclusion criteria are severely disfigured posttraumatic cases, revision cases, and cases with a nontitanium implant in the opposite leg because there are too many metal artifacts in the CT scan. However, we have seen no problems using the pinless system on patients with a cementless titanium implant in the opposite leg.

Compared to an average planning time of about 15 min per case for the pin-based system, the pinless system requires about 25 min of planning time per case as the pinless surface model needs to be generated in addition to the planning of the implant. For a surgeon who performs the pinless planning procedure regularly, even cases with severe osteophytes in the region of the femoral neck are no contraindication for the pinless procedure. Such cases, however, add quite a lot of additional time to the planning procedure because every single slice of the CT scan needs to be carefully inspected and the surface model needs to be corrected when necessary. We believe that any surgeon who has just started using the pinless system should select only patients with minor osteophytes as the first cases to become familiar with the system. Gradually, this restriction can be removed after the surgeon has acquired a planning routine.

Our average planning time for the pinless system has decreased from 55 min on average to about 25 min on average after the learning phase. At our hospital, 152 patients were operated on using the pinless system before its official release on a clinical trial basis using a beta version of the software. When the system was released to all users, we also received a new Orthodoc workstation and the new, modified software at the end of October 1998. In the period between October 28th, 1998, and May 12th, 1999, 423 patients were operated on using Robodoc, 253 of them with the pinless system; 230 were men and 193 were women. We operated on 202 right and 221 left hips. The number of pinless procedures has risen steadily since October. In November 1998 we had 26 pinless cases, 28 in December, 38 in January 1999, 40 in February 1999, 56 in March 1999, and from April 1999 after the arrival of two new pinless robots all patients were done pinless, with only a few exceptions.

Postoperative knee pain was eliminated almost completely compared to the pin cases. Because we are now using a spiral CT for the pinless cases as well, the radiation exposure is not higher than for the pin cases. We also save much OR time and money by not having to do a second operation for the pin implantation. At the beginning we could only use the Howmedica Osteolock implant for our pinless plannings. The introduction of a new software that enabled us to also use an anatomical implant, the Howmedica ABG prosthesis in January 1999, showed a sharp increase in the use of this anatomic prosthesis (25 pinless cases compared to 15 Osteolock pinless cases in February 1999). Similar numbers apply for the pin-based cases.

By January 2000, the pinless procedure had become everyday routine at BGU just as is the pin-based procedure. At the end of January 2000, we had performed more than 2500 Robodoc operations since the introduction of the system in 1994, more than 600 of which were performed with the pinless system.

References

1. Kazanzides P, Mittelstadt B, Musits B, et al (1995) An integrated system for cementless hip replacement: robotics and medical imaging technology enhance precision surgery. IEEE Eng Med Biol, pp 307–313
2. Mittelstadt B, Paul H, Kazanzides P, et al (1993) Development of a surgical Robot for cementless total hip replacement. Robotica 11:553–560
3. Mittelstadt BD, Kazanzides P, Zuhars J, et al (1994) The evolution of a surgical robot from prototype to human clinical use. In: Proceedings, first international symposium on medical robotics and computer assisted surgery, Pittsburgh, 1:36–41

4. Bargar WL, Bauer A, DiGioia A, et al (1999) Robodoc clinical trial status. Center for Orthopaedic Research, *http://www.cor.ssh.edu/projects/robodoc/status.html*
5. Lahmer A, Boerner M, Bauer A (1997) Experiences with an image directed workstation(Orthodoc) for cementless hip replacement. In: Proceedings, 11th international symposium and exhibition on computer assisted radiology and surgery (CAR' 97), pp 939–943
6. Börner M, Bauer A, Lahmer A (1997) Computerunterstützter Robotereinsatz in der Hüftendoprothetik. Unfallchirurg 100:640–645
7. Börner M, Bauer A, Lahmer A (1997) Rechnerunterstützter Robotereinsatz in der Hüftendoprothetik. Orthopäde 26:251–257
8. Bargar W, Bauer A, Boerner M (1998) Primary and revision total hip replacement using the Robodoc system. Clin Orthop 354:82–91
9. Boerner M, Wiesel U (1999) Einsatz computerunterstützter Verfahren in der Unfallchirurgie. Trauma Berufskrank 1:85–90
10. Bauer A, Boerner M, Lahmer A (1997) Tierstudie: Roboterassistierte vs. Handgeraspelte Endoprothese. Langenbecks Arch Chir I (Forumband 1997):465–469
11. Integrated Surgical Systems (1998) DigiMatch user manual international edition: Robodoc surgical assistant system and Orthodoc preoperative planning workstation. ISS, Davis, CA
12. Lahmer A, Wiesel U, Boerner M (1999) Experiences in using the Robodoc system without pins. In: Proceedings, 4th international symposium on computer assisted orthopaedic surgery, Davos
13. Wiesel U, Lahmer A, Boerner M, Skibbe H (1999) Robodoc® at Berufsgenossenschaftliche Unfallklinik Frankfurt (BGU): experiences with the pinless system. CAS6(4):342

Part 6 Computer Assisted Evaluation in Joint Replacement Surgery

Intraoperative Analysis for Soft Tissue Balancing with Total Knee Arthroplasty

Makoto Kawakubo, Takahiro Koyanagi, and Masanori Takahashi

Summary. Soft tissue balancing of the tibiofemoral joint during total knee arthroplasty (TKA) was evaluated in 23 patients. To evaluate soft tissue balance, the Nitta pressure distribution measurement system (I-SCAN) was used in this study. I-SCAN can calculate a contact pressure and a contact area during the operation so that the pressure distribution and a contact center between the medial compartment and lateral compartment of the tibiofemoral joint can be displayed in real time. Further, changes in contact pressure during knee flexion can be recorded and displayed in a graph simultaneously. When the contact pressure of the medial compartment was demonstrated to be much higher than that of the lateral compartment after fitting the trials, with reference made to the changes in contact pressure during knee flexion, medial soft tissue release was performed until the soft tissue balance was equalized between the medial and the lateral compartments. This method, using I-SCAN, has a great advantage in that it enables us to evaluate the soft tissue balancing at any angle during knee passive motion and to determine the optimum amount of soft tissue release.

Key words. Total knee arthroplasty, Soft tissue balancing, Pressure distribution, Soft tissue release, Intraoperative monitoring

Introduction

Total knee arthroplasty (TKA) has become the primary procedure for severe deformity of the knee. Recently, advances in implant design, operative instruments, and surgical technique have contributed to significant improvements in clinical results. However, it is still difficult to determine adequate soft tissue balance in knees with severe valgus or varus deformity. Since 1997, we have evaluated the soft tissue balance using a pressure distribution measurement system. The purpose of this study is to introduce a new method of intraoperative evaluation of soft tissue balancing with TKA and to discuss the clinical significance of this method.

Department of Orthopaedic Surgery, Tokyo Dental College, Ichikawa General Hospital, 5-11-13 Sugano, Ichikawa, Chiba 272-8513, Japan

Materials

Twenty-three patients were involved in this study. Their mean age at the time of operation was 70 years. The original diagnoses were osteoarthritis in 16 patients and rheumatoid arthritis in 7 patients. The prostheses used in this study were NexGen (Zimmer Inc., Warsaw, IN, USA) in 18 patients and Deltafit (Stryker Co., Kalamazoo, MI, USA) in 5 patients.

Methods

The Nitta pressure distribution measurement system (I-SCAN) was used to evaluate soft tissue balance during TKA. I-SCAN consisted of a thin and flexible sensor sheet, PC-AT-compatible computer, interface, and its software (Fig. 1). Pressure distribution can be measured with this system and the results displayed on the computer screen.

A contact pressure and contact area can be calculated simultaneously with this software so that the pressure distribution and a contact center between the medial and lateral compartments of the tibiofemoral joint can be displayed in real time during the operation. Further, changes in contact pressure during knee flexion were recorded and displayed in a graph (Fig. 2).

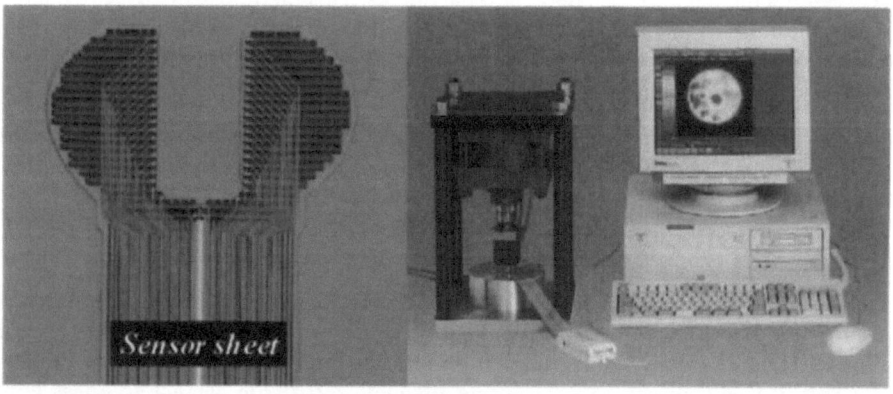

FIG. 1. Nitta pressure distribution measurement system (I-Scan)

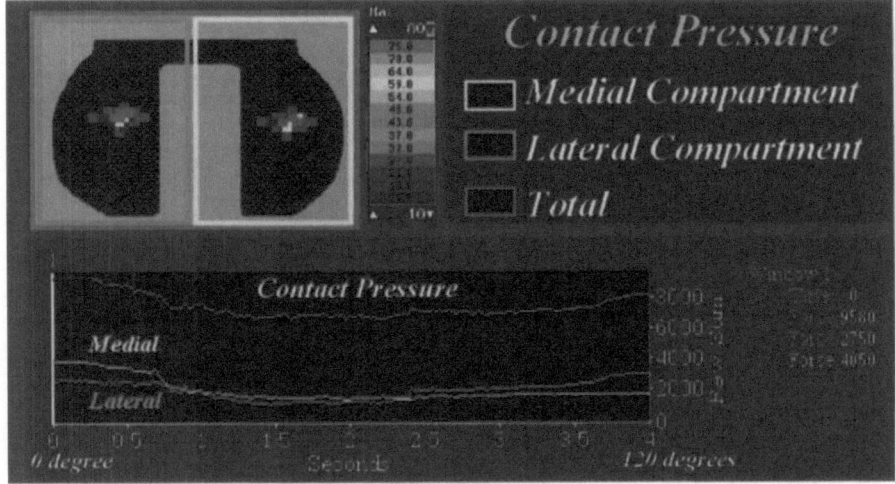

FIG. 2. Changes in pressure distribution of the tibiofemoral joint during knee flexion

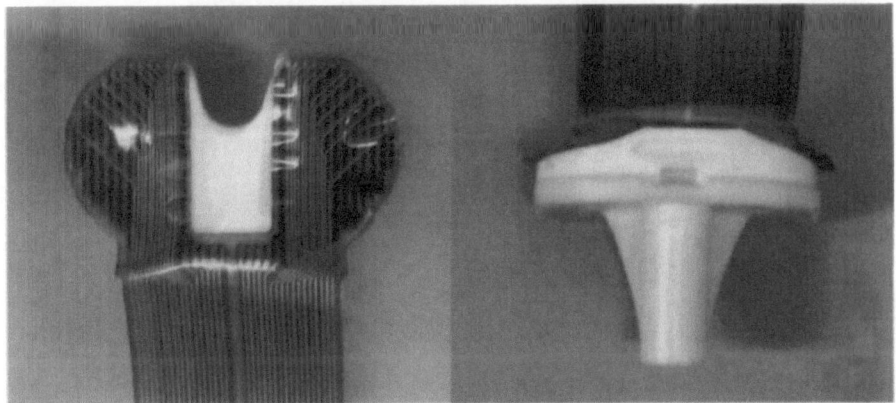

FIG. 3. The sensor sheet is taped onto the tibial insert

Method for Intraoperative Monitoring of Soft Tissue Balancing

After fitting the trials of the artificial joint, the sensor sheet was taped onto its tibial insert (Fig. 3) and inserted between the femoral and tibial components (Fig. 4). When passive knee motion was applied from 0° to full flexion, pressure distributions of the contact area and contact center of the tibiofemoral joint were displayed on a computer screen in real time. When the soft tissue balance was equalized between the medial and the lateral compartments, both medial contact pressure, indicated by a yellow line,

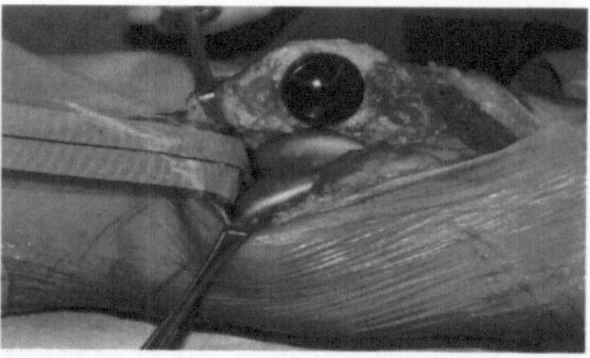

FIG. 4. Passive knee motion is applied

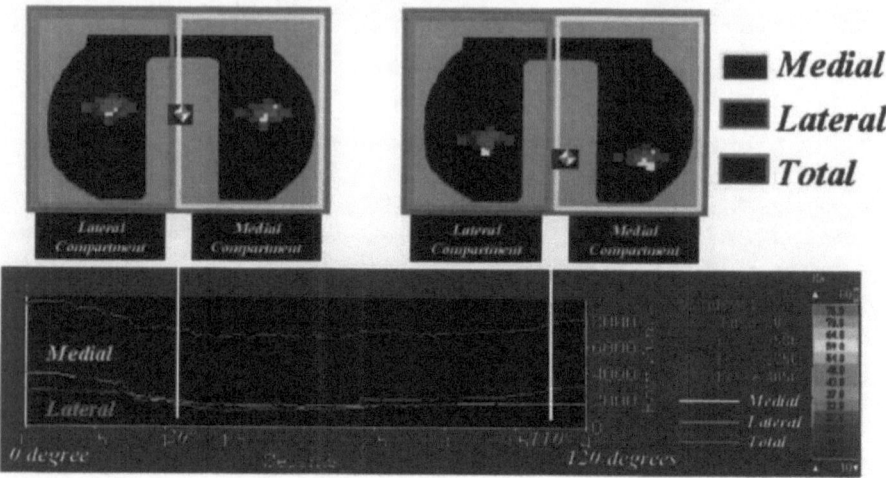

FIG. 5. Pressure distribution of the contact area and contact center of the tibiofemoral joint. When the soft tissue balance was equalized between the medial and the lateral compartments, both medial contact pressure and lateral contact pressure changed similarly with knee flexion. The contact center was positioned at the center of the tibofemoral joint

and lateral contact pressure, by a green line, changed similarly with knee flexion. The contact center was also positioned at the center of the tibofemoral joint (Fig. 5).

Results

As the aim of this article is to introduce a new method to evaluate soft tissue balancing, typical results obtained from one case are presented here.

A 78-year-old woman with a severe varus deformity of the knee underwent TKA. The femoral and the tibial components were properly positioned, and the

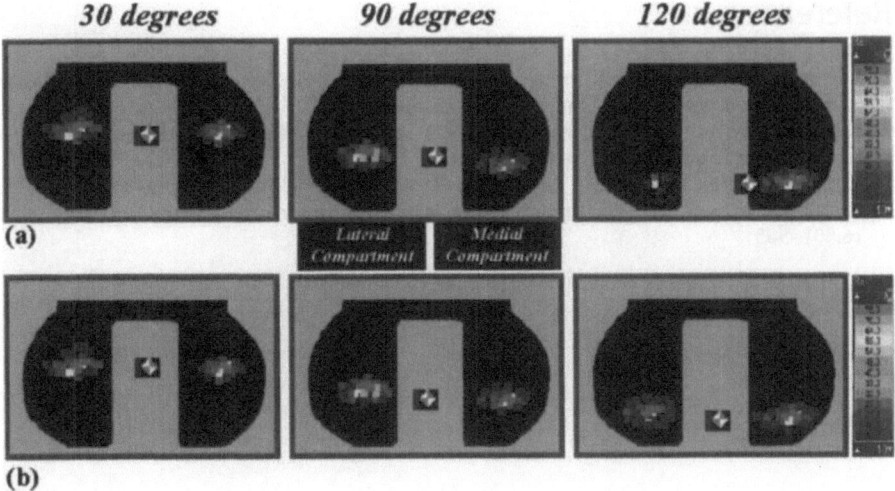

FIG. 6a,b. Analysis for soft tissue balancing before soft tissue releasing (a) and after soft tissue releasing (b)

ligament balance seemed to be equalized between medial and lateral at both 0° and 90°. However, when soft tissue balancing was analyzed using I-SCAN after the trials were placed, much higher contact pressure was demonstrated in the medial compartment than in the lateral compartment at the flexion range from 95° to 120° (Fig. 6a). After releasing the medial collateral ligament and the soft tissue at the posteromedial corner, optimum balancing was obtained through 0° to 120° of knee flexion (Fig. 6b).

Discussion

Recently, many improvements in operative instruments have contributed to well-aligned, properly positioned prostheses. However, it is still difficult to determine soft tissue balance and to achieve optimum ligament balance, especially in patients with a severe valgus or varus deformity of the knee [1].

The conventional method to evaluate soft tissue balance was to check the thickness and alignment of the planes of femoral and tibial cuts only at 0° and 90° of knee flexion using the Spacer/Alignment Guide [2] or a special instrument [3]. However, this method does not allow us to evaluate the ligament balancing objectively. Further, even if ligament balancing was performed and equalized between the medial and lateral compartments at 0° or 90° of knee flexion, optimum ligament balance at other knee flexion angles was not always achieved.

This method, using I-Scan, enables us to evaluate soft tissue balance and find the causes of imbalance at any angle of knee flexion, so that we can determine how much and also where to release the ligament and soft tissue easily during the operation. Therefore, it would be a useful new method to evaluate soft tissue balancing during TKA.

References

1. Edwards E, Miller J, Chan K (1988) The effect of postoperative collateral ligament laxity in total knee arthroplasty. Clin Orthop 236:44–51
2. Wilton TJ, Wilton TJ, Pratt DJ, et al (1944) Soft-tissue balancing at the time of knee replacement: rationale and method. Knee 1:111–116
3. Attfield SF, Warren-Forward M, Wilton T, et al (1994) Measurement of soft tissue imbalance total knee arthroplasty using electronic instrumentation. Med Eng Phys 16:501–505

Preoperative Computer Simulation Using a 3-D Template

Nobuhiko Tanaka, Nobuo Matsui, Yoichi Taneda, Yukio Yoshida, Hirotaka Iguchi, and Toshiyuki Kawanishi

Summary. In total hip arthroplasty, a two-dimensional (2-D) template on plain X-ray is usually used for preoperative planning, but deformity and contracture can cause malpositioning and measurement error. To reduce those problems, a 3-D preoperative simulation system was developed. Two methods were compared in this study: one is to create very accurate AP and ML images that can be used for a standard 2-D template, and the other is a fully 3-D preoperative template system. Because helical scanning CT is an excellent method to extract 3-D geometry of the bone, our system provides 3-D geometries using helical scanning CT. Accurate AP and ML surface-cutting 3-D images of the femur were created. Ordinary 2-D templates were compared to the surface-cutting 3-D image, and preoperative measurement was done. For the full 3-D simulation, axial images were converted to the 3-D geometry data using the STL (stereolithography) format. The extracted 3-D geometry was displayed on a personal computer using "magics" (STL data visualization software; Belgium Materialise), and 3-D geometry of the stem was then superimposed upon it. The full 3-D simulation system made it possible to observe the bone and stem geometry from any direction and by any section view. This 3-D template system was very useful for very accurate preoperative measurement and better selection of the prosthesis.

Key words. 3-D CT, Preoperative simulation, THA, 3-D template

Introduction

A standard way of preoperative planning of total hip arthroplasty (THA) has been to use plain X-rays and 10% enlarged transparent 2-D template sheets. Exact anterior and lateral images of the femur (after reduced anteversion angle) are necessary for measurement of stem type and size. However, to obtain exact A-P and M-L X-rays is very difficult because of the joint deformity and contracture. For those cases it is impossible to say that the conventional way is accurate enough. 3-D computer simulation methods using CT images had been reported but were not popular yet [1,2],

Department of Orthopaedic Surgery, Nagoya City University Medical School, 1 Kawasumi, Mizuho-cho, Mizuho-ku, Nagoya 467-8601, Japan

because 3-D preoperative simulation needs a particular computer and software and the data format of a 3-D model was not yet standardized.

Our 3-D preoperative simulation system for custom THA was already in practical usage and reported [3]. Stereolysographic (STL) models have been also used for pre-operative planning. Femur STL model data were converted from 3-D CT data, and STL model data of the stem were offered by the implant maker. The STL data format has become the standard 3-D geometry data format in the industrial field. Many more stem STL model data may be offered from the implant maker in the future. In the present study, the preoperative simulation system for the ZCHW (Zimmer custom hip workstation) custom stem [4] was expanded to be used for an off-the-shelf (OTS) stem also. It is very difficult to do 3-D simulation for all THA, however, because 3-D simulation requires much time. A simpler and quicker version of the system has been also developed, which obtains accurate A-P and M-L images from 3-D CT and 2-D templates superimposed. Those two methods are reported.

Materials and Methods

Template Method Using the 3-D Model

From August 1999 to January 2000, 3-D simulation was done in 15 cases (7 hips from 6 cases in which ZCHW custom prostheses were used and 10 hips from 9 cases which OTS prostheses were used). A helical CT scanner (GE Yokogawa high-speed advantage SG) is used for scanning of the hip joints and femora.

Scanning and reconstruction conditions were beam width, 3.0 mm; table speed, 3.0 mm/cycle; 120 kV; 120 mA; and reformation slice thickness, 1.5 mm. Cortical and canal models of femora were made using Mimics (converting software axial CT data to STL data; Belgium Materialise). In the prior three cases of ZCHW, the appropriate threshold was checked for each case in comparison with plain X-ray, and it was found that about 500 Hounsfield units (HU) is the best threshold for detection of cortical bone and canal. Thus, the same threshold was used for the other cases. The distal reaming was observed to cut in above 1000 HU, but the distance between 1000 HU and 500 HU was about 0.6 mm, so it had hardly any effect on the precision of the simulation.

The thickness of cortical bone was not great enough to use the same threshold around the greater and lessor trochanteric area. If the same threshold, 500 HU, was used, the continuity of the geometry was lost. To avoid this, 160 HU was applied to this area. As for the OTS stem geometry, two stem makers could provide STL data to us. Using magics (which is the software for processing the STL data), the femoral geometry and stem geometry were placed at the same axis. Cross-sectional images from many directions were observed, and the best type and size of the stem was selected. Osteotomies on the femoral geometries were done as in the real operation, then adaptation in the neck was also confirmed (Figs. 1, 2, 3b).

Template Method Using a 3-D CT Surface-Cutting Image

The 3-D CT image of volume-rendering method was made using a GE Yokogawa Advantage workstation. The gradation conditions from transparent to opaque were from 100 to 700 HU. After reducing the anteversion, adduction, and external rotation,

FIG. 1a,b. Case 1: 75-year-old woman, total hip arthroplasty (THA) using Omnifit-c size #7. **a** Preoperative simulation using 3-D CT surface-cutting image and 2-D stem template. **b** Preoperative 3-D simulation using femur and stem model

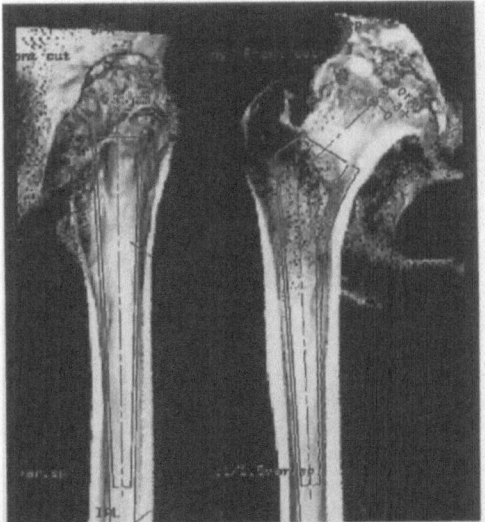

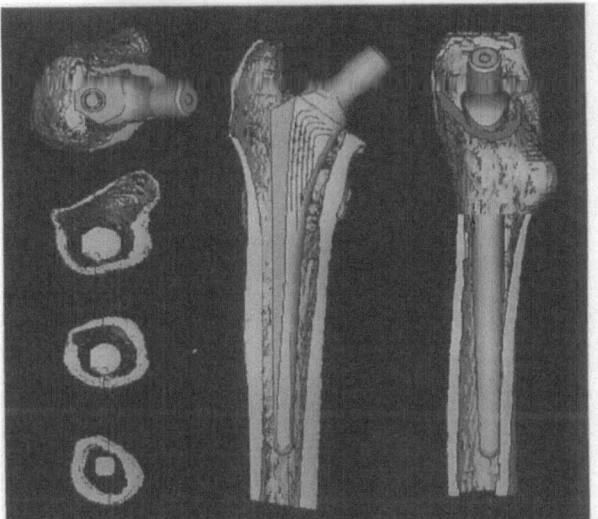

surface-cutting images from anterior and lateral direction were made. The images were resized 10% larger and printed to film, then 10% enlarged transparent 2-D template sheets were compared (Figs. 1, 2, 3a). The expansion rate was very exact, because it was calculated based on ROI (range of interest). This simulation method was easy and exact but could remove the measurement error caused by wrong positioning.

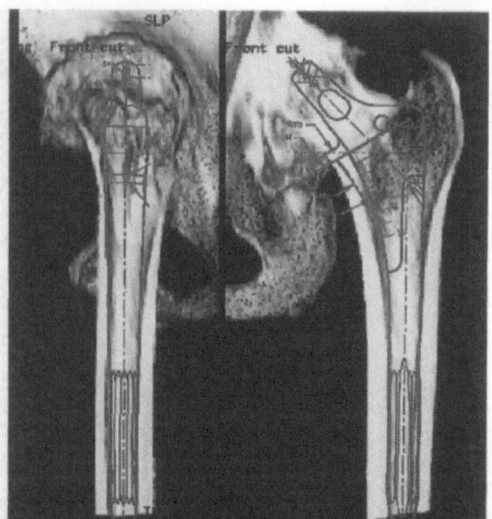

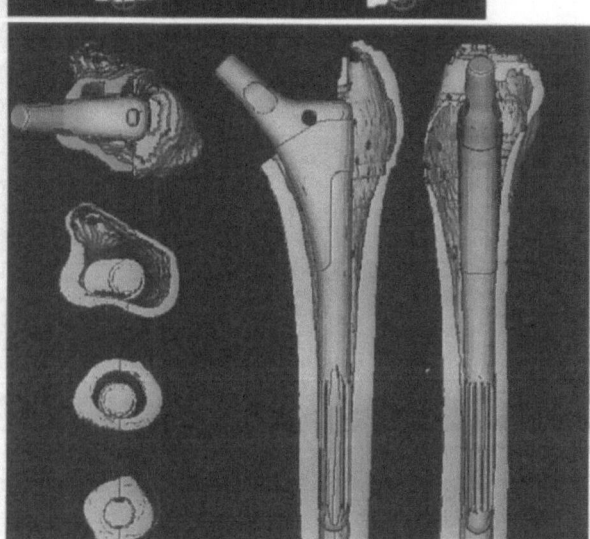

FIG. 2a,b. Case 2: 53-year-old woman, THA using VerSys size #12. **a** Preoperative simulation using 3-D CT surface-cutting image and 2-D stem template. **b** Preoperative 3-D simulation using femur and stem model

Case Reports

Case 1: 75-year-old woman; THA was done using Omnifit-c stem (Fig. 1).
Case 2: 53-year-old woman; THA was done using a VerSys pressfit stem (Fig. 2).
Case 3: 49-year-old woman; THA was done using a ZCHW stem because of severe femoral deformity (Fig. 3). Secondary osteoarthritis was caused by acetabular

FIG. 3a,b. Case 3: 49-year-old woman, THA using custom ZCHW. Severe femoral deformity because of post-valgus osteotomy. **a** Preoperative simulation using 3-D CT surface-cutting image and 2-D stem template. **b** Preoperative 3-D simulation using femur and stem model

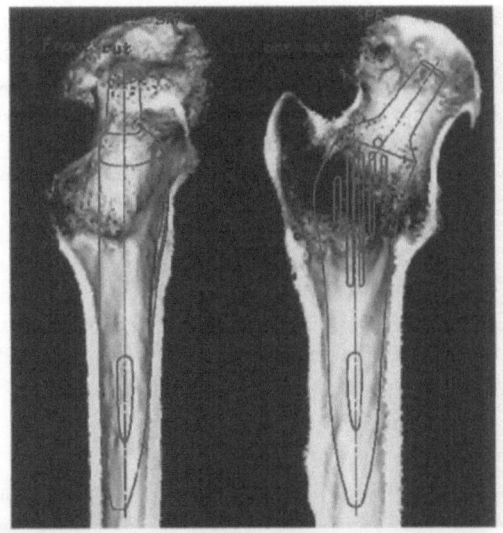

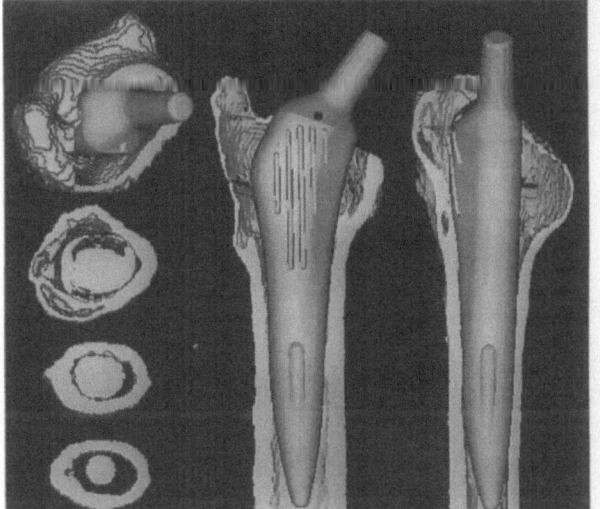

dysplasia; valgus osteotomy had been done to the right femur and varus osteotomy to the left femur.

Results and Conclusions

In eight of ten OTS hips, the same size stems were selected intraoperatively compared with the expected size using surface-cutting 3-D CT images. In the other two hips, stems smaller 1 size were selected intraoperatively. In those cases, it is revealed that stems tended to be inserted to a slightly posteriorly rotated position because of the anterior bow of the midproximal femur by the full 3-D simulation system. It is also revealed that smaller stems tended to be selected intraoperatively when not enough posterior rasping around the neck cut level was done.

Because ZCHW custom stems have anterior and lateral flares to obtain a tight proximal fit, posterior rasping around the neck cut level should be done so as to remove a small part of the cortical bone in most cases. From this point of view, in ZCHW custom stems full 3-D simulation was very important to confirm the exact rasping area. In a severely deformed case (such as post valgus osteotomy and valus osteotomy), a detailed preoperative simulation using full 3-D data is indispensable. To make those three-dimensional preoperative simulations popular, it is essential that many more makers of the OTS stem provide 3-D geometry data.

References

1. Izumida R, Iida M, Ishinada Y, et al (1993) Simulation of total hip replacement (THR) using 3-DCT images. Hip Joint 19:164–167
2. Ohneda Y, Kakihana T, Kawade K, et al (1993) CT assisted canal measurement and computer simulation of uncemented THA. Hip Joint 19:168–171
3. Yoshida Y, Kawanishi T, Tanaka N, et al (1999) Preoperative computer simulation for total hip arthroplasty. J Joint Surg 18:23–29
4. Iguchi H, Matsui N, Taneda Y, et al (1999) Peter Walker Custom Hip System (ZCHW) and its preoperative simulation. J Joint Surg 18:55–65

Virtual Implantation Using the ROBODOC Preoperative Planning Workstation

Tsuyoshi Koyama[1], Nobuhiko Sugano[1], Takashi Nishii[1],
Takashi Sakai[1], Keiji Haraguchi[1], Shunsaku Nishihara[1],
Keisuke Hagio[1], Nobuo Nakamura[3], Kenji Ohzono[1], and
Takahiro Ochi[2]

Summary. The purpose of this study was to determine the influence of curvature of femoral components on fit and fill of the femoral canal using ORTHODOC, a preoperative planning workstation of the ROBODOC system. CT data of 18 cases with developmental dysplasia of the hip (DDH) were used for simulation of implantation. Osteolock as a straight type and the ABG as an anatomic type were used. The canal fill ratio and the canal fit ratio were calculated on the cross-sectional images at five levels. The length of the proximal posterolateral femoral cortex removed by milling at the neck cut level was also measured. ABG showed significantly greater canal fit ratio at the proximal portions above the lesser trochanter than Osteolock. In addition, Osteolock showed significantly greater length of the proximal posterolateral femoral cortex removed at the neck cut level than ABG. These results show that to achieve good fit and fill in cases with DDH, the straight type requires greater range of removal of cortex at the posterolateral femoral neck in implanting than the anatomic type, and that the anatomic type is more advantageous in improving the canal fit ratio at the proximal portions above the lesser trochanter than the straight type.

Key words. ROBODOC, ORTHODOC, Fit, Fill, Curvature

Introduction

ORTHODOC is the preoperative planning workstation associated with the ROBODOC system (developed by Integrated Surgical Systems [ISS], Davis, CA, USA) [1]. It can simulate implantation of different femoral components into any femur reconstructed from CT data and assist us in determining which design of femoral component fits better. The purpose of this study is to determine, using ORTHODOC, the influence of the lateral curvature of femoral components on fit and fill in the femoral canal.

[1] Department of Orthopaedic Surgery, Osaka University Medical School, 2-2 Yamadaoka, Suita, Osaka 565-0871, Japan
[2] Division of Computer Integrated Orthopaedics, Osaka University Graduate School of Medicine, Suita, Osaka, Japan
[3] Joint Reconstruction Center, Kyowakai Hospital, Suita, Osaka, Japan

Materials and Methods

Preoperative CT scans of 18 patients with developmental dysplasia of the hip (DDH) (male, 2 hips; female, 16 hips) were used for simulation of implantation. The average age of the patients was 49 years (range, 20–75 years). The femoral components used for simulation were the straight Osteolock (Howmedica, Rutherford, NJ, USA), and the anatomic ABG (Howmedica).

Femoral components were implanted as follows. The center of the femoral head was determined by fitting a circle to the femoral head contour on the coronal, sagittal, and axial views of the workstation display. The femur was reoriented on the workstation to obtain the coronal plane that passed through the head center and the proximal femoral medullary axis. Then, the sagittal plane through the medullary axis was obtained. Stems of the maximum size that would not penetrate the cortical bone on the workstation display were selected and implanted into the femoral canal by referring to the fit and fill of the stem in the coronal and sagittal planes.

After the stem was planted, the canal fill ratio and the canal fit ratio were calculated on the cross-sectional images at the following five levels: the lower corner of the femoral neck cut, the center of the lesser trochanter, 1 cm distal from the lesser trochanter, the middle of the stem, and 1 cm proximal from the stem tip. The canal fill ratio was defined as the ratio of stem area to the total medullary cavity area, at each cross-section level. The canal fit ratio was defined as the ratio of the length of stem–endosteal contact to the total endosteal length, at each cross-section level. The length of proximal posterolateral femoral cortical bone removed by milling at the neck cut level was also calculated.

The paired t-test was used for statistical analysis, and differences were considered significant when the P value was less than 0.05.

Results

Canal Fill Ratio

At the middle of the stem, the Osteolock showed significantly greater canal fill than the ABG. On the other hand, at the center of the lesser trochanter and at 1 cm proximal from the stem tip, the ABG showed significantly greater canal fill than the Osteolock. No significant differences were found at the femoral neck cut level and at 1 cm distal from the lesser trochanter (Fig. 1).

Canal Fit Ratio

At the middle of the stem, the Osteolock showed greater canal fit than the ABG. At 1 cm distal from the lesser trochanter, no significant difference was found. At the lower corner of the femoral neck cut, the center of the lesser trochanter, and 1 cm proximal from the stem tip, the ABG showed significantly greater canal fit than the Osteolock (Fig. 2).

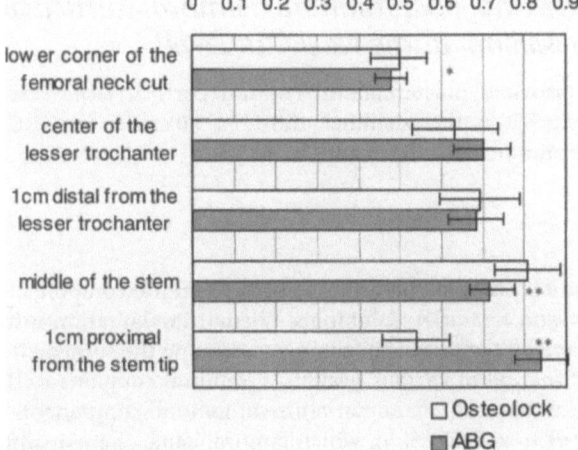

FIG. 1. Canal fill ratio. *$P < 0.05$; **$P < 0.001$

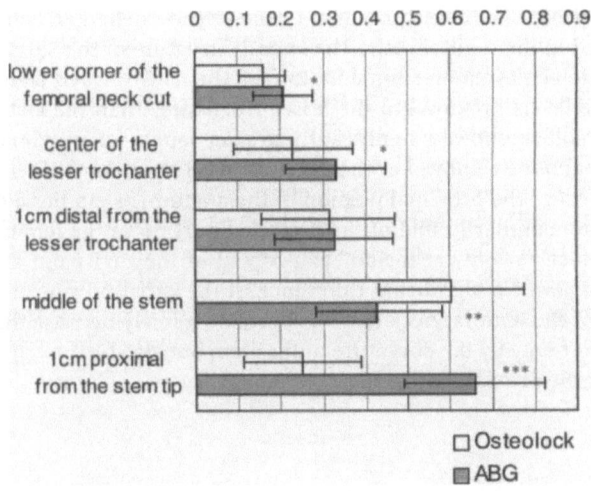

FIG. 2. Canal fill ratio. *$P < 0.05$; **$P < 0.005$; ***$P < 0.001$

Length of Proximal Posterolateral Femoral Cortical Bone Removed by Milling at the Neck Cut Level

The length of proximal posterolateral femoral cortical bone removed was 6.0 ± 4.3 mm (average ± SD) in the Osteolock and 1.3 ± 3.0 mm in the ABG. This difference was statistically significant.

Discussion

The canal fit and fill ratios are determined by the femoral component design, femoral canal geometry, and operative techniques. Virtual implantation using ORTHODOC can eliminate some of the technical factors by assisting the surgeon in visualizing and assessing the fit and fill of various designs of femoral components. In this study, we focused on the influence of lateral curvature of femoral components on canal fit and fill ratios in patients with DDH, in which femoral canal shape is different from that of the normal femur [2]. The Osteolock is a tapered straight stem, whereas the ABG consists of a posteriorly bowed proximal portion and a straight cylindrical distal portion. The reason that the canal fit and fill ratios of the ABG are higher 1 cm proximal from the stem tip is thought to be the difference of the distal design. The distal cylindrical design decreases both the canal fit and fill ratios at the middle of the stem because the cylindrical distal portion results in proximal undersizing as the result of tight distal fit in cases with a high canal flare index.

On the other hand, at levels proximal to the lesser trochanter, where the proximal femur is bowed in the sagittal plane, the lateral curvature of the stem is considered to be important to achieve better canal fit. In fact, the ABG showed significantly greater canal fit at the levels proximal to the lesser trochanter than the Osteolock. Furthermore, the Osteolock showed significantly greater length of proximal posterolateral femoral cortical bone removed at the neck cut level than the ABG. This difference is most likely because the proximal portion of the anatomic stem has a curvature in the sagittal direction similar to that of the proximal portion of the femur, and has better endosteal contact not only at the anterior aspect of the cavity but also at the posterior aspect (Fig. 3). No significant difference in the canal fill ratio was found at the lower corner of the femoral neck cut, however, most likely because the canal fill ratio is influenced not only by the curvature of the stem but also by the cross-sectional area of the stem in the proximal portion.

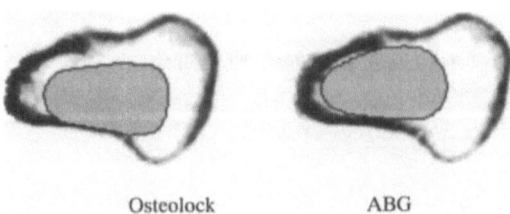

Osteolock   ABG

FIG. 3. Examples of cross-sectional images at the lower corner of the femoral neck cut

Conclusion

To achieve good fit and fill in cases with DDH, implantation of a straight stem type requires removal of cortical bone at the posterolateral femoral neck to a greater degree than required by an anatomic stem type. The anatomic stem type results in a higher canal fit ratio at levels proximal to the lesser trochanter than the straight stem type.

References

1. Bargar WL, Bauer A, Borner M (1998) Primary and revision total hip replacement using the Robodoc system. Clin Orthop Relat Res 354:82–91
2. Sugano N, Noble PC, Kamaric E, et al (1998) The morphology of the femur in developmental dysplasia of the hip. J Bone Joint Surg Br Vol 80(4):711–719

Part 7 Current Topics in Total Knee Arthroplasty

Lateral Parapatellar Approach for Total Knee Arthroplasty in Valgus Knee or Patellar Subluxation

Hwa-Chang Liu, Jih-Horng Wang, Chang-Chou Yen, and Ting-Kuo Yao

Summary. In patients with valgus deformity of the arthritic knee, the contracted lateral soft tissue structures must be released before performing total knee arthroplasty (TKA). In subluxation of the patellar, release of the lateral patellar retinaculum must be carried out to keep the patella in the central part of the patellar sulcus of the femoral component and then to have good patellar tracking. Otherwise, inadequate patellar tracking will remarkably reduce the longevity of the knee prosthesis. In a series of more than 1000 consecutive TKA, 120 knees were operated on by means of the lateral parapatellar approach (LPPA). The knee joints were exposed after releasing the contracted lateral tissues, such as the retinaculum, joint capsule, and iliotibial band. The advantages of this approach include less damage to the blood supply of the patella and better tracking of the patella. In all these cases, the TKA was performed without difficulty. Excellent patellar tracking was observed immediately after each operation and at a later follow-up visit as well. Muscle power of the quadriceps recovered satisfactorily. Short-term functional results as rated by the Hospital for Special Surgery scoring system were excellent. Also, no peroneal nerve palsy or herniation of the joint capsule was found.

Key words. Total knee arthroplasty, Lateral parapatellar approach, Valgus knee, Patellar subluxation

Introduction

On selecting an approach for a operation, orthopaedic surgeons should consider whether the approach could provide not only wide exposure but also complete correction of the deformity in a simple fashion. A simplified lateral parapatellar approach (LPPA) has been used by the senior author for more than 15 years to correct lateral soft tissue contracture in the valgus knee as well as to provide ample space for performing total knee arthroplasty (TKA). Recently, the author expanded its indication to include the knee with a normal femorotibial (FT) angle but with subluxation of the patella, so that lateral retinacular release can be omitted.

Department of Orthopaedic Surgery, National Taiwan University Hospital, No. 7 Chung-Shan S. Rd, Taipei, Taiwan, ROC

Patients and Methods

From January 1991 to January 1999, the senior author performed more than 1000 TKA for patients with osteoarthritis (OA) of the knee. In this series, 120 knees with either valgus deformity or simply subluxation of the patella were exposed through the lateral approach. These 120 knees were classified into three groups according to the severity of valgus deformity, i.e., the FT angle: group 1, FT angle 173°–160°, 87 knees; group 2, FT angle 160°–140°, 32 knees; group 3, FT angle <140°, 1 knee. Different extents of soft tissue release were used in different groups during TKA. The age of the patients ranged from 45 to 87 years.

Operational Procedures

Stage 1

After a middle longitudinal incision over the knee, arthrotomy was carried out by making an incision on the middle line of the quadriceps tendon separating the vastus lateralis from the remainder of the quadriceps, downward to and then around the lateral board of the patella and finally along the lateral side of the patellar tendon. The contracted lateral retinaculum was released by this incision. The distal end of the incision was ended at the level of the tibial tuberosity or even downward distally if necessary. The proximal part of the tibia was exposed anterolaterally by subperiosteal elevation. At this stage, the ilotibial band (ITB) was released from Gerdy's tubercle. Then, the knee was extended completely and the balance between medial and lateral collateral ligaments was checked. If the valgus deformity is less than 10°–20° (normal FT angle is 173°), i.e., in patients of group 1 or group 2, this procedure can restore the FT angle to normal.

Stage 2

If the iliotibial band was still tight and the valgus deformity persisted, the iliotibial band was then resected 5 cm above the knee joint. The iliotibial band may be elongated by Z-plasty or by multiple punctures. Normal FT angle was usually restored by this stage in patients of group 2.

Stage 3

Resection of the popliteal tendon and detachment of the femoral attachment of the fibular collateral ligament might be performed for patients of group 3, i.e., for those with FT angle <140°. The proximal 1 cm of the tibia was also exposed by releasing soft tissue attaching to the lateroposterior rim of the plateau. We advise exposing the common peroneal nerve after resection of the iliotibial band and before detaching the popliteal tendon and the fibular collateral ligament from the femur. The patella was then everted medially and the knee flexed for resection of the anterior cruciate ligament (ACL) and lateral meniscus. If the patella was difficult to evert, it might be displaced laterally by a Hoffman retractor so that the knee could be flexed for resection of ACL. The lateral meniscus was resected, and femoral osteotomy was carried out. The medial meniscus could be resected following femoral osteotomy.

This recommended sequence of operation is very helpful in cases of difficult exposure of the medial meniscus. Tibial and patellar osteotomies were carried out as usual. After installation of the prosthesis with cement for all three components, the patellar tracking was checked with the no-thumb test before closing the arthrotomy. Drain tubes were then placed. The vastus lateralis was sutured back to the quadriceps. However, the lateral retinaculum of the patellar remained open, and the wound was closed in three layers without a covering of fat pad for the defect.

Follow-Up

Following the operation, 3–5 months later, standing triple films or standing anteroposterior (AP) and supine lateral radiographs were taken. A 45° Merchant view was also obtained. Postoperative FT angle was measured on AP films, and patellar position was measured as described by Gomes et al. [1].

Knee function was assessed with the Hospital for Special Surgery (HSS) knee rating system before and every 6 months after surgery. All the knees have been followed up at least 1 year after operation.

Results

Patellar tracking was checked by the no-thumb test after all three components were installed with cement. It was excellent even before closing the wound (Fig. 1).

Postoperative FT angles are shown in Table 1. The valgus deformity has been corrected satisfactorily.

Postoperative patellar positions of 21 knees after TKA carried out through LPPA were compared with those of 25 knees after TKA utilizing medial parapatellar approach (MPPA) and with 30 normal nonoperated knees (Table 2). The tilting or displacement of the patella appears less in the lateral approach group than in the medial approach group, but the difference is not of statistical significance.

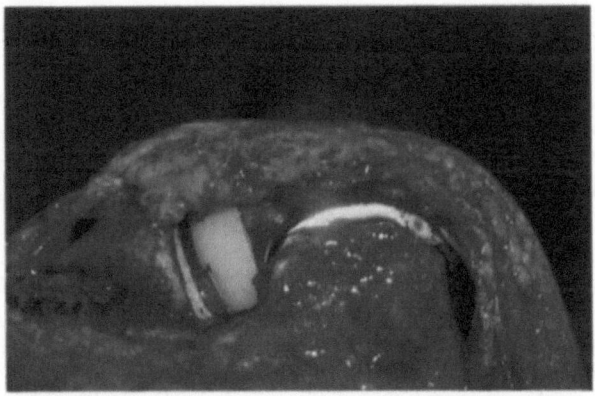

FIG. 1. Excellent patellar tracking is evident even before closing the wound

TABLE 1. Femorotibial angle in degrees on standing antero-posterior (AP) films

Number of knees	87 (Group 1)	32 (Group 2)	1 (Group 3)
Preoperation	173–160	160–140	<140
Postoperation	175.1 ± 2.2	173.7 ± 2.5	172

TABLE 2. Patellar position after operation

Number of knees	21 (Lateral approach)	25 (Medial approach)	30 (Normal, nonoperation)
Tilting (degree)	3.2 ± 1.5	4.5 ± 1.7	3.2 ± 1.2
Displacement (mm)	2.2 ± 1.2	2.3 ± 1.4	2.0 ± 1.3

As checked by the manual method, muscle power was normal in 120 knees 6 months after operation. Range of motion (ROM) of 120 knees ranged from 0°–5° to 100°–125°. The Hospital for Special Surgery Score was 54.5 ± 5.2 before operation and 90.1 ± 6.5 after the operation.

In this series, no patient sustained peroneal palsy. Only one patient, with valgus deformity of 40°, had numbness at the lateral side of the leg after TKA. Skin dimpling at the lateral side of the patella was noted in seven patients but there was no significant morbidity. Lateral skin flap numbness was found in two patients.

Discussion

The vascularization of the patella was studied in detail in 21 cadaver knees by Kayler and Lyttle [2] in 1986. They demonstrated the influence of the operation on the intraosseous flow. Prepatellar cauterization disrupted the intraosseous flow but left the vascular ring intact. Vascular filling was absent following a medial arthrotomy incision made too close (<1 cm) to the patella, radical excision of the fat pad, lateral retinacular release performed too close (<1.5 cm) to the patella, and the cauterization of the prepatellar vessels.

In contrast, if the medial approach was made more than 1 cm from the patella, if the fat pad was excised partially, or if lateral release of retinaculum was made more than 1.5 cm far from the patella, blood flow would remain normal. Bonutti et al. [3] also demonstrated that a medial parapatellar approach and a lateral release would incur a 75% decrease in total patellar perfusion. Damage to the central 50% of interosseous bone or anterior soft tissue cuff because of a central fixation post or anterior cruciate ligament graft also increases the risk for segmental devascularization. Therefore, in the case of valgus knee or a knee with subluxed patella, lateral release of retinaculum has to be carried out in addition to making the incision for arthrotomy, we recommend the LPPA to combine arthrotomy and lateral release in one incision.

Several approaches for TKA have been commonly used [4]. The popular medial parapatellar approach (MPPA) has the advantages of easy eversion of the patella laterally and releasing the medial contracted soft tissue in varus deformity. The disadvantages of MPPA include that additional lateral release for poor patellar tracking would jeopardize the patellar blood supply. In addition, in MPPA patellofemoral complication would occur at a rate of 5%–30% [5–7]. The subvastus approach described in 1929 and reported by Hofmann et al. [8] in 1990 has the advantage of not disturbing the patella and the quadriceps, i.e., there is excellent recovery of extension mechanism and reduced pain postoperatively. However, the surgical exposure is poor and difficult in obese patients.

Engh et al. [9–11] reported that the midvastus approach could reduce lateral retinacular release from 50% in cases of MPPA to 3% in midvastus approach. However, the exposure is still not good in the obese patient. For the knee with valgus deformity, only LPPA seems ideal for good exposure and good tissue balance [12]. Buecjel [13] described a sequential three-step lateral release for correcting fixed valgus knee deformities. We think it is not necessary to release the iliotibial band (ITB) from the Gerdy tubercle in addition to resecting it in the case of severe valgus deformity. Resection of only the ITB 5 cm proximal to the knee joint is enough to have satisfactory release. We also extend the indication of lateral approach to the knee with normal FT angle but with subluxation of the patellar.

In our series of 120 knees, FT angle has been restored to normal as shown in Table 1 even in patients with valgus deformity as great as 40°. In addition, peroneal nerve palsy did not occur in this series. Patellar position is satifactory (see Table 2), along with excellent patellar tracking noted before closure of the wound (Fig. 1). Postoperative knee function is excellent, as the average HSS score is 90.1 compared to 54.5 before operation. In conclusion, we think LPPA is helpful in TKA for OA knee with valgus deformity or with patellar subluxation to lessen vascular injury of the patella and to obtain good patellar tracking.

References

1. Gomes LS, Bechtold JE, Gustilo RB (1988) Patellar prosthesis positioning in total knee arthroplasty: a roentgenographic study. Clin Orthop 236:72–81
2. Kayler DE, Lyttle D (1988) Surgical interruption of patellar blood supply by total knee arthroplasty. Clin Orthop Relat Res 229:221–227
3. Bonutti PM, Miller BG, Cremens MJ (1998) Intraosseous patellar blood supply after medial parapatellar arthrotomy. Clin Orthop Relat Res 352:202–214
4. Insall JN (1984) Surgical approaches to the knee. In: Insall JN (ed) The knee. Churchill Livingstone, New York, p 41
5. Hungerford DS, Krackow KA (1985) Total joint arthroplasty of the knee. Clin Orthop 192:23
6. Leblanc JM (1989) Patella complications in total knee arthroplasty: a literature review. Orthop Rev 18:296
7. Merkow RL, Soudry M, Insall JN (1985) Patellar dislocation following total knee replacement. J Bone Joint Surg 67:1321
8. Hofmann AA, Plaster RL, Murdock LE (1991) Subvastus (southern) approach for primary total knee arthroplasty. Clin Orthop Relat Res 269:70–77
9. Engh GA, Parks NL, Ammeen DJ (1996) Influence of surgical approach on lateral retinacular release in total knee arthroplasty. Clin Orthop Relat Res 331:56–63
10. Engh GA, Holt BT, Parks NL (1997) A midvastus muscle-splitting approach for total knee arthroplasty. J Arthroplasty 12(3):322–331

11. Engh GA, Parks NL (1998) Surgical technique of the midvastus arthrotomy. Clin Orthop Relat Res 351:270–274
12. Keblish PA (1991) The lateral approach to the valgus knee. Surgical technique and analysis of 53 cases with over two-year follow-up evaluation. Clin Orthop Relat Res 271:52–62
13. Buecjel FF (1990) A sequential three-step lateral release for correcting fixed valgus knee deformities during total knee arthroplasty. Clin Orthop Relat Res 260:170–175

Soft Tissue Balancing in Total Knee Arthroplasty

Leo A. Whiteside

Summary. Most ligament balancing problems in total knee arthroplasty can be solved by first resecting the distal femur at 5°–7° valgus and the proximal tibia perpendicular to its long axis. The next step is to remove osteophytes and release adhesions, then to insert the trial components and release tight structures. It rarely is necessary to tighten loose structures. The operative treatment principles of varus and valgus knees are the same. The most prominent surface of the joint is used as a point of reference for resection, and bony defects on the deficient side of the knee are grafted with either morselized or block autograft. Because ligament balancing in flexion is dependent on rotational alignment of the femoral component, 3°–4° of external rotation of the femoral component usually provides correct varus–valgus balance in flexion and also places the patellar groove laterally and helps to stabilize patellar tracking. Finally, the tibial component thickness is adjusted to achieve proper balance between the medial and lateral sides of the knee. Anteroposterior stability and femoral rollback are assessed, and steps are taken to achieve acceptable posterior stability.

Key words. Ligament balancing, Varus, Valgus, Total knee arthroplasty, Rotational alignment

Introduction

Ligament balancing is an integral part of total knee arthroplasty and is highly dependent on correct alignment of the knee in flexion and extension. Since the mid-1970s, the rudimentary concepts of releasing the medial collateral ligaments in knees with varus deformity and the lateral ligaments in knees with valgus deformity have been widely taught and practiced [1]. Various schemes have been proposed to achieve ligament balancing. The earliest technique was simply to release tight ligaments before the bone cuts were made, and then to resect the distal and posterior surfaces of the femur to create equal flexion and extension spaces [1]. This method improved ligament balance over simple replacement in situ, but left little leeway for final precise ligament balancing and also provided no means to align varus–valgus in flexion.

Missouri Bone and Joint Center, 10 Barnes West Drive, Suite 100, St. Louis, MO 63141, USA

Another ligament balancing scheme involves the use of tensioners to tension the ligaments in flexion, allowing the ligaments to dictate the rotational position of the femoral component and thus the varus–valgus position in flexion as well as alignment of the patellar groove. Although this technique can result in equal ligament tension on the medial and lateral sides of the knee in flexion, it also can rotationally malalign the femoral component in flexion, creating a varus or valgus deformity in the flexed position, and tilt the patellar groove so that it does not lie in the same plane as the long axis of the tibia during flexion and extension.

The technique proposed in this chapter begins with correct alignment of the articular surfaces of the femur in both flexion and extension so that the joint surfaces are perpendicular to the anteroposterior plane of the lower extremity. This alignment is done separately on the femur and tibia in extension and flexion, irrespective of ligament contracture or stretching. Once alignment, sizing, and positioning of the implants are correct, the ligaments can be assessed. Only ligaments that are tight need to be released, thus minimizing trauma and maximizing the stability of the knee.

Alignment

The cornerstone to correct ligament balancing is correct varus and valgus alignment in flexion and extension. For alignment in the extended position, fixed anatomic landmarks such as the intramedullary canal of the femur and long axis of the tibia are accepted [2,3] (Fig. 1). When the joint surface is resected at an angle of 5°–7° valgus to the medullary canal of the femur and perpendicular to the long axis of the tibia, the joint surfaces are perpendicular to the mechanical axis of the lower extremity and roughly parallel to the epicondylar axis of the femur (Fig. 2). In the flexed position, anatomic landmarks are equally important for varus and valgus alignment. Incorrect varus and valgus alignment in flexion not only malaligns the long axes of the femur and tibia but also incorrectly positions the patellar groove in both flexion and extension.

Finding suitable landmarks for varus and valgus alignment has led to efforts to use the posterior femoral condyles [4], epicondylar axis [5], and anteroposterior axis of the femur [6,7]. The posterior femoral condyles provide excellent rotational alignment landmarks if the femoral joint surface has not been worn or otherwise distorted by the arthritic process [4,8–14] (Fig. 3). However, as with the distal surfaces, the posterior femoral condylar surfaces are sometimes damaged or hypoplastic (more commonly in the valgus than in the varus knee) and cannot serve as reliable anatomic guides for alignment [9].

The epicondylar axis is anatomically inconsistent and, in all cases other than revision total knee arthroplasty with severe bone loss, is unreliable for varus and valgus alignment in flexion just as it is in extension. The anteroposterior axis, defined by the lateral border of the posterior cruciate ligament posteriorly and the deepest part of the patellar groove anteriorly, is highly consistent, and always lies within the median sagittal plane that bisects the lower extremity, passing through the hip, knee, and ankle [6,7]. When the articular surfaces are resected perpendicular to the anteroposterior axis, they are perpendicular to the anteroposterior plane, and the extremity can function normally in this plane throughout the flexion and extension arc [7].

FIG. 1. The centers of the hip, knee, and ankle lie approximately in a straight line—the mechanical axis of the lower extremity. The mechanical axis of the femur is collinear with the mechanical axis of the lower extremity. The long axis of the femur (the anatomic axis) aligns in approximately 5° valgus to the mechanical axis of the lower extremity. The long axis of the tibia is collinear with the mechanical axis of the lower extremity. The patellar groove is collinear with the mechanical axis of the extremity and perpendicular to the epicondylar axis. The mechanical axis of the lower extremity becomes a plane when flexion and extension are considered. The centers of the hip, knee, and ankle remain within this plane through the flexion–extension arc. The patellar groove (AP axis of the femur) is coplanar with this plane so that the patella is drawn smoothly through the groove as a rope is pulled smoothly through a well-aligned pulley. The epicondylar axis is perpendicular to the AP plane, and the tibia swings through this axis, staying in the AP plane throughout the flexion–extension arc. (From [24], with permission)

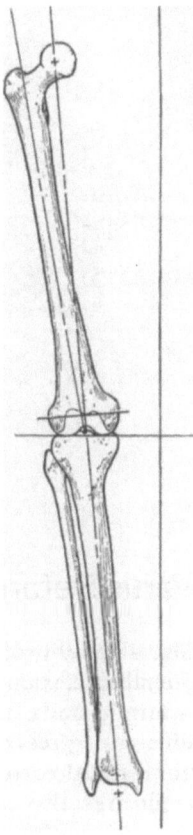

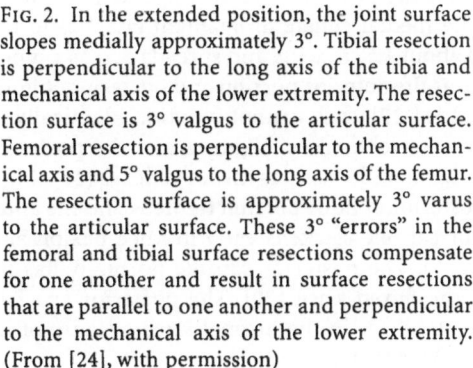

FIG. 2. In the extended position, the joint surface slopes medially approximately 3°. Tibial resection is perpendicular to the long axis of the tibia and mechanical axis of the lower extremity. The resection surface is 3° valgus to the articular surface. Femoral resection is perpendicular to the mechanical axis and 5° valgus to the long axis of the femur. The resection surface is approximately 3° varus to the articular surface. These 3° "errors" in the femoral and tibial surface resections compensate for one another and result in surface resections that are parallel to one another and perpendicular to the mechanical axis of the lower extremity. (From [24], with permission)

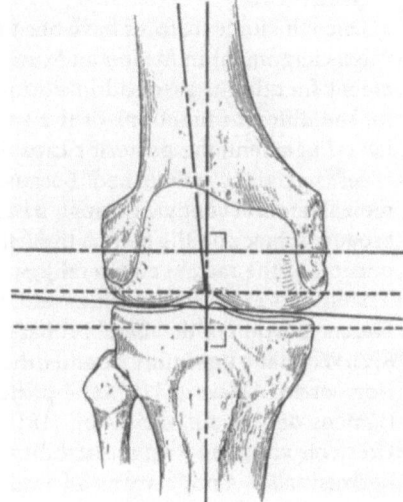

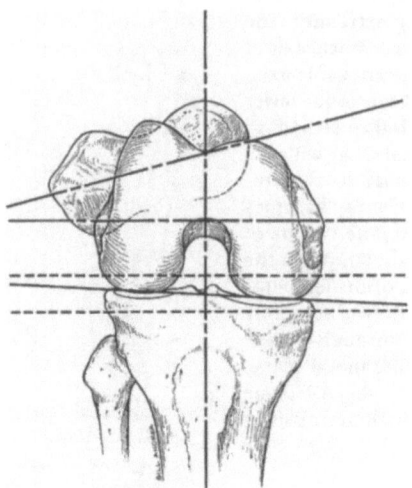

FIG. 3. With the knee flexed 90°, the joint surface resections are parallel to the epicondylar axis and perpendicular to the AP axis of the femur. The femoral neck is anteverted approximately 15° to the epicondylar axis. When the knee is in functional position in flexion (walking up stairs or standing from a seated position), the positions of the femoral neck and epicondylar axis remain unchanged, and in the normal knee the tibia is vertical. (From [24], with permission)

Varus Deformity

Medial stability of the knee is a complex issue and involves ligaments that behave differently in flexion and in extension. The contracture and stretching that occur due to deformity and osteophytes affect these ligament structures unequally and often cause different degrees of tightness or laxity in flexion and extension after the bone surfaces are resected correctly for varus and valgus alignment. The distortion of alignment landmarks also can cause varus and valgus alignment to differ in the flexed and extended positions, and the knee may thus require adjustment of portions of the medial stabilizing complex that affects stability either in flexion or extension [15] (Figs. 4A–C, 5).

Once the joint surfaces have been resected correctly to establish normal varus and valgus alignment in flexion and extension, the trial components are inserted and ligament function is assessed in flexion and extension (Figs. 6, 7). The anatomic basis for the different functions of the anterior and posterior portions of the medial collateral ligament, the posterior capsule, and the posterior cruciate ligament has been at least partially established. Because the medial collateral ligament attaches to the medial femoral condyle through a band about 1.5 cm wide and spreads across a much broader surface on the medial tibial flare as the anterior portion and posterior oblique portion of the medial collateral ligament [16,17], each cannot function identically in flexion and extension [18]. Instead, the anterior portion tightens and the posterior oblique portion of the medial collateral ligament loosens as the knee flexes [18] (Figs. 8, 9). When the knee fully extends, the posterior oblique portion tightens and the anterior portion slackens [19]. The posterior capsule slackens early in knee flexion and tightens only in full extension [18] (Fig. 9). The posterior capsule normally has no effect on varus and valgus stability in the flexed knee [20]. The posterior cruciate ligament also is not a varus and valgus stabilizer in the normal knee because of its distance from the medial and lateral condylar surfaces [20].

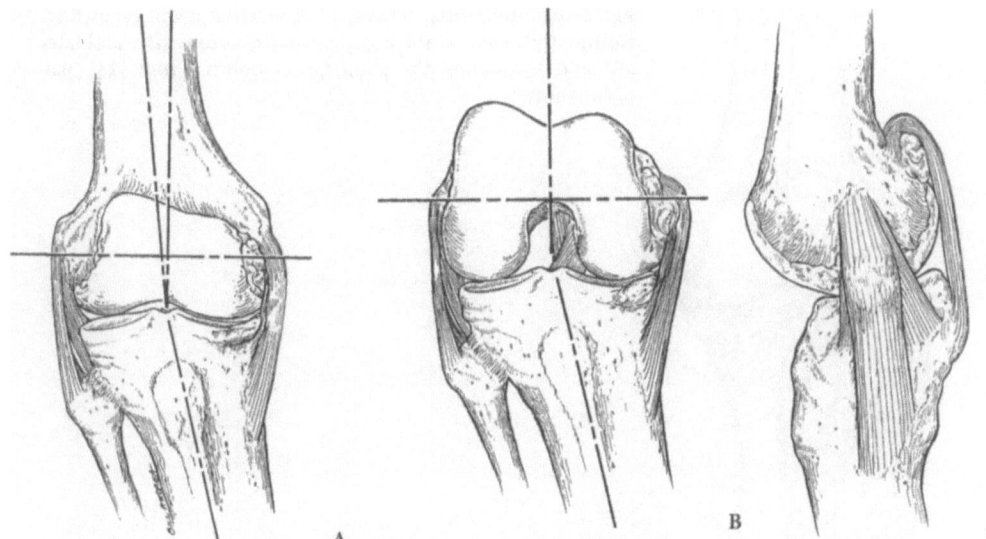

FIG. 4. **A** The mechanical axis of the femur is tilted medially relative to the long axis of the tibia. The distal femoral surface usually remains in valgus alignment to the long axis of the femur. Resection of the distal surface of the femur at a 5° valgus angle aligns the distal surface perpendicular to the mechanical axis of the femur. Approximately equal thickness of bone is removed from medial and lateral surfaces. Most of the varus deformity is caused by deficiency in the medial tibial plateau. Resection of the tibial bone surface perpendicular to the long axis of the tibia often leaves a defect in the medial tibial plateau. The deep and superficial medial collateral ligaments are contracted and deformed by osteophytes. **B** The varus knee has a group of bone and ligament abnormalities that must be addressed to correct the deformity. The anteroposterior axis of the femur tilts medially relative to the long axis of the tibia. The deep and superficial medial collateral ligaments are contracted, and the posterior cruciate ligament, being a medial structure, often is contracted as well. **C** The osteophytes may deform the medial collateral ligament and posterior capsule enough to cause flexion contracture. (**A, B, C** from [24], with permission)

With this information, the medial ligament structures of the knee can be released individually according to the position in which excessive tightness is found: release of the anterior portion of the medial collateral ligament to correct inappropriate medial ligament tension in flexion (Figs. 10, 11), release of the posterior oblique portion of the medial collateral ligament (Fig. 12) and the posterior medial capsule (Fig. 13) to correct inappropriate medial ligament tension in extension, and release of the posterior cruciate ligament to correct any remaining medial tightness in flexion (Fig. 14). The posterior cruciate ligament is an important secondary varus and valgus stabilizer in flexion and, in the absence of the medial collateral ligament, also is likely to function as an important medial stabilizing structure in extension.

Once the surgeon has determined with certainty which ligaments are contracted, limited releases can be done, releasing only the ligaments that are tight and leaving alone those that are not. A knee that is aligned correctly after total knee arthroplasty and tight medially only in flexion first should have the anterior portion of the medial

176   L.A. Whiteside

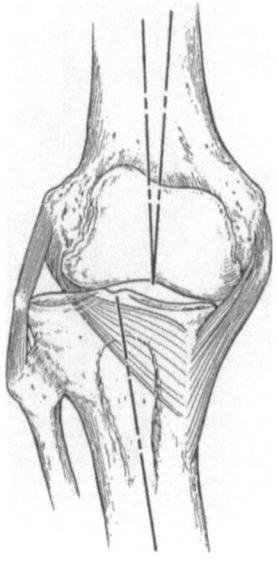

FIG. 5. The tibia often is subluxed laterally in the varus knee, shifting the origin of the popliteus muscle proximally and laterally and shortening the popliteus complex. (From [24], with permission)

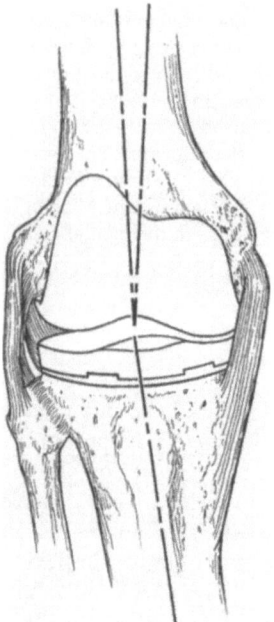

FIG. 6. After all the osteophytes are removed and the bone surfaces are finished, the trial components are inserted to act as tensioners throughout the entire flexion arc. A 10-mm tibial component is used. In this illustration the knee is tight medially and gapes spontaneously laterally. It also has a 10° flexion contracture. (From [24], with permission)

FIG. 7. The knee is tight medially in flexion as well. The lateral side gapes spontaneously, and the medial femoral condyle rolls to the posterior edge of the tibial spacer. The entire superficial medial collateral ligament (MCL), when palpated, feels tight in the flexed and extended positions. At this stage it is impossible to know if all medial structures are tight, but it is clear that at least the anterior and posterior portions of the MCL are tight. (From [24], with permission)

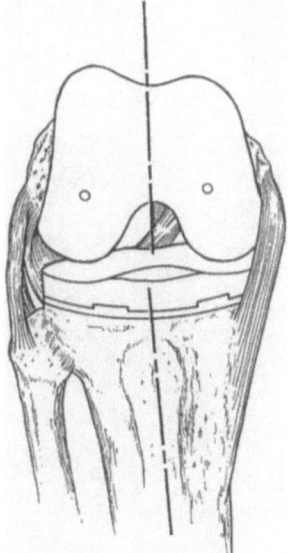

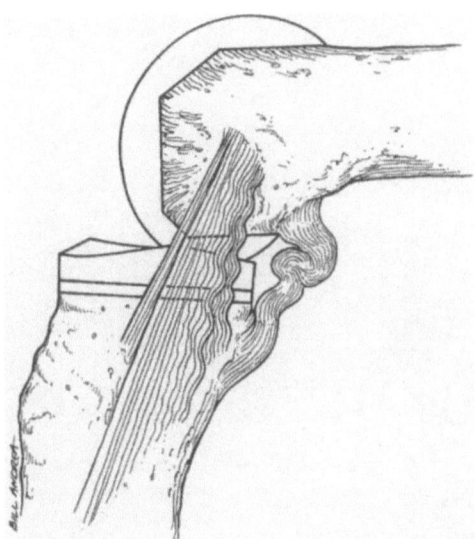

FIG. 8. Normally, the anterior portion of the MCL is tight in flexion and the medial portion is loose. The posterior capsule also is loose in flexion. (From [15], with permission)

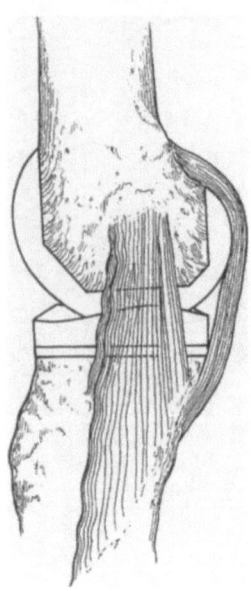

FIG. 9. The posterior portion of the medial collateral ligament becomes taut in extension, and the anterior portion slackens so that the knee has normal ligament balance in extension. (From [15], with permission)

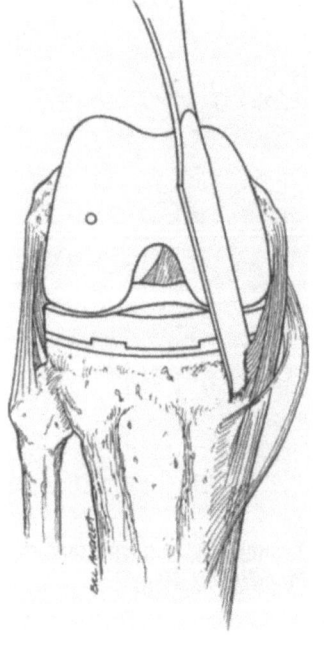

FIG. 10. The knee is flexed to 90° and a curved 1/2-in. osteotome is used to elevate the anterior portion of the deep and superficial medial collateral ligament while leaving the attachment of the pes anserinus intact. (From [24], with permission)

FIG. 11. The taut anterior fibers are released sub-periosteally, leaving the posterior fibers intact. The attachment of the pes anserinus also is left intact. (From [15], with permission)

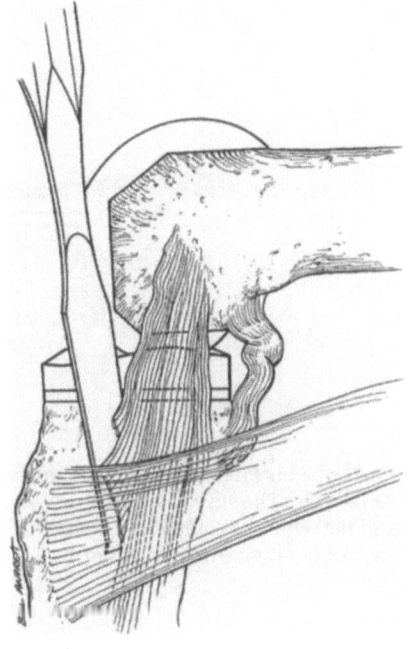

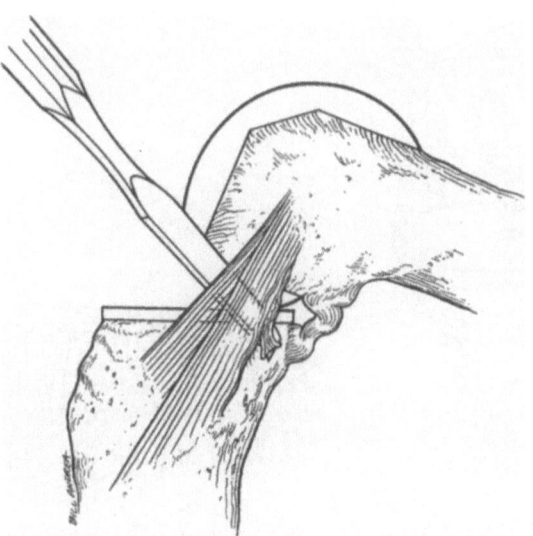

FIG. 12. A curved 1/2-in. osteotome is used to elevate the posterior portion of the medial collateral ligament. (From [15], with permission)

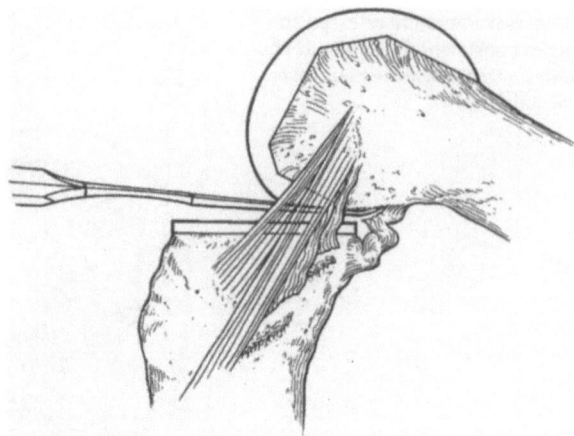

FIG. 13. If the knee still is too tight medially in extension, then the medial posterior capsule can be released. The curved 1/2-in. osteotome is used to gently elevate the capsule from the femur, and the release is completed by elevating the capsule from the posterior surface of the tibia as well. (From [24], with permission)

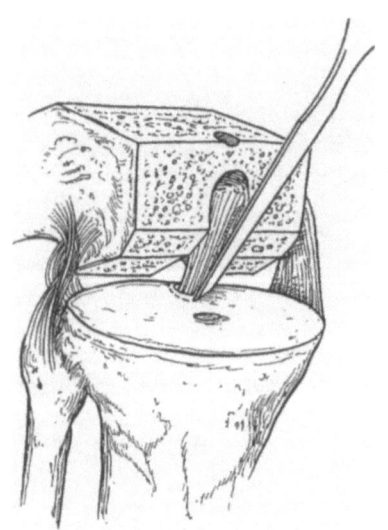

FIG. 14. The tight posterior cruciate ligament (PCL) is released along with its tibial bone attachment. Here a 1/4-in. osteotome is used to elevate a small fragment of bone with the attached ligament. When this bone segment is pried loose, it slides proximally 5–10 mm, slackening the PCL. (From [24], with permission)

collateral ligament released; this leaves the posterior oblique portion intact to provide stability in both flexion and extension. Knees that are tight only in extension after total knee arthroplasty should have release first of the posterior oblique fibers of the medial collateral ligament, and then release of the posterior capsule if medial contracture persists in extension. This procedure leaves the anterior portion of the medial collateral ligament intact to stabilize the knee. The results of posterior cruciate release suggest that major destabilization of the knee may occur if this ligament is released after full release of the medial collateral ligament, posterior oblique fibers of the medial collateral ligament, and posterior capsule has been done.

This conclusion is in close agreement with other studies that evaluated the effect of posterior cruciate ligament release on varus and valgus and rotational stability after release of either collateral ligament. These studies demonstrated a major role for the posterior cruciate ligament in both varus and valgus and rotational stability after either collateral ligament was released [21,22]. Knees requiring full release of the medial collateral ligament and release of the medial posterior capsule will be highly dependent on the posterior cruciate ligament for both valgus and rotational stability. Sacrifice of the posterior cruciate ligament in knees with major varus deformity should be done rarely, if at all.

Valgus Deformity

Correction of alignment and elimination of articular surface deformity now can be achieved with modern instruments and alignment devices even in the most difficult valgus knees. Using the anteroposterior axis of the distal femoral surface or the epicondylar axis of the femur has virtually eliminated the rotational alignment problem of the femoral component and has paved the way to a rational approach to ligament balancing in the valgus knee [7]. Using the central axis of the femur and tibia as reference lines for valgus angle ensures highly reproducible alignment in the frontal plane [6,7] (Fig. 15). Using the distal surface of the medial femoral condyle as the point of reference for distal femoral resection ensures that the distal surface of the femur will be in correct position relative to the medial ligaments and the patella. This approach ensures that the patellar groove, intercondylar notch, and condylar surfaces are all positioned correctly.

For alignment in flexion, either the anteroposterior axis or the epicondylar axis of the femur is used as anatomic reference for resection of the anterior surfaces of the femur. The posterior femoral condyles are unreliable as references for femoral component alignment because of lateral femoral condylar deficiency (Fig. 16). Correct resection of the femoral surfaces before ligament balancing produces a laterally conveying joint space in flexion (Fig. 17).

With the surfaces in correct alignment, ligament balancing requires a rational approach for correct balance in flexion and extension. Consideration of the effects of the functions of the lateral stabilizing structures throughout the arc of flexion offers a basis from which to formulate this approach [23]. The lateral collateral ligament is regarded as a stabilizing structure in both flexion and extension and has rotational as well as valgus stabilizing effects [20] (Figs. 18, 19). The popliteus tendon complex also has passive varus stabilizing effects in flexion and extension and a prominent role in external rotational stabilization of the tibia on the femur. These two structures would be appropriate to release for a knee that is excessively tight laterally both in flexion and in extension.

The iliotibial (IT) band is aligned perpendicular to the joint surface when the knee is extended and therefore can provide lateral knee stability when the knee is extended.

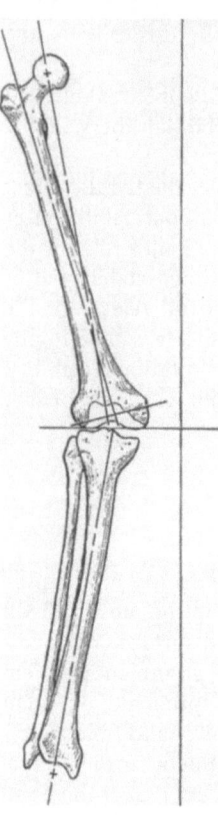

FIG. 15. In the valgus knee the lateral femoral condyle is deficient, usually distally and posteriorly, so that the knee is in valgus in extension and flexion. A valgus curvature usually is found in the midshaft of the femur and tibia, so a line down the midshaft diaphyseal medullary canal crosses the joint medial to the center. Entry points into the joint for intramedullary alignment rods should be medialized 5–10 mm to accommodate and correct this valgus curvature. (From [24], with permission)

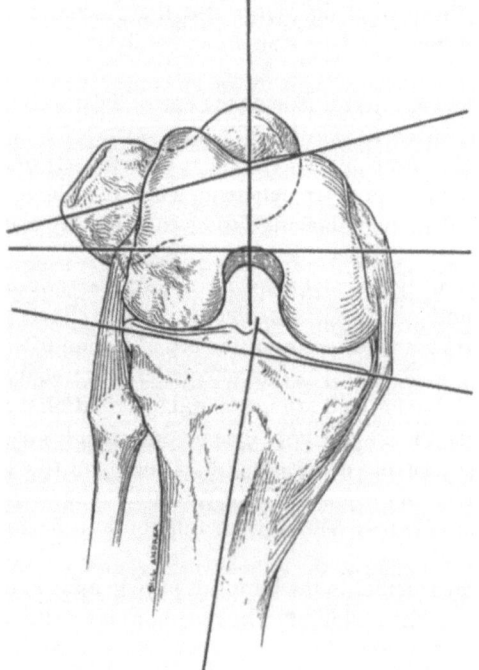

FIG. 16. Viewed from the distal end of the femur, the AP axis of the knee is no longer collinear with the long axis of the tibia but is tilted laterally as is the mechanical axis of the femur on the anterior view. (From [23], with permission)

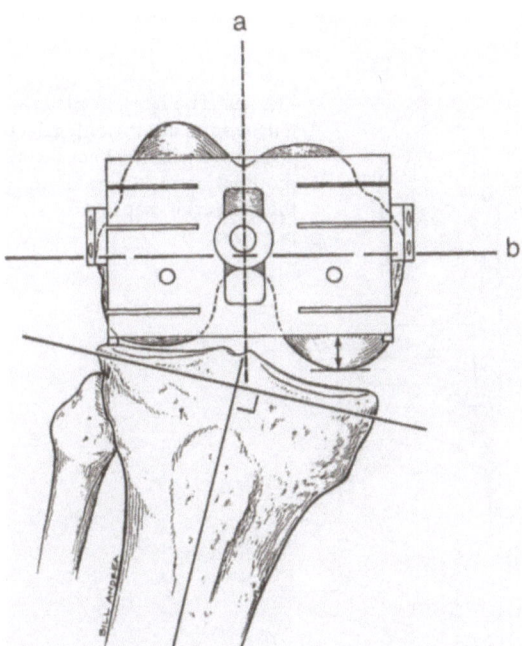

FIG. 17. The cutting guide for femoral resection is aligned so the surfaces are resected perpendicular to the AP axis of the femur (*a*) and parallel with the epicondylar axis (*b*), resecting the thickness of the implant from the intact medial femoral condyle, and much less from the deficient lateral side. This step places the joint surfaces in anatomic position to correct the valgus position in flexion and places the patellar groove correctly with the mechanical axis of the lower extremity. The tibial surface is resected perpendicular to the long axis of the tibia. The lateral ligaments are still tight, and the femur is held in an externally rotated valgus position by the ligament contractures. (From [23], with permission)

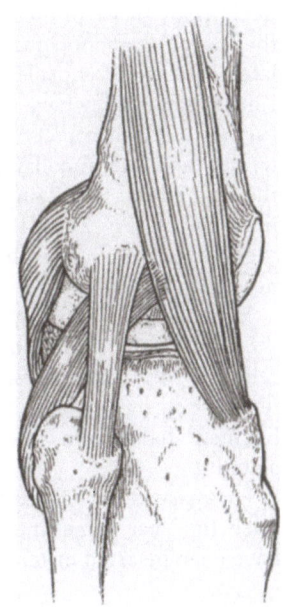

FIG. 18. The lateral collateral ligament, lateral posterior capsule, popliteus tendon, and iliotibial band all cross the joint perpendicular (or nearly so) to its surface, and are capable of stabilizing the knee in the extended position. (From [23], with permission)

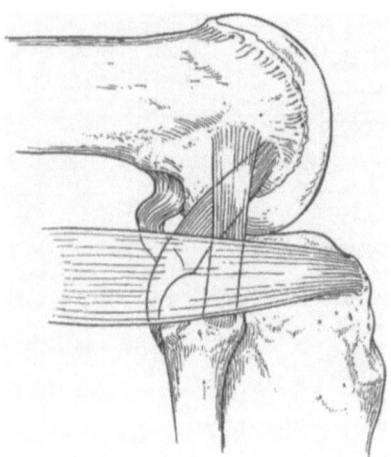

FIG. 19. The lateral collateral ligament and popliteus tendon are the only effective lateral stabilizing structures with the knee flexed to this position. The iliotibial band is parallel to the joint surface, and the posterior capsule is slack. (From [23], with permission)

When the knee is flexed to 90°, however, the IT band is parallel to the joint surface and cannot stabilize the knee to varus stress. The lateral posterior capsular structures are tight only in full extension and are slack when the knee is flexed. Release of either the posterior capsule or the IT band would have a rational basis only for a knee that is tight laterally in extension. Release of either would have little effect on lateral knee stability in the flexed position.

Thus, after total knee arthroplasty, the knee that is tight laterally in flexion and extension will be almost completely corrected by release of the lateral collateral ligament and popliteus tendon (Fig. 20). No other structures afford lateral stability in flexion, so release of these two structures is all that is needed to correct the effects of the lateral ligament contracture in flexion. However, in extension the IT band and the lateral posterior capsule are effective lateral stabilizers and may still need release. Knees that initially have tight lateral structures in flexion and extension often require further work to correct lateral tightness in extension after release of the popliteus tendon and lateral collateral ligament. Because the IT band is easily accessible, it is the next lateral stabilizing structure to be released if the knee remains tight laterally in extension (Fig. 21). If the knee remains tight laterally even after the IT band release, then the posterior capsule can be released to finish correcting lateral ligament tightness (Fig. 22).

Because knee stability in extension is absolutely necessary for good function, these two extension stabilizers (IT band and lateral posterior capsule) should be released only as a last resort. If they are released first, before lateral laxity is tested in flexion, and the lateral collateral ligament and popliteus tendon are released to achieve ligament balance in flexion, then nothing remains to provide crucial extension stability.

For reasons probably related to differences in deformity of the lateral side of the knee, the knee sometimes is tight laterally only in extension after the trial implants have been inserted or tensioners applied. In these cases the lateral collateral ligament

FIG. 20. Because this knee is tight on the lateral side in flexion, one or both of these structures require release. If the tibia has internal rotation contracture and the knee is tight laterally as well, the popliteus tendon almost certainly will require release. If the contracture is strictly lateral without a rotational component, then only lateral collateral release should be tried first, followed by release of the popliteus tendon if necessary. (From [23], with permission)

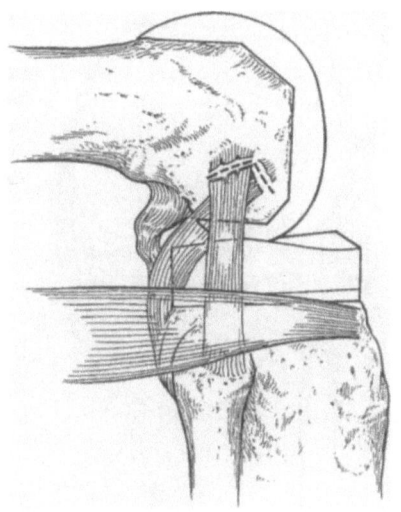

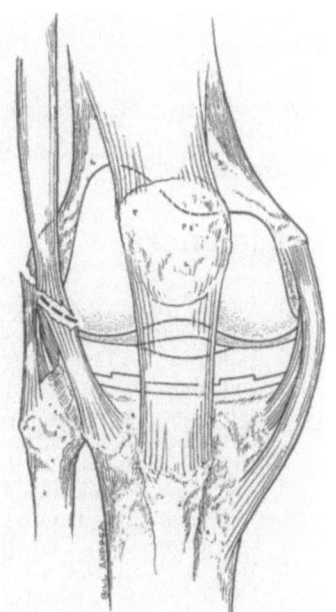

FIG. 21. The iliotibial band has been released, leaving it adherent to the underlying synovial membrane. The knee is still tight laterally, but no longer gapes spontaneously medially. (From [23], with permission)

and the popliteus tendon should not be released, but only the IT band and the lateral posterior capsule should be released to achieve ligament balance. Uncommonly, valgus knees require all static lateral stability structures to be released to adequately correct the deformity and ligament imbalance. In these cases, the biceps femoris muscle, gastrocnemius muscle, and deep fascia provide support for the lateral side of the knee until capsular healing occurs.

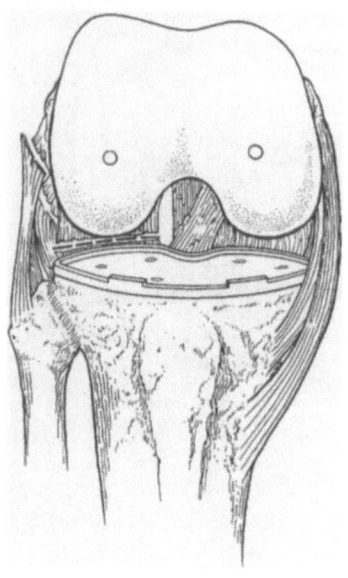

FIG. 22. When the posterior capsule must be released, access is achieved by removing the tibial spacer and distracting the joint with the knee flexed 90°. The capsule either can be transected at the joint line or released from the posterior surface of the femur with a curved osteotome, as illustrated for the varus knee. (From [24], with permission)

Acknowledgment. This article is reprinted with permission from Whiteside LA (2000) Positioning the femoral component: the effect of proper ligament balance. Am J Knee Surg 13:173–180.

References

1. Insall J, Ranawat CS, Scott WN, Walker P (1976) Total condylar knee replacement. Preliminary report. Clin Orthop 120:149–154
2. Whiteside LA (1989) Intramedullary alignment of total knee replacement. A clinical and laboratory study. Orthop Rev (Suppl), pp 9–12
3. Whiteside LA, McCarthy DS (1992) Laboratory evaluation of alignment and kinematics in a unicompartmental knee arthroplasty inserted with intramedullary instrumentation. Clin Orthop 274:238–247
4. Anouchi YS, Whiteside LA, Kaiser AD, Milliano MT (1991) The effect of axial rotational alignment of the femoral component on knee stability and patellar tracking in total knee arthroplasty. Clin Orthop 287:170–177
5. Yoshioka Y, Siu D, Cooke TDV (1987) The anatomy and functional axes of the femur. J Bone Joint Surg 69A:873–880
6. Arima J, Whiteside LA, White SE, McCarthy DS (1995) Femoral rotational alignment in the valgus total knee arthroplasty based on the anterior-posterior axis: a technical note. J Bone Joint Surg 77A:1331–1334
7. Whiteside LA, Arima J (1995) The anteroposterior axis for femoral rotational alignment in valgus total knee arthroplasty. Clin Orthop 321:168–172
8. Martin JW, Whiteside LA (1990) The influence of joint line position on knee stability after condylar knee arthroplasty. Clin Orthop 259:146–156
9. Matsuda S, Matsuda H, Miyagi T, et al (1998) Femoral condyle geometry in the normal and varus knee. Clin Orthop 349:183–188

10. Whiteside LA (1993) Correction of ligament and bone defects in total arthroplasty of the severely valgus knee. Clin Orthop 288:234–245
11. Whiteside LA (1995) Ligament release and bone grafting in total arthroplasty of the varus knee. Orthopedics 18:117–122
12. Whiteside LA, Kasselt MR, Haynes DW (1987) Varus and valgus and rotational stability in rotationally unconstrained total knee arthroplasty. Clin Orthop 219:147–157
13. Whiteside LA, Summers RG (1983) Anatomical landmarks for an intramedullary alignment system for total knee replacement. Orthop Trans 7:546–547
14. Whiteside LA, Summers RG (1984) The effect of the level of distal femoral resection on ligament balance in total knee replacement. In: Dorr LD (ed) The knee: papers of the first scientific meeting of the Knee Society. Baltimore, University Park Press, pp 59–73
15. Whiteside LA, Saeki K, Mihalko WM (2000) Functional medial ligament balancing in total knee arthroplasty. Clin Orthop 380:45–57
16. Warren LF, Marshall JL (1979) The supporting structures and layers on the medial side of the knee. J Bone Joint Surg 61A:56–62
17. Warren LF, Marshall JL, Girgis F (1974) The prime static stabilizer of the medial side of the knee. J Bone Joint Surg 56A:665–674
18. Burks RT (1990) Gross anatomy. In: Daniel D, Akeson W, O'Connor J (eds) Knee ligaments: structure, function, injury, and repair. New York, Raven Press, pp 59–76
19. Hull ML, Berns GS, Varma H, Patterson HA (1996) Strain in the medial collateral ligament of the human knee under single and combined loads. J Biomech 29:199–206
20. Grood ES, Noyes FR, Butler DI, Suntay WJ (1981) Ligamentous and capsular restraints preventing straight medial and lateral laxity in intact human cadaver knees. J Bone Joint Surg 63A:1257–1269
21. Grood ES, Stowers SF, Noyes FR (1988) Limits of movement in the human knee. J Bone Joint Surg 70A:88–97
22. Nielson S, Ovesen J, Rasmussen O (1985) The posterior cruciate ligament and rotatory knee instability. An experimental study. Arch Orthop Trauma Surg 104:53–56
23. Whiteside LA (1999) Selective ligament release in total knee arthroplasty of the knee in valgus. Clin Orthop 367:130–140
24. Whiteside LA (2000) Positioning the femoral component: The effect of proper ligament balance. Am J Knee Surg 13:173–180

HA-Coated Total Knee Arthroplasty: A 9-year HA Omnifit Experience

Jean-Alain Epinette

Summary. In joint arthroplasty, a lasting, stable implant fixation without the use of acrylic cement, by means of a bioactive bond between implant and host bone, is a goal as important in the knee as it is in the hip. We would like to report on a personal experience of 345 hydroxyapatite-coated (HA) cruciate-retaining (CR) knees operated on since 1990. Of this number, no patient has been lost to follow-up. The average age was 70.52 years. The type of surgery was primary in 324 cases (93.9%) and revision in 21 cases. Osteoarthritis remains as usual the main etiology (85%). We recorded 0.9% of typical mechanical failures. The mean IKS values at 5yr were 95.3 and 85.1 points regarding "knee score" and "function score," respectively. In such a way, we recorded 98% (knee score) and 73% (function score) of excellent and good results. Radiographically, we had no mechanical loosening, and radiographic changes demonstrated a very good HA–bone interface for both femoral and tibial components. The cumulative survival rate at 5 years reaches 0.9935 ± 0.0106. The very encouraging results reported in the current study make us very confident about the ultimate outcome of bioactive coatings in knee arthroplasty.

Key words. Hydroxyapatite, HA joint replacement, Cruciate-retaining knee arthroplasty, Omnifit, Bioactive coatings

Introduction

Hydroxyapatite-coated (HA-coated) joint replacements have come a long way. For many years, they had been lumped together with the "cementless" devices generally; among so many others, they were no more than a fad and passing fancy. Then, step by step, the picture changed, and now HA-coated devices are recognized as an implant "family" in their own right. As a matter of fact, lasting, stable implant fixation without the use of acrylic cement, by means of a bioactive bond between the implant and the host bone, is a goal as important in the knee as it is in the hip. The preservation of bone stock, the elimination of a "third component," and better resistance to bacterial attack are all arguments in favor of a hydroxyapatite (HA) interface. However, looking

Orthopaedic Surgery, Clinique Medico-Chirurgicale, 62700 Bruay-la-Buissière, France

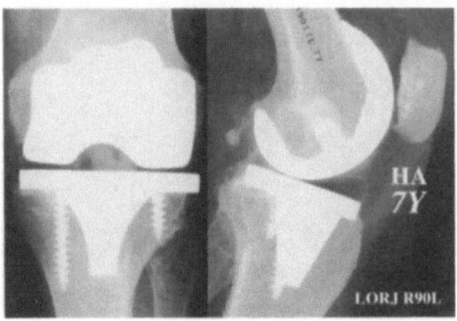

FIG. 1. HA Omnifit 3000 knee; A 7-year case

at the considerable number of large-scale studies of HA-coated hips in the literature and the paucity of similar studies in the knee, it would appear that the knees are lagging a shaft's length behind.

One should say that HA-coated knee prostheses remain a bit confidential. Despite excellent histological findings proving the real efficiency of "biological" bone bonding, and despite excellent HA-hip results during 10 years of follow-up (FU), the HA line wavers insofar as knees are concerned. Nevertheless, for years some papers have reported promising results with HA-coated knees. Verhaar [1] and Epinette [2] published good clinical reports in 1995. More recently, Nilsson et al. [3] published, in the *Journal of Arthroplasty*, a prospective randomized comparison of HA-coated and cemented tibial components with 5 years of FU using RSA and concluded that greater long-lasting stability was possible in the HA group.

We began using HA knees in 1990 with the Omnifit Knee (Osteonics, Allendale, NJ, USA). Since that first implantation, we have operated on 345 HA knees in the Clinique Medico-chirurgicale of Bruay-Labuissiere, France (Fig. 1). We report here on these 9-year HA-coated knees from our personal experience with a prospective study led by the CRDA (Center of Orthopaedic Research in Arthroplasty) and using the OrthoWave outcome study software.

Material and Methods

The Series

From 1990 to the present, 345 knees have been operated on in 66 men and 279 women (81%) by the author in the same clinic and using the same operative procedure. Of this number, 309 knees remain "on file" (90%), 20 (5.8%) patients died of unrelated causes, 5 (1.5%) were retrieved for septic problems, 5 (1.5%) were assessed as "out of study" because of major disabling non-knee-related problems, 4 knees (i.e., 1.2%) underwent a revision for mechanical failure, and no patient was lost to follow-up. The mean follow-up delay is 2.33 years (SD, 1.931), and 49 knees (16.3%) are past 5 years of FU. The average age is 70.52 (range, 54–86) years; 167 patients were more than 70 and 36 over 80 years. Conversely, only 23 knees (7%) were of patients under 60 years of age. As far as weight is concerned, only 8% were considered as "regular," whereas obesity was "mild" in 41%, "medium" in 44%, and "severe" in the remaining 7%.

The mean value for body mass index was 30.97 (range, 20.2–41.7). The Charnley classification indicated only 17% of cases belonging to the "A" group (i.e., no other disabling problem except the operated knee), while 40% were "B" (other knee affected) and 43% were "C" (significant non-knee-related disabling problem). The type of surgery was primary in 324 cases (93.9%) and revision in 21 cases. Osteoarthritis remains, as usual, the main etiology (85%); rheumatoid arthritis was only 6.2%, necrosis was 1.7%, 1 case was posttraumatic, and 1 was neurometabolic disease.

Type of Implants

The type of implant was, in all cases, a HA-coated knee for both femoral and tibial components; in 12 cases, however, either the HA tibial tray was matched to a cemented femur (9 cases) or a cemented tray to a HA femoral component (3 cases). The first implanted femoral component was the partial HA-coated 3000 Omnifit knee in 58 cases (17%), then the one with HA on beads in 26 cases (8%), followed by the HA fully coated HA 3000 Omnifit in 135 cases (39%), and finally the HA 7000 Omnifit in 77 cases (22%). In all these knee replacements, the posterocruciate ligament was retained. According to the work of Tom Schmalzried and Mark Kester, we recently moved to using PS (posterocruciate-substituting) knees with the use of the HA Scorpio Knee in 39 cases to date (11%). The cemented components (3%) were either a CR (posterocruciate-retaining) Omnifit in a single case (severe rheumatoid arthritis), or 9 posterostabilized ones with stems (revision cases). In more than 50% (187 of 345 cases), the femur size was the #7 size.

Considering the tibial component, 12 trays were coated with HA on beads (3%), 102 tibial components were the regular HA 3000 cruciate keel (30%), and 228 were the new HA fully coated delta keel (66%), which is currently matched with the Scorpio femoral component. Only 3 tibiae were cemented (less than 1%), due to a revision procedure. The more commonly used height for the PE (polyethylene) tibial insert was 8 mm. Four screws are routinely used to enhance the mechanical fixation of the tray.

The patellar replacement using a cemented PE nonmetal-backed button was performed in 127 cases (37%), mainly in the early procedures. No patellar-related procedure was done in 38 cases (11%). At the current time, we prefer routinely to make a patelloplasty by doing a double facetectomy of the patella in "upside-down ridge roof" shape to obtain better congruency across the patellar groove. In all cases, a release of the lateral parapatellar tendon is performed as a routine procedure.

Partial weight-bearing (WB) is immediately allowed. Early mobilization and physiotherapy and the use of CPM are performed. Total WB is generally obtained at 2–3 months.

Methods

All patients are included in this nonselective series. Preoperative status, surgical details, and postoperative management are systematically recorded. Postoperative clinical and radiological evaluations are performed at the 6th week, then at 4–6 months, and then yearly. The secretary systematically addresses all patients who do not attend the 5-year visit. Data are input in the global OrthoWave database, allowing us to access clinical status, radiological evaluation, X-rays, image cataloger, statistics, cumulative survival curves, and finally crossed comparisons using the related statistical tests.

All cases are taken into account for complication rates. At the given delay, all cases for which we previously ensure there is neither retrieval nor clinical or radiological non-reoperated-on failure are included in the survivorship analysis. Some cases with non-knee-related very disabling problems, which make us unable to really assess their functional abilities, are considered as "out of study." Of the remaining cases, only reviewed patients affording complete clinical and radiological evaluation are included in the clinical result study. Assessment is performed by using the IKS global score, including on one hand the 100 points knee score and on the other hand the 100 points function scores. On the whole, assessment could be achieved for 283 knees according to "knee score" and 230 according to "function score." Results are distributed in three groups: global series, 2-year group, and 5-year group.

Results

Complications

As regards complications, we recorded no perioperative adverse effect in the whole series. Conversely, we recorded numerous postoperative complications (Table 1). Some of these complications led to reoperation. The 16 reoperations (4.6%) are listed in Table 2. Finally, of 345 knees, we recorded less than 5% of reoperation, of which 3 cases were typical mechanical failures (0.9 % of cases) including 1 primary knee and 2 revision cases. We had no explanation for the severe pain in the primary knee. Considering the 2 revision cases, we may confirm the use of a nonstemmed tibial component was not convenient in case of severe bone loss. The patellar pain following a single patelloplasty, and thus leading to secondary fit of a button, occurred in 2% of cases. These 7 cases all belong to the group of knees in which we simply left the patella in situ without any facetectomy. As we routinely perform the double facetectomy of the patella in "upside-down ridge roof" shape, no patient experienced any patellar pain.

TABLE 1. Complications

Problem	Number	Percent
DVT: Phlebitis	37	10.7
Pulmonary embolism	4	1.2
Manipulation under anesthesia	17	4.9
Hematomae	6	1.7
Wound delayed healing	20	5.8
Infection: subcutaneous	2	0.6
Deep infection	6	1.8
Traumatic fracture	8	2.4
Patellar fracture	6	1.8
Secondary patellar button	8	2.3

TABLE 2. Reasons for reoperation

Reoperations	n	Cases	Comments
Pain (no loosening)	1 (0.3%)	Primary case: retrieval at 2 years; stiffness, inflammatory synovitis (rheumatoid)	
Mechanical failure	2 (0.6%)	Two revision cases: two retrievals (replaced by stemmed cemented implants)	Poor indication of nonstemmed implants on revision cases with severe bone loss
Deep infection	4 (1.2%)	Three primary knees (in two patients) secondarily infected due to a distal severe wound infection. One revision case (MG1 knee with patellar implant fracture and severe allergy)	The three primary implants were retrieved and replaced by three stemmed cemented knees; the revision case finally had to undergo a fusion because of severe pain and functional failure
Patellar traumatic fracture	1 (0.3%)	Only one patella had to be reoperated on of a total of six traumatic patellar fractures	The reoperated patella had primarily a cemented button
Synoviectomy	1 (0.3%)	Primary case: severe stiffness due to a very curious phenomenon of "frozen knee" caused by a postop retraction of the joint capsule with major nonseptic inflammatory synovitis	Good result following the synoviectomy: no pain and good ROM (flexion >90°). We had similar cases in shoulders and hips: perhaps a sympathic dystrophy reaction?
Secondary patellar button	8 (2.3%)	Of these eight cases, one had a previous button; seven had a single patelloplasty	A typical failure of single patelloplasty was recorded in 2% of cases

Clinical Results

We report first on clinical status according to knee-related parameters such as pain or range of motion and to functional abilities such as walking distance or stairs, with 276 knees enrolled in this "knee" result. Conversely, we took into account for the "function" status only the knees belonging to the Charnley class "A," i.e., with no other significant disabling problem, to not bias the clinical evaluation; 55 knees were assessed in class "A." Second, clinical scores based upon the Knee Society Rating system will be displayed according to the preoperative ($n = 321$), 2 years+ of FU ($n = 175$), and 5 years+ of FU ($n = 46$ knees), taking into account both the "knee score" and the "function score." Finally, survivorship analysis is calculated at 5 years of FU, including 324 knees, of which 50 remain at risk at 5 years.

Descriptive Analysis

Pain within the whole series was "none" in 94.2% of cases, "mild" (stairs or walking) in 4.7%, "moderate-occasional" in 1 case (0.4%), and "moderate-continual" in 2 cases (0.7%). No patient experienced "severe" pain postoperatively. This lack of pain remains over the years, as pain was "none" in 94.4% at 2 year+ and in 94.1% at 5 year+. For patellar pain, we report "no pain" in 97.5% of cases, "mild" in 1.8%, and "moderate" in 0.7%. Only 1 patient experienced "severe" patellar pain. When categorizing the patellar results according to the surgical procedure, patellar pain was none in 75% within the "patella left in situ" cohort (1 case of severe pain in that group), whereas results were better in the two remaining groups with "no patellar pain" in 82.4% (patelloplasty) and 90.6% (PE cemented button).

Stability was recorded as complete in 97% for mediolateral and in 98% for anteroposterior. It is interesting that less than 2% of AP instability was seen in these PCL-retaining knees. Observed median value for flexion was 120° (range, 35° to 160°; SD, 20.7°). Only 4% of cases were less than 80°; 7% were recorded as between 80° and 89°, 38% between 90° and 119°, and finally 51% over 120°. No flexion contracture was recorded in 96%, and only three knees experienced a flexion contracture greater than 16°. Observed median value for mechanical axis was ideal at 0° (i.e., femoral-tibial omega angle at 7° valgus) with a SD of 2.18, ranging from valgus 10° to 8° varus, while 88.5% of mechanical axis ranged between 3° valgus and 2° varus.

Considering *functional abilities* in the "Charnley A" group, (1) walking distance was "unlimited" in 76%, and limited for more than 10 blocks in 18% and less than 10 blocks in 4%. (2) Stairs were climbed up and down normally in 50%, "normal up, rail down" in 34%, "up-and-down rail" in 14%, and "up rail, unable down" in the remaining 2%. (3) Support was none in 90%; one cane was needed by 10%. (4) Limp was none in 86%, moderate in 14%. (5) Unipodal standing was normal in 88%, with "slight difficulty" in 10% and "extreme difficulty" in 2%. Finally, "activity" was recorded as "strenuous" in 6%, "ADL" in 88%, and "independent" in 6%. Nevertheless, when breaking down the results by age this "activity" is significantly different (mean age at 60.7 years for "strenuous," 70.2 years for "ADL," and 76.5 years for "independent"); i.e., $P = 0.05$ according to ANOVA and Kruskall–Wallis tests. Similarly, the level of activity was better in men as compared to women (chi square and Pearson tests: $P = 0.01$). No statistical test was available as far as etiology is concerned because of an insufficient number of rheumatoid cases.

IKS Results

The mean values of "knee score" were noted preoperatively as 23.4 of a possible 100 points (0–59 points), up to 94.8 at 2 years (20–100), and 95.3 at 5 years (61–100). Grouping results by categories ("excellent," 95; "good," 80–94; "fair," 60–79; and "poor" <60 points), IKS knee results were preoperatively 100% poor, while recorded on the one hand at 2 years as "excellent" in 69%, "good" in 27%, "fair" in 3%, and "poor" in 1%, and on the other hand at 5 years as "excellent" in 65%, "good" in 33%, "fair" in 2%, and "poor" in 0%.

The mean values of "function score" related to all classes of patients (Charnley A, B, C), were noted preoperatively as 34.8 of a possible 100 points (0–80 points), up to 88.6 at 2 years (0–100) and 85.1 at 5 years (45–100). Grouping results by categories ("excellent," 95; "good," 80–94; "fair," 60–79; "poor" <60 points), IKS function results were 89% poor and 11% fair preoperatively, while recorded on the one hand at 2 years as "excellent" in 51%, "good" in 34%, "fair" in 7%, and "poor" in 8%, and on the other hand at 5 years as "excellent" in 47%, "good" in 26%, "fair" in 14%, and "poor" in 12%.

No significant difference was reported when crossing both knee and function results with sex, obesity, age, and patellar replacement. When crossing etiology and function score, there is no significant difference, while we found a significant difference (ANOVA, $P = 0.05$; Kruskall–Wallis, $P = 0.02$) when comparing knee score and etiology.

Radiological Results

We systematically checked the lines at the HA–bone interface on the components at 5 years+ of follow-up (Fig. 2). Great attention was given to obtain tangential beams in lateral films of femoral components, as well as AP and lateral views of tibial components. Results were recorded in accordance with the IKS radiographic areas.

Results were excellent with no line regarding the HA-coated zones of the Omnifit 3000 femoral components, which were at the beginning only coated on zones 2 and 3 (Fig. 3). Conversely, both reactive and lucent lines were commonly recorded on non-coated zones 1 and 4, whereas these lucencies were never grading down to coated zones thanks to the ultimate bone–metal seal afforded by HA. Nevertheless, the current femoral components, Omnifit 7000, then Scorpio, are fully coated, and never experienced any line on the whole surface.

Regarding the tibial components, the over-5-year prostheses were Omnifit 3000, having a non-HA-coated keel (Fig. 4a,b). Thus, we might expect some changes, especially around these keels. As a matter of fact, we had only 12% of reactive lines at the

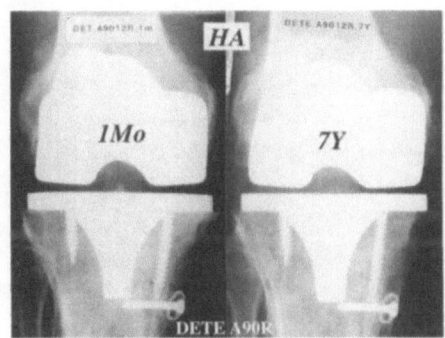

Fig. 2. Comparison of radiological results postoperatively and at 7 years: no change and excellent long-lasting fixation

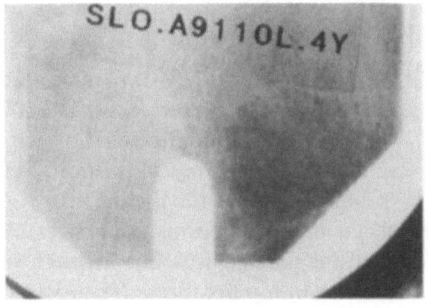

Fig. 3. Close view at 4 years of femoral hydroxy apatite-(HA-) coated interface: intimate bony ongrowth

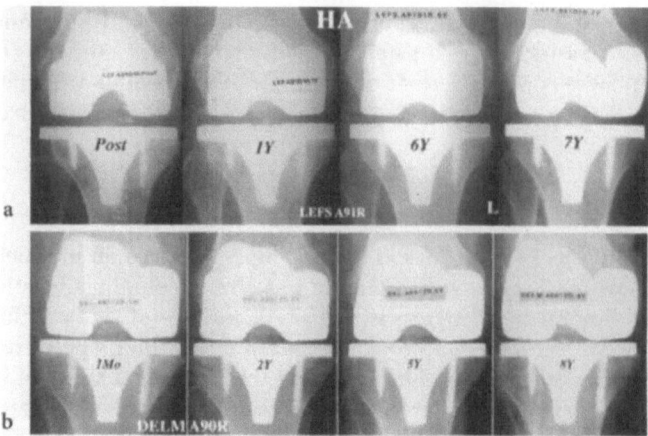

FIG. 4a,b. Two serial X-ray results demonstrating the stability of images over years: no lines, no lysis, no subsidence

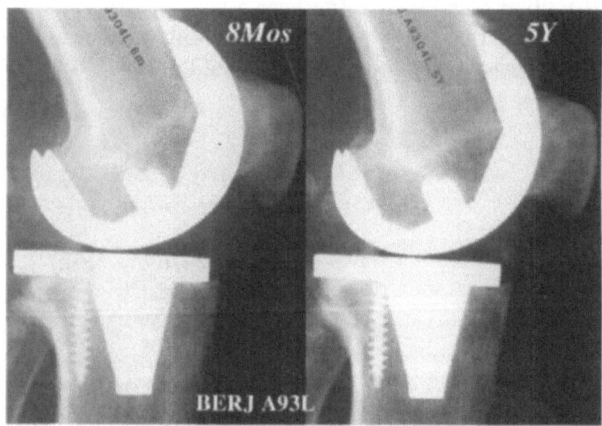

FIG. 5. A case of "scalloping" anteriorly and medially. The lytic zone appeared soon after the operation (8 months) and did not change over the years until after 8 years, perhaps because of the "seal" afforded by HA. No extensive lysis, especially around screws, is observed

tip of the cruciate keel. We are interested in comparing these figures to the fully coated delta keels of the current Omnifit 7000 tibial components, as to date we have never recorded any change around this new design of keel, affording a potential better mechanical and biological fixation. Furthermore, lines or lucencies were recorded in 16% beneath either the medial aspect of the plateau in AP films (i.e., zone C1) or the anterior one in Lat films (i.e., zones L1 and L2), that we often defined as a "scalloping" of the plateau, in a like manner to that we call limited lysis at the upper part of the femur in hip prostheses (Fig. 5).

The origin of these lines may be related to some lytic action of the joint fluid under pressure, as well documented by Schmalzried and Whiteside [4,5,6]. However, neither extensive lysis nor mechanical loosening was demonstrated in the whole series. In addition, comparison between immediate postop and 5-9 years later confirmed no change, especially beneath the tibial plateau, around screws, or around the keel.

Finally, the most important finding as regards the HA biological interface was demonstrated by the ability for bone to fill in the previous lucent line resulting from the fibrous tissue layer. In some cases we had, between the first year and up to the third year, a lucent line beneath the tibial plateau. In all these cases, the radiological evaluation over years demonstrated an evolutive pattern, i.e., formation of new bony bridges between bone and metal and a progressive new bony structure filling in the gap (Fig. 6a–c). The explanation can be found in Soballe's works, demonstrating that the fibrous tissue beneath a HA interface contains collagen fibers regularly assembled

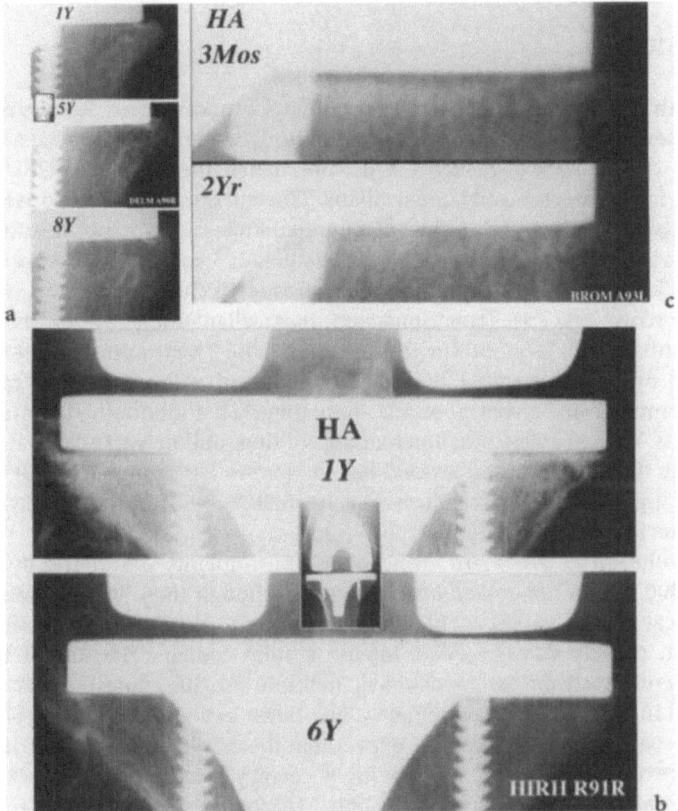

FIG. 6a–c. Three images demonstrating the ability of HA to fill in gaps over years. a Lysis under the tibial plateau, with bony bridges and new bone formation at 5 years, leading to a close contact at 8 years. b Tangential beams at 1 year and 6 years showing a large gap caused by osteolysis, secondarily filled in by new bone until an intimate contact is obtained. c Postoperative and control at 2 years demonstrating the new bone filling in the previous gap at 2 years

in a perpendicular axis to the metallic surface and able to guide a secondary bony ongrowth. Conversely, the random distribution of collagen fiber in the case of a porous coating does not enable the bone to fill in the gap. This finding is striking, and this ability to fill in gaps has to be seen as a tremendous benefit in favor of HA as compared to porous coatings as well as cemented interfaces.

Survivorship Analysis

Cumulative survival rate, according to Kaplan–Meier analysis, was calculated for primary cases ($n = 324$) with 50 knees remaining on file at 5 years. The number of knees is too low in the following years, up to 9 years, to allow a correct analysis. When taking into account all retrievals (failures + traumatic + deep infection cases), the cumulative survival rate at 5 years is 0.9820 ± 0.0146. For all failures (retrievals for mechanical failures + nonreoperated clinical and radiological failures), the cumulative survival rate is 0.9935 ± 0.0106.

Discussion

Results with HA are very encouraging as compared to cemented. Results in this study may represent an interesting counterpoint to both cemented and porous-coated knee series. HA-coated knee experience will soon reach the 10 years of FU milestone; however, a few midterm results are available. The current series is a nonselective one; the main age is 70 years, and of the 345 operated knees at 9 years of maximum FU, no patient was lost to follow-up. The mean IKS values at 5 years were 95.3 and 85.1 points regarding "knee score" and "function score," respectively. In such a way, we recorded 98% (knee score) and 73% (function score) of excellent and good results (80 points). These promising results stood the test of time, as the 2-year examination is similar to the 5-year+ one. Radiographically, we had no mechanical loosening, and radiographic changes demonstrated a very good HA–bone interface for both the femoral and tibial components. We had a very small percentage of lines and no extensive lysis, especially beneath the tibial plateau and around keel or screws. The cumulative survival rate at 5 years, taking into account all failures, reaches 0.9935 ± 0.0106, which is a very encouraging midterm result (Fig. 7a,b).

As to evolution in prosthetic design, the first implants were partially HA-coated Omnifit 3000 with a noncoated cruciate keel. Although these first implants afforded good clinical results, radiographic changes led us to ask for a fully coated femoral component, namely Omnifit 7000, having a fully coated delta keel that seems to provide significantly better mechanical fixation. We may question having a fully coated keel in case of retrieval, but as we had never experienced any need for retrieving a fully coated delta keel, we may expect that the excellent fixation provided by this keel will prevent any retrieval from being necessary. Nevertheless, the very first delta keels were partially coated (having a 8-mm HA-coated zone at the upper part of the keel), and we did not record any difference. Maybe this partial HA-coated zone at the upper aspect of the keel represents an interesting compromise, affording a sound fixation and minimizing problems in case of retrieval.

Conversely, screws never demonstrated any clinical or radiological problem. We recorded no lysis around the screws in the whole series except in an isolated

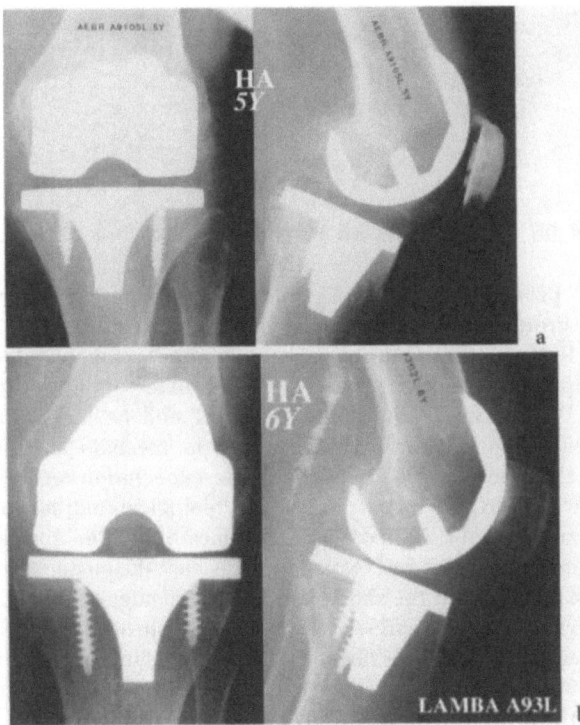

FIG. 7a,b. Two typical X-rays at 5 and 6 years with HA Omnifit 3000 CR knee show excellent results, both clinical and radiological

case, and if subsidence of the tibial tray occurs, causing damage to the polyethylene insert because of the screws, a reoperation must be scheduled whether we have screws or not. In addition, no evidence of PE wear due to the head of screws was ever shown. Thus, we consider that screws are of estimable help to enhance the mechanical fixation of the tibial component, and we remain sincere advocates of screws in knees.

Should patellar resurfacing be used or not? The patellar procedure in TKR is a controversial concern. Most of us seem to agree that metal-backed patellar buttons are to be avoided. Conversely, the question of patelloplasty versus cemented PE remains unanswered (Fig. 8). In our experience, we started resurfacing all patellae, then we moved to doing a double facetectomy of the patella in "upside-down ridge roof" shape to get better congruency across the patellar groove, whereas a lateral parapatellar tendon is performed as a routine procedure. Our current results did not show any significant difference between these two options, while results were significantly lower if we leave the patella in situ without any patelloplasty or resurfacing. Secondary patellar buttons (2.3%) had to be performed mainly in the "patella left in situ" cohort, and the patelloplasty seems to prevent such a potential risk, especially since we moved to the Scorpio knee, which seems to afford a much better designed patellar groove. Within the 39 cases belonging to the Scorpio

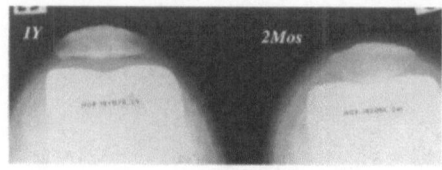

Fig. 8. Patellar resurfacing versus patello-plasty in a same patient: no clinical difference in results

group, we had no patellar pain, no patellar fracture, and zero secondary patellar button.

X-rays show promising results. RSA studies by Nilsson et al. [3] recently demon-strated a very promising outcome in HA knees if a sound primary stability can be achieved after the operation. Our radiographic findings seemed to demonstrate a very good bone–implant interface, as proved by the intimate bony apposition onto the HA-coated zones. We had no radiographic loosening and no lucent lines leading to a pending lack of stability. We may consider that the mechanical fixation afforded by these Omnifit and now Scorpio knees meets our expectation regarding primary sta-bility and allows HA to play its role in a sound biological long-lasting fixation. Some of our knees experienced a limited lytic area beneath the tibial plateau, mainly medi-ally and anteriorly. We had no real explanation because the postoperative films showed a very intimate contact, and the short delay could not suggest any PE wear or debris-related problem. We were impressed by the theory proposed by Schmalzried and Whiteside about the lytic properties of the joint fluid, and our findings seem to suit this explanation. Fortunately, in all these cases the radiological evaluation over years demonstrated the formation of new bony bridges between bone and metal and a pro-gressive new bony structure filling in the gap. This ability to fill in gaps has to be seen as a tremendous benefit in favor of HA as compared to porous coatings as well as cemented interfaces.

As we had good results with retaining knees, why move to PS Scorpio? The final concern has to address our behavior regarding the PCL: do we have to retain or to sacrifice it? For the past 14 years, with the porous Miller–Galante Knee, then with the HA Omnifit design, we were used to retaining the PCL. As a matter of fact, results are quite good and very satisfying as demonstrated in the current study, whereas almost 95% of our knees were PR TKR. Thus, why did we move to the HA Scorpio knee, which is to date a PS knee?

Some studies comparing PR results to PS results have reported for a year's identi-cal results. Retaining the PCL is a very demanding surgical procedure to obtain a rig-orous balance. Additionally, in many cases, the PCL looks a bit loose, and we may expect, especially in heavy persons, some instability. Our first findings seem to demon-strate that in bilateral cases, PR on one side, Scorpio on the other one, patients sub-jectively speak of faster functional recovery and better subjective stability on the Scorpio side. Consequently, and following some actual trends, we were convinced by Tom Schmalzried and remain satisfied with the Scorpio knee (Fig. 9). We have to bear in mind that this new Scorpio design affords very interesting features, including the epicondylar axis allowing a single radius for the femoral curve, and a very well designed patellar groove. A PR version of this knee should be soon available, and perhaps in the future this Scorpio femoral component should be matched with a rotat-ing platform.

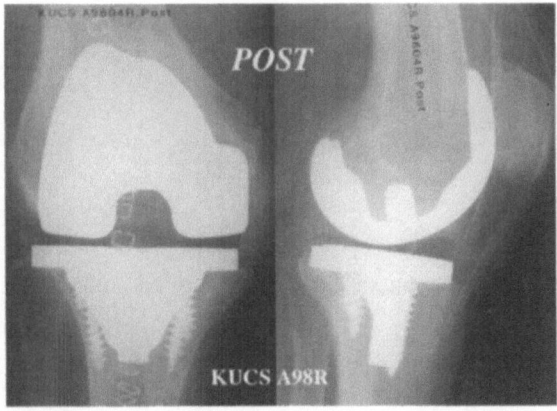

FIG. 9. The Scorpio PS knee: postoperative control

Conclusion

We like to say that HA is not a magic powder. Surely, more in knees than in hips, HA models have to prove their assets versus cemented or porous design. Technical skills and appropriate design are certainly more important than the interface. Nevertheless, the current study may demonstrate that we obtain, with hydroxyapatite in these Omnifit knees, excellent results, as good and sometimes better than the best-cemented or porous studies at 5–9 years of follow-up. Radiographic findings are encouraging and confirm the excellent intimate contact between bone and metal with no difference between the 2-year and 5-year examination. Furthermore, the HA coating over years enables bone to fill in gaps, which should be seen as a critical benefit in favor of bioactive coatings.

Thus the current study serves as a reference for the coming new models. We have to follow up these patients to obtain long-term results with this "basic PR HA knee," and each new development or improvement, regarding design or bioactive coating, will have to prove a real benefit as compared to the actual findings.

Naturally, the current study has to be continued on with further examination over 10–15 years to confirm the actual excellent cumulative survival rates. An appropriate use of survivorship analysis, taking into account all the clinical and radiological failures, whether they underwent a revision, having a significant number of patients remaining at risk at 10 or 15 years, and a minimum of patients lost to follow-up, is an absolute need if we want to compare different series in a way as objective as possible.

So far, so good, and the use of HA knees has become a routine procedure in our daily practice. The very encouraging results reported about the current study make us very confident about the ultimate outcome of bioactive coatings in knee arthroplasty (Fig. 10).

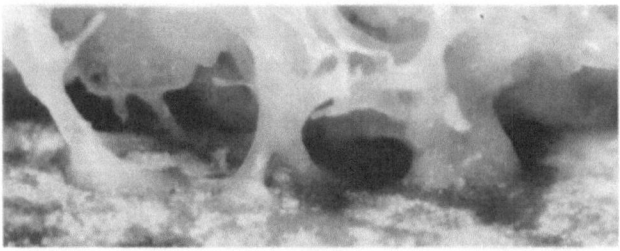

FIG. 10. Intimate bone–metal contact without any fibrous tissue from an histological view in a HA-coated tibial tray

References

1. Verhaar J (1995) HA coating in knee arthroplasty. principles, importance and results. In: Cahiers d'enseignement de la SOFCOT: Hydroxyapatite coated hip and knee arthroplasty, vol 51 (English volume), Expansion Scientifique Française, Paris, pp 319–322
2. Epinette J-A (1995) Hydroxyapatite and TKR: the HA Omnifit knee prosthesis. In: Cahiers d'enseignement de la SOFCOT: Hydroxyapatite coated hip and knee arthroplasty, vol 51 (English volume). Expansion Scientifique Française, Paris, pp 323–332
3. Nilsson KG, Kärrholm J, Carlson L, Dalen T (1999) Hydroxyapatite coating versus cemented fixation of the tibial component in total knee arthroplasty. J Arthroplasty 14:9–20
4. Schmalzried TP, Jasty M, Harris WH (1992) Periprosthetic bone loss in total hip arthroplasty. Polyethylene wear debris and the concept of the effective joint space. J Bone Joint Surg Am 74:849–863
5. Schmalzried TP, Akizuki KH, Fedenko AN, Mirra J (1997) The role of access of joint fluid to bone in periarticular osteolysis. A report of four cases. J Bone Joint Surg Am 79:447–452
6. Whiteside LA (1995) Effect of porous-coating configuration on tibial osteolysis after total knee arthroplasty. Clin Orthop 321:92–97

Part 8 PCL Resection Versus PCL Retention in Total Knee Arthroplasty

Cruciate-Retaining Versus Posterior-Stabilized Total Knee Arthroplasty: The Argument for Posterior Cruciate Substitution

ALFRED J. TRIA, JR.

Summary. Posterior cruciate-retaining and posterior-stabilized total knee designs have been competing with each other since the early 1980s. Preservation of the posterior cruciate ligament is said to produce a knee with a more natural feeling for the patient and with better function on stair climbing. The posterior-stabilized knee is said to be an easier knee surgery to perform, and the results are said to be the same or better than the cruciate-retaining designs with better range of motion. The arguments for each design are both convincing. In the United States, the number of posterior-stabilized knee surgeries continues to increase versus the posterior-retaining designs. The majority of the total knee arthroplasties are performed by surgeons who implant 15–20 per year. The publications concerning the two designs are written by surgeons who perform hundreds of implants each year. The surgeon performing the operation must call upon his own experience and not that of the authors who write the articles. The surgeon must feel comfortable with the implant design and the technique. If the results are quite similar, the posterior-stabilized knee surgery is easier to perform and duplicate from case to case. The posterior-stabilized knee continues to gain in popularity and probably will continue to do so over the next few years.

Key words. Knee, Total knee replacement, Knee ligaments, cruciate ligaments, Posterior cruciate ligament

Introduction

The argument for and against preservation of the posterior cruciate ligament (PCL) in total knee arthroplasty dates back to the early 1980s when the Porous Coated Anatomic knee and the Insall–Burstein Posterior Stabilized knees were developed. Andriacchi's paper in 1982 discussed the knee designs from biomechanical aspects and favored PCL retention [1]. The first paper compared a cruciate-retaining design to the total condylar knee (which sacrificed both the anterior and posterior cruciate

The Orthopaedic Center of New Jersey, 1527 State Highway 27, Suite 1300, Somerset, NJ 08873, USA

ligaments). The paper concluded that the PCL-retaining knee had better range of motion on stair climbing and felt more like a normal knee. Many authors criticized this paper because it did not compare the cruciate-retaining design to a design that included a substitution for the PCL. The follow-up paper, published in 1988, compared the cruciate-retaining design to the Insall–Burstein I design, which did substitute for the PCL [2]. The conclusions once again favored the PCL-retaining design.

In 1995, Tullos published a cadaveric study that compared the PCL-retaining design to the PCL-substituting knee [3]. In the laboratory, he showed that the PCL-substituting design had better biomechanics and better function.

Dennis contributed a new technique to evaluate the total knee with computerized interpretations of lateral fluoroscopies [4,5]. The results, thus far, have been very encouraging; and he is able to see rollback of the components and liftoff. The data for the cruciate-retaining knees show that many of the knees have limited flexion and that rollback is not predictable in every knee, with some actually rolling forward through the range of motion. The posterior-stabilized knees do show rollback with flexion in most cases.

Surgical Technique

The clinical problems with cruciate-retaining knees include loss of range of motion and late subluxation. Both these problems are related to the difficulty of tensioning the PCL in the operating room. If the PCL is left too loose, the knee will have paradoxical anterior motion with flexion. This abnormal motion will lead to sliding upon the polyethylene insert, excess wear, and failure of the prosthesis. The natural tendency in the operating room is to tension the PCL as much as possible. The surgeon looks for stability, and oftentimes fails to appreciate the associated tightness in flexion. The excessive PCL tension leads to loss of range of motion, possible loosening of the components, and pain. Lotke has published data that the ligament must be tensioned within 1 mm to produce proper kinematics [6]. In ten consecutive cases, his group was unable to tension the ligament perfectly. If the tibial cut is made deeper than 10 mm, the bone island that is left on the posterior tibial plateau may fracture during the operation or fatigue some time after the procedure is completed, leading to instability of the total knee arthroplasty.

There are several clinical tests that can be performed during the operation to properly tension the PCL. The knee can be flexed with the trial components in place. If the tibial tray lifts off anteriorly before the knee reaches 90°, the PCL is too tight. The PCL is also too tight if there is excess posterior rollback, if the knee has limited flexion, or if the femoral component pulls off the femur before full flexion is obtained. The PCL can also be palpated to evaluate the tension, but this technique tends to be too subjective.

The posterior-stabilized designs also require attention to the surgical technique. If the knee is left too loose in flexion, the post of the tibial component can sublux beneath the cam of the femoral component and dislocate behind the cam. This problem can be avoided by making sure the knee is tight in flexion. Although excess tightness is not recommended, it is less dangerous to make the posterior stabilized knee tight in flexion. The design can be left slightly looser in extension, and this will permit full extension. The posterior-stabilized knee is also criticized because it can lead to elevation of the joint line and patella baja. If the space in extension is stuffed tightly, that is, with an abnormally thick component, it is possible to elevate the joint line. However, this is usually associated with increased tightness in extension and with a subsequent flexion contracture. The flexion contracture should be visible on the operating room table and should be corrected. This is another reason to leave the posterior-stabilized knee slightly loose in extension.

The surgeon should be familiar with the particular posterior-stabilized knee he is implanting because some designs allow the cam of the femur to move superiorly on the tibial polyethylene post and encourage dislocation in deep flexion. Other designs keep the cam of the femur low in deep flexion and, thus, give greater stability to the implant.

Both the PCL-retaining and the posterior-stabilized designs still require proper ligament balancing, correction of deformity, an equal flexion-extension spacing, and an extensor mechanism that tracks in the midline throughout the full range of motion. Neither prosthetic design will allow for inappropriate surgical technique.

Clinical Results

The results of the two designs are well documented in the literature. Richard Scott is one of the strong proponents of cruciate retention. He reported his favorable 12-year experience with the cruciate-retaining designs but did not formalize the results in his paper [7]. Rand reported his results with the Kinematic Condylar Knee, a posterior cruciate-sparing design; 119 of 168 knees were available with an average of 10 years of follow-up [8]. Six knees were revised (four for a loose patella); the mean knee score was 81, and the survival rate at 10 years was 96%. Stulberg reported less desirable results with the Microloc cruciate-retaining design [9]. The knee score was 84% in the knees that did not go on to revision. However, he did report cases of polyethylene failure and of catastrophic wear. The tibiofemoral articulation failed in 21.5% of the knees. Ochsner reported a case of late instability in the cruciate-retaining design [10]. He studied the tibial cuts in the cadaveric knee and concluded that rupture was associated with a tibial cut that was greater than 7–10 mm in depth.

Insall has been the strongest supporter of the posterior-stabilized design. His group has reported the longest term follow-up with results that have set a standard for total knee replacement. Colizza and Insall reported a mean score of 92% with a minimum of 10 years of follow-up in 101 of 165 posterior-stabilized knees [11]; there were only 4 revisions. Stern and Insall reported 9- to 12-year follow-up of 194 of 289 knees with excellent or good results in 97% of the patients [12]. They reported a 94% success rate at 13 years. Lombardi [13] and Booth [14] have both published reports of dislocation in the posterior-stabilized knees and related it to the design of the stabilizer post, to laxity in flexion, to increased range of motion, and to excessive lateral release in the valgus knee.

The next step in the analysis includes bilateral surgeries with a posterior-stabilized knee on one side and a cruciate-retaining knee on the other. Shoji reported 28 patients with no difference in the clinical results [15]. Becker and Insall reported on 30 patients, also with no difference in the clinical results [16].

The earlier results of gait analysis and cadaver lab studies are conflicting in their final conclusions. The author is presently completing a study of a comparison of 100 patients with a PCL-retaining knee on one side and a PCL-substituting on the other. The components are identical, from the same company, with the only variable being the PCL ligament. The surgeries were performed in three centers with random assignment of the sides and with identical surgical techniques. The clinical results are just passing 2 years and are identical. The valuable data will be the gait analysis, which is just now undergoing completion.

Summary

The clinical results of the PCL-retaining and the PCL-substituting total knees are similar. Insall's reports are slightly better than most others with longer-term follow-up and an increase in the final range of motion of the knee. Both designs have a reported incidence of instability, which does appear to be avoidable with proper surgical techniques.

The reports in the literature are from major groups that have very significant experience and a large volume of surgery each year. The senior authors of each of the papers are all talented surgeons with surgical experience performing both types of total knee arthroplasty. Two of the papers concerning the bilateral surgery report similar results in the hands of the same surgeon performing a PCL-retaining and a posterior-stabilized knee in the same patient.

In the United States, surgeons who do 15–20 replacements per year do the majority of the knee arthroplasties that are performed in the country. Therefore, most of the total knees are performed by surgeons who do not have the experience of the authors who write the articles. It would be best to gather the results of 50–100 of the typical surgeons and publish those data as a more meaningful reference. Each orthopaedic surgeon must look at their own experience and comfort level with the knee implant. It is not a foregone conclusion that the results of both designs will be similar in the hands of the proven experts and in the hands of the practicing orthopaedic surgeons; this is not meant as a criticism of the abilities of the practicing orthopaedic surgeon, but rather as a comment on the best approach to the surgical procedure for the majority of surgeons.

In any event, the practicing orthopaedic surgeon must choose the implant system that they are going to use for those 15–20 knee arthroplasties they will perform each year. Because the results of both designs are somewhat similar, the surgeon should choose the device that is easiest for him or her to implant. Most authors agree that the posterior-stabilized total knee is an easier procedure. Excision of the PCL makes collateral ligament balancing easier and permits better surgical exposure. As the deformity increases in varus and valgus, it becomes more difficult to save the PCL, adequately correct the deformity, and obtain proper collateral ligament balance.

Conclusions

At the present time, in the year 2000, there are two major designs for total knee replacement: PCL sparing and PCL substituting. As the designs continue to develop, there may come the day when we return to sparing both cruciates and to implanting a design that truly resurfaces the existing knee. With the present technology, the PCL-sparing designs are the most popular knees for implantation according to the actual numbers. However, the PCL-substituting arthroplasties are becoming more popular every year. The numbers continue to increase, and the surgical technique is simpler for the practicing orthopaedic surgeon. The posterior-stabilized total knee represents the best compromise for knee replacement surgery.

References

1. Andriacchi TP, Galante JO, Fermier RW (1982) The influence of total knee replacement design on walking and stair climbing. J Bone Joint Surg 64:1328–1335
2. Andriacchi TP, Galante JO (1988) Retention of the posterior cruciate in total knee arthroplasty. J Arthroplasty 3(suppl):s13–s19
3. Mahoney OM, Noble PC, Rhoads DD, et al (1994) Posterior cruciate function following total knee arthroplasty: a biomechanical study. J Arthroplasty 9(6):569–578
4. Stiehl JB, Komistek RD, Dennis DA, et al (1995) Fluoroscopic analysis of kinematics after posterior cruciate retaining knee arthroplasty. J Bone Joint Surg 77(6):884–889
5. Dennis DA, Komistek RD, Hoff WA, Gabriel SM (1996) In vivo knee kinematics derived using an inverse perspective technique. Clin Orthop Relat Res 331:107–117
6. Hirsch H, Lotke P, Morrison L (1994) The posterior cruciate ligament in total knee surgery. Save, sacrifice, or substitute? Clin Orthop Relat Res 309:64–68
7. Scott RD, Volatile TB (1986) Twelve years' experience with posterior cruciate-retaining total knee arthroplasty. Clin Orthop Relat Res 205:100–107
8. Malkani AL, Rand JA, Bryan RS, Wallrichs SL (1995) Total knee arthroplasty with the kinematic condylar prosthesis. A ten-year follow up study. J Bone Joint Surg 77(3):423–431
9. Feng EL, Stulberg SD, Wixson RL (1994) Progressive subluxation and polyethylene wear in total knee replacement with flat articular surfaces. Clin Orthop Relat Res 299:60–71
10. Ochsner JL Jr, McFarland G, Baffes GC, Cook SD (1993) Posterior cruciate ligament avulsion in total knee arthroplasty. Orthop Rev 22(10):1121–1124
11. Colizza WA, Insall JN, Scuderi GR (1995) The posterior stabilized total knee prosthesis. Assessment of polyethylene damage and osteolysis after a ten-year minimum follow up. J Bone Joint Surg 77(11):1713–1720
12. Stern SH, Insall JN (1992) Posterior stabilized prosthesis. Results after follow-up of nine to twelve years. J Bone Joint Surg 74:980–986
13. Lombardi AV, Mallory TH, Vaugh BK, et al (1993) Dislocation following primary posterior-stabilized total knee arthroplasty. J Arthroplasty 8(6):633–639
14. Galinat BJ, Vernace JV, Booth RE Jr, Rothman RH (1988) Dislocation of the posterior stabilized total knee arthroplasty. A report of 2 cases. J Arthroplasty 3(4):363–367
15. Shoji H, Wolf A, Packard S, Yoshino S (1994) Cruciate retained and excised total knee arthroplasty. A comparative study in patients with bilateral total knee arthroplasty. Clin Orthop Relat Res 305:218–222
16. Becker MW, Insall JN, Faris PM (1991) Bilateral total knee arthroplasty. One cruciate retaining and one cruciate substituting. Clin Orthop Relat Res 271:122–124

Choice of PCL Substituting in HA Knee Arthroplasty

Jean-Alain Epinette[1], Mark A. Kester[2], and Avram A. Edidin[3]

Summary. "The issue of retention versus sacrifice of the Posterior Cruciate Ligament [PCL] remains an enigma for the Orthopaedic Surgeon." While reviewing the literature, it is difficult to anticipate some sound benefit afforded by one of these two options. Biomechanical studies have demonstrated that the theoretical benefit of retention of the PCL unfortunately does not remain consistent in vivo, and thus it is more a theoretical than a practical advantage to retain the PCL. Clinically speaking, posterior substituting (PS) and cruciate retaining (CR) results look similar. However, each surgeon must bear in mind the outcome of this ligament in the long run, and any potential late rupture of the PCL owing to some traumatic disease or extension over years of inflammatory lesions. Furthermore, after more than 15 years of successful PCL-retaining experience, it seemed to us that substituting knees are easier to fit. As far as hydroxyapatite-coated (HA) implants are concerned, we have refrained for years from using PS knees to avoid any potential increase of shear forces at the bone–implant interface. The novel design afforded by the HA Scorpio model decreases shear forces and increases contact area and thus led us to move to the HA Scorpio PS knee.

Key words. PCL substituting, PS total knee replacement, Epicondylar axis, Hydroxyapatite-coated Scorpio prosthesis

Introduction

"The issue of retention versus sacrifice of the PCL [posterior cruciate ligament] remains an enigma for the Orthopaedic Surgeon," noted Clifford W. Colwell [1]. While reviewing the literature, it is difficult to anticipate some sound benefit afforded by one of these two options. Peirera et al. [2] carried out a comparative study between PCL-sparing and PCL-sacrificing arthroplasty and of the functional results using the same prosthesis and concluded that "The data revealed no difference in clinical or early radiographic outcome between PS [posterior-substituting] and CR [cruciate-

[1] Orthopaedic Department, Clinique Medico-Chirurgicale, 62700 Bruay Labuissière, France
[2] Ridge Road, Saddle River, NJ 07458, USA
[3] 217 Cupsaw Drive, Ringwood, NJ 07456, USA

retaining] knees." Similarly, Huang et al. [3] compared muscle strength of PCL-retained versus cruciate-sacrificed total knee arthroplasty (TKA) and concluded: "The results showed that in all testing conditions, the hamstring to quadriceps ratios did not significantly differ among the tested prostheses even after long-term functional adaptation." Another study was carried out by Vinciguerra et al. [4] concerning total knee replacement (TKR) with or without preservation of the PCL: "The functional outcome seems to be the same whether a PS or CR knee was used." Finally, as a conclusion of a comparative study in patients with bilateral TKA, Shoji et al. [5] found no significant difference between the retained or excised PCL in terms of HSS score.

Biomechanical Concerns in the PCL Procedure

We have first to define well what is usually called "PS" knees. As a matter of fact, because current femoral designs provide a cam mechanism, PS knees are no longer "sacrificing" and have become "substituting" because the cam is supposed to play the role, more or less, of a regular posterior cruciate ligament.

Advocates for the cruciate-retaining procedure often speak about the need for making replacement joints kinematically equivalent to their natural counterparts. However, most contemporary total knees make no provision to preserve the anterior cruciate ligament. Thus, CR knees become ACL-deficient knees! ACL excision and the need for a posterior slop led to some biased biomechanics in the knee because of the posterior displacement of the femur (Fig. 1). Two solutions are proposed to avoid wear and laxity due to the lack of rollback: (1) get the right tension in the PCL (but it is difficult to balance), or (2) increase the AP conformity (but this increases shear forces). Consequences of ACL excision were well defined further by fluoroscopic evaluation and retrieval analysis [6]. Fluoroscopic evaluation has confirmed posterior femoral

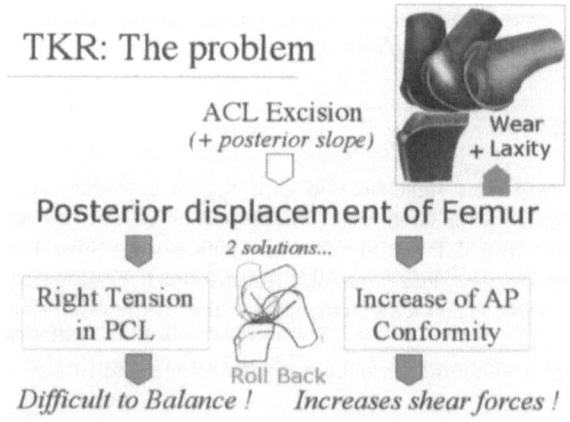

FIG. 1. Total knee replacement (TKR): a critical biomechanical problem furthered by anterior cruciate ligament (ACL) excision

ACL excision: findings

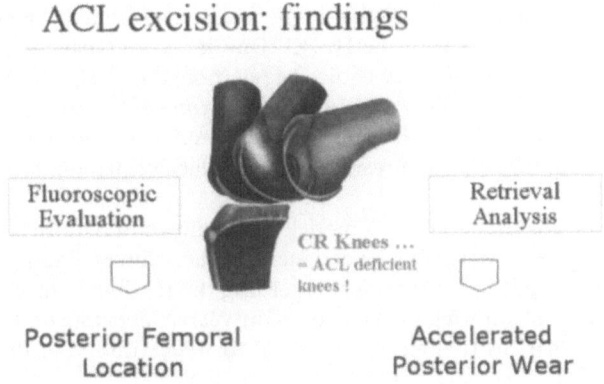

Fluoroscopic
Evaluation

Retrieval
Analysis

CR Knees ...
= ACL deficient
knees !

Posterior Femoral
Location

Accelerated
Posterior Wear

FIG. 2. ACL excision: experimental findings

location, and retrieval analysis confirmed accelerated posterior wear (Fig. 2). According to these authors, fluoroscopic findings demonstrated that in the case of cruciate retention, motion is more erratic and paradoxical, and there is a larger midrange sagittal translation and a larger axial rotation. Conversely, in case of cruciate substitution, they could demonstrate controlled rollback-deep flexion and a smaller midrange sagittal translation and finally less axial rotation.

Thus, it is a difficult challenge to obtain the right tension in the PCL and control the compressive forces on the joint surface, as demonstrated by Peter Walker [7]. The challenge addresses the femoral component geometry, as well as the placement of the contact point and the location of the bottom of the dish, and finally the tilt of the tibial component. Finally, and considering the biomechanical studies, the role of PCL was analyzed by Colwell [1] as follows:

— There is a more theoretical than a practical advantage to retaining the PCL.
— Based on contact center data, there are advantages to maintaining the isometry of the PCL in nonloaded knees, but minimal benefit is obtained when the knee is loaded.
— Strain gauge data indicate it is extremely difficult to maintain isometry of the PCL in TKA.
— Unless the joint line is maintained, the PCL is a disadvantage anatomically in TKA.
— Finally, gait analysis in monoarticular disease is similar regarding PS or CR knees.

Clinical Concerns Regarding PCL-Substituting Versus PCL-Retaining HA Knees

In addition to these theoretical concerns regarding biomechanics, we wish to explain why we moved to HA PS total knees as a routine procedure after having had an excellent 9-year experience with hydroxyapatite-coated CR knee arthroplasty. We started our HA experience in knees in 1990 and reported in a dedicated chapter of this book our very promising results with the HA CR Omnifit Knee (Osteonics, Allendale, NJ, USA). The reason for this primary choice of retaining the PCL could be explained by this simple statistic: 99% of PCL are present at the time of the surgery! As a matter of fact, surgeons generally dislike excising intact ligaments. In addition, during the past 9 years, we had continuous good results regarding lack of pain and recovery of functional abilities.

At the time of this CR surgery, PS models were known to require large bone resection and, above all, they were supposed to increase shear forces. This potential increase of shear forces was particularly critical regarding the HA–bone interface and caused us to refrain from substituting the PCL for many years. Reporting on 12 years of experience with CR TKA, Scott et al. [8] explained that substitution of the PCL with the addition of prosthetic constraint will increase bone–cement reaction forces and, additionally, these prostheses require significant intercondylar femoral bone stock resection. Interestingly, the HA knee retrievals demonstrated direct bony apposition of bone onto the metallic substrate, and we may remain extremely cautious about these fragile bony bridges in case of any significant increase of shear forces.

Nevertheless some questions arose considering the fate of our prosthetic knees:

1. We were happy with CR results. However, in all published series, results of PS and CR knees are similar.
2. We have to bear in mind the outcome of this ligament in the long run, as well as any potential late rupture of the PCL owing to some traumatic disease or extension over years of inflammatory lesions.
3. The CR procedure is a more demanding and challenging surgery.
4. Finally, we may expect for the long run a better stability in heavy patients when PS knees are used.

The Critical Assets Afforded by the HA PS Scorpio Knee

Due to Scott's arguments against substitution or sacrifice of the PCL [8], for years we had refrained for using PS owing to a potential increase of bone–HA reaction forces on the one hand and the need for a significant intercondylar femoral bone stock resection on the other hand. Interestingly, two major features came up a few years ago with the Scorpio Knee (Osteonics, Allendale, NJ, USA) and led us to change our minds about these potential problems of PS knees in HA-coated replacement: first, the transepicondylar axis and, second, the specific Scorpio cam mechanism.

The basic motion of the femur across the tibia was first studied by Rouleux in 1880. He determined that the instant center of rotation of the femur varied as the knee was flexed. Thus, in space-fixed coordinates, the femur appeared to simultaneously rotate and slide across the tibia; the combination of rolling and sliding could be mapped to body-fixed coordinates using a series of instantaneous centers of rotation. The locus of points describing the path of these instantaneous centers formed a path that looked somewhat like the English letter "J." Thus, knees designed with this kinematic description were sometimes called "J-curve" knees. In practice, the theoretical J-curve description was generally reduced to two or three finite radii describing the distal geometry of the femoral component.

In the mid-1980s, researchers at Tulane University took another look at the function of the knee. In particular, they hypothesized that the complicated sliding and rolling motion of the femur over the tibia leading to the J-curve description might be an artifact of the plane of reference of the description. Often a combination of rolling and sliding can be transformed into pure rotation in another plane or set of planes. They determined that in fact the knee had two primary axes of rotation, one with an axis running nearly exactly through the epicondyles, and a second parallel to the anatomic axis of the knee offset to the medial side of the trochlear groove. A description of the kinematics of the knee through the transepicondylar axis [9] permitted a single axis of rotation to allow for 90° of flexion (Fig. 3a,b). Ultimate posterior slide was still found to be controlled by the PCL or the cam of a replacement arthroplasty. In such a way, the transepicondylar-based design used in the HA PS Scorpio knee leads

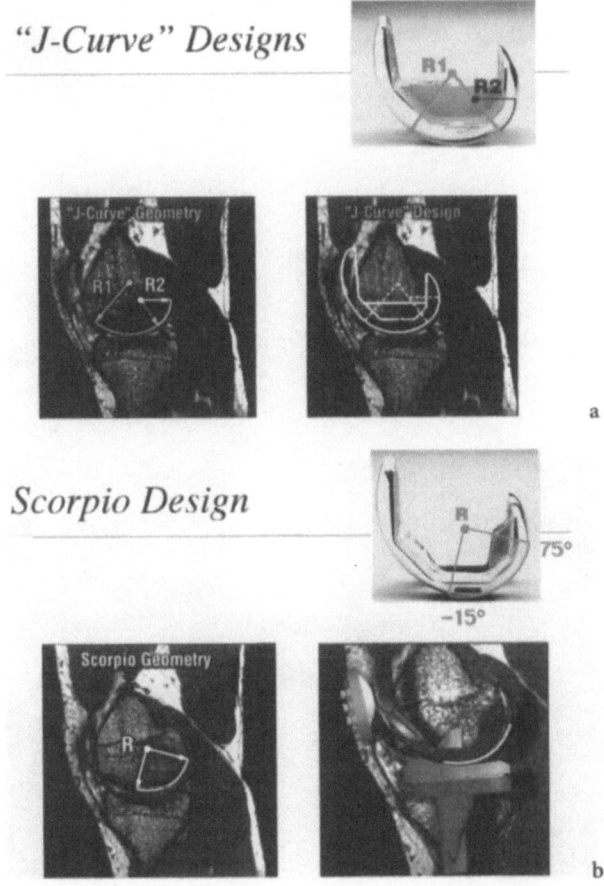

FIG. 3a,b. Knee replacement femoral design: "J-curve" designs (a) versus "epicondylar" designs (b)

to a more conforming sagittal geometry, providing both an increased contact area and a decrease of the shear forces. The increased contact area decreases wear while the decreased shear forces prevents loosening (Fig. 4).

The second argument against PS knees provided by Scott was a "significant inter-condylar femoral bone stock resection." Interestingly, bone-conserving measures were also employed by situating the posterior stabilizing cam mechanism of the Scorpio knee in a narrow open box, which on a radiograph looks very similar to a cruciate-retaining design (Fig. 5). Additionally, this open box prevents the classical problem of "clunk" syndrome.

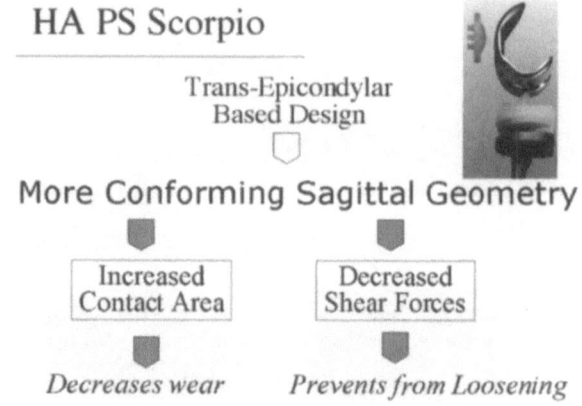

FIG. 4. Critical assets afforded by the Scorpio design, thanks to a more conforming sagittal geometry

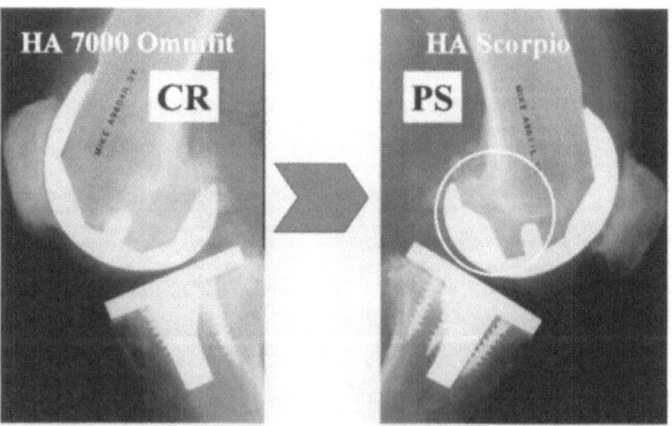

FIG. 5. Minimal bone stock resection with the "open box" of the HA PS Scorpio design as compared to the previous HA CR 7000 Omnifit model

Discussion

Even if "the issue of retention versus sacrifice of the PCL remains an enigma for the Orthopaedic Surgeon," we may currently gain some more precise ideas regarding this personal surgical choice. First, it is a real utopia to think about restoring a "normal knee" following a joint replacement. All current designs sacrifice the anterior cruciate ligament, and subsequently any TKR becomes an anterior cruciate ligament- (ACL-) deficient knee. We no longer are allowed to speak about any "normal knee" after the surgery, and the theoretical benefit of retaining the PCL is no more consistent at the time the ACL is sacrificed. Additionally, we have to speak about PCL substitution, which is different from PCL sacrificing in sofar as restoration of efficient kinematics is concerned. Some biomechanical studies have clearly demonstrated that the theoretical benefit of the retention of the PCL unfortunately does not remain consistent in vivo, and thus it is more a theoretical than a practical advantage to retain the PCL.

Clinically speaking, it seems evident that in the long run PS and CR results look similar. In our personal experience, we have obtained excellent midterm results with an HA CR knee. However, each surgeon must bear in mind some assets for the future afforded by PS versus CR procedures, which may contend with some adverse effects in the long run. In this matter, we must bear in mind the outcome of this ligament in the long run and any potential late rupture of the PCL owing to some traumatic disease or extension over years of inflammatory lesions. Additionally, a better stability in heavy patients is expected when PS knees are used. Results of joint replacement mainly depend on the surgical expertise. An easier procedure certainly will lead to better results. In our hands, after more than 15 years of successful retaining experience, we have to confirm that substituting knees are easier to fit. The surgical protocol seems to be faster and safer, and this concern may be of major interest for senior surgeons as well as for residents.

So far as HA-coated implants are concerned, we have refrained for years from using PS knees to avoid any potential increase of shear forces at the bone–implant interface, and additionally to prevent a "significant" bone stock resection due to the intercondylar box used for previous models. The novel design afforded by the HA Scorpio model decreases shear forces and increases contact area thanks to the epicondylar axis, and additionally allows bone-conserving measures by situating the cam mechanism in a narrow and open box. These critical assets caused us to change our mind and move to HA PS knees.

Our HA PS Scorpio experience is too recent to allow us to speak about any results because the maximum follow-up to date is 2 years with 71 operated cases. Of this series, 16 were bilateral with an HA CR Omnifit on one side and HA PS Scorpio on the other side. Comparative studies on these specific cases will certainly be of major interest, and these studies are currently carried out.

References

1. Colwell CW Jr (1966) The role of the posterior cruciate ligament in design: clinical aspects. In: Insall JN, Scott N, Scuderi GR (eds) Current concepts in primary revision total knee arthroplasty. Lippincott-Raven, Philadelphia, pp 19–27

2. Pereira DS, Jaffe FF, Ortiguera C (1998) Posterior cruciate ligament-sparing versus posterior cruciate ligament-sacrificing arthroplasty: functional results using the same prosthesis. J Arthroplasty 13:138–144
3. Huang C-H, Lee Y-M, Liau J-J, Cheng C-K (1998) Comparison of muscle strength of posterior cruciate-retained versus cruciate-sacrificed total knee arthroplasty. J Arthroplasty 13:779–783
4. Vinciguerra B, Pascarel X, Honton JL (1994) Comparative results of total knee replacement with or without preservation of the posterior cruciate ligament. Rev Chir Orthop 80:620–625
5. Shoji H, Wolf A, Packard S (1994) Cruciate retained and excised total knee arthroplasty: a comparative study in patients with bilateral total knee arthroplasty. Clin Orthop 305:218–222
6. Banks SA, Markovich GD, Hodge WA (1997) In vivo kinematics of cruciate-retaining and substituting knee arthroplasties. J Arthroplasty 12:297–304
7. Walker PS (1996) The role of the posterior cruciate ligament in total knee design. In: Insall JN, Scott N, Scuderi GR (eds) Current concepts in primary revision total knee arthroplasty. Lippincott-Raven, Philadelphia, pp 9–18
8. Scott RD, Volatile TB (1986) Twelve year's experience with posterior cruciate-retaining total knee arthroplasty. Clin Orthop 205:100–107
9. Berger RA, Rubash HE, Seel MJ, et al (1993) Determining the rotational alignment of the femoral component in total knee arthroplasty using the epicondylar axis. Clin Orthop 286:40–47

The Bisurface Total Knee Prosthesis: A New Design with Posterior Stabilization

Masao Akagi, Eiichi Kaneda, Toshihiro Mata, Taiyo Asano, and Takashi Nakamura

Summary. Under weight-bearing conditions, femorotibial contact points in a sagittal plane were determined in vivo by computer-assisted video fluoroscopy. With the components mounted in a test machine according to in vivo positional data, a 300-kg force was applied with pressure-sensitive film placed between the components. Contact points were defined as central points of the colored areas; areas of total contact and high pressure were measured using the NIH image. Intrinsic stability of the articular geometry was assessed as a horizontal reaction force arising when the tibial component was translated horizontally on the fixed femoral component under a 10-kg vertical force. In both prostheses, contact points in the sagittal plane moved posteriorly as much as 8mm during knee flexion from 0° to 130°. Contact area of the I/B II was large (>300 mm^2) at 0° but decreased with increasing flexion. Contact area of the Bisurface knee was >200 mm^2 at flexion from 0° to 90° but increased to >250 mm^2 in deep flexion because the cam functions as a bearing surface. The intrinsic stability test demonstrated that the Bisurface prosthesis has sufficient posterior stabilization compared to I/B II. The Bisurface knee has a sufficient rollback to improve range of flexion, wide contact area and low contact stress in flexion position, and sufficient posterior stabilizing ability.

Key words. Total knee arthroplasty, The Bisurface knee, Contact point, Contact area, Intrinsic stability

Introduction

To retain or to substitute the posterior cruciate ligament (PCL) in total knee arthroplasty is still controversial. Recently, in vivo kinematic analyses of the PCL-retaining total knee prosthesis have demonstrated postoperative insufficiency of the PCL [1]. Abnormal kinematics may be related to abnormal wear characteristics of this PCL-retaining design. Accordingly, many manufacturers are developing new PCL-substituting designs. In our institute, a new posterior stabilizing prosthesis called the Bisurface knee has been developed and used clinically since 1989. Follow-up study of

Department of Orthopaedic Surgery, Faculty of Medicine, Kyoto University, 54 Kawahara-cho, Shogoin, Sakyo-ku, Kyoto 606-8507, Japan this prosthesis revealed that arthroplasties with the Bisurface prosthesis resulted in an excellent range of motion, a high level of satisfaction with the operation, and promising durability of the prosthesis [2,3]. The purpose of the present study is to investigate the functional properties of this prosthesis (type 3 plus) with a series of basic experiments compared to the Insall/Burstein 2 (I/B 2) knee.

The Bisurface knee is a PCL-substituting prosthesis and has a unique ball-and-socket joint in the midposterior portion of the femorotibial (FT) joint. The femoral component is made of alumina ceramic. This ball-and-socket joint causes femoral rollback to improve range of flexion and works as a posterior stabilizer, a load-bearing surface, and an axial rotation center on the tibia [2,3]. The I/B 2 knee is also a PCL-substituting knee. Interaction of the tibial post with the femoral transverse cam causes the rollback. The condylar surface of the tibial insert has a posterior slope. Clinical follow-up studies of this prosthesis have demonstrated better range of motion and excellent long-term durability [4,5].

Materials and Methods

In Vivo Contact Point Study

In vivo position of the components in the sagittal plane was determined for ten implanted knees using the lateral view of the fluoroscopic image, five with the Bisurface and five with the I/B 2, at 0°, 30°, 60°, 90° of flextion. Contact of the cam was assumed at 110° and 130° of flexion. Knee motion when climbing up a step was recorded on video. The video was taken into a personal computer, and then the mean relative positions of the components on still images were determined at 30° increments up to 90° of flexion. Posterior translation was measured as a distance from anterior edge of the femoral component to that of the tibial component. Mounting the components on a test machine according to the in vivo positional data, a 300-kg force was applied with pressure-sensitive film placed between the components. Contact points were defined as centers of the colored areas, and the distance from the anterior edge of the articular surface to the contact point was measured at each flexion angle.

Contact Area Study Based on In Vivo Contact Point Data

Images of colored films were taken into a personal computer using an image scanner and analyzed using the image-analyzing software NIH image to measure areas of total contact and high pressure. With the super low scale film, total contact area of the condylar parts and the cam part were measured separately. With the medium-scale film, contact areas 20 to 40 Mpa and more than 40 Mpa were measured separately. Contact areas less than 20 Mpa were calculated by subtracting areas more than 20 Mpa from total contact areas.

Intrinsic Stability Test

Using an experimental system (see following), anteroposterior stabilizing properties of the articular geometry and the cam mechanism were assessed. A horizontal reaction force, which was detected with a load cell attached under the tibial tray, was produced by horizontal translation of the tibial component under a 10-kg vertical force. Relative position of the tibial components was detected with a position sensor. According to these two parameters [horizontal reaction force (kg) and translation of the tibial component (mm)], a curve was depicted on a CRT. The tibial tray was moved slowly (a few minutes per cycle) under monitoring with the CRT as far as the FT joint was subluxated or interaction of the cam mechanism produced steep reaction force.

Dislocation Safety Factor Study

Vertical and horizontal dislocation safety factors of both prostheses were assessed using computer simulation of the knee motion. The vertical dislocation safety factor (DSF) was defined as a distance from the top of the tibial post to the bottom of the femoral cam according to Kocmond et al. [6,7]. The horizontal DSF was defined as a distance from the posterior aspect of the tibial cam to the perpendicular passing through the most inferior point of the femoral cam.

Results

In Vivo Contact Point Study

In the I/B 2, contact points in the sagittal plane translated anteriorly 4 mm at flexion of 60° and translated posteriorly to about 12 mm during deep flexion of the knee. In the Bisurface knee, the posterior translation was 8 mm (Fig. 1).

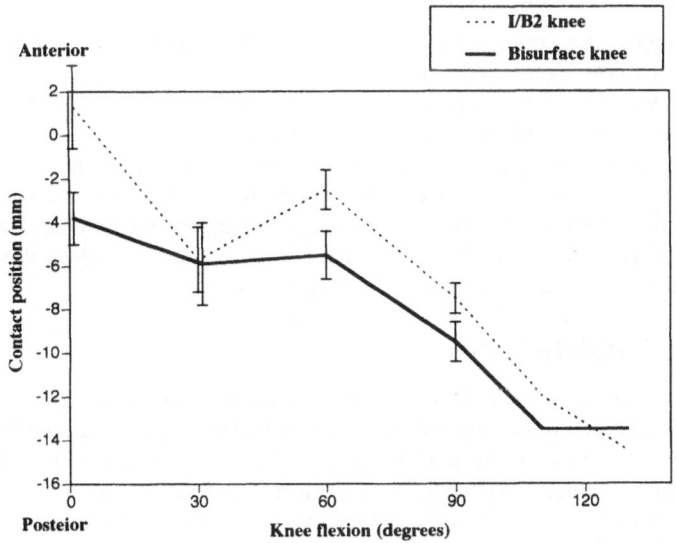

FIG. 1. In vivo contact point study comparing Bisurface and I/B 2 (Insall/Burstein) prostheses

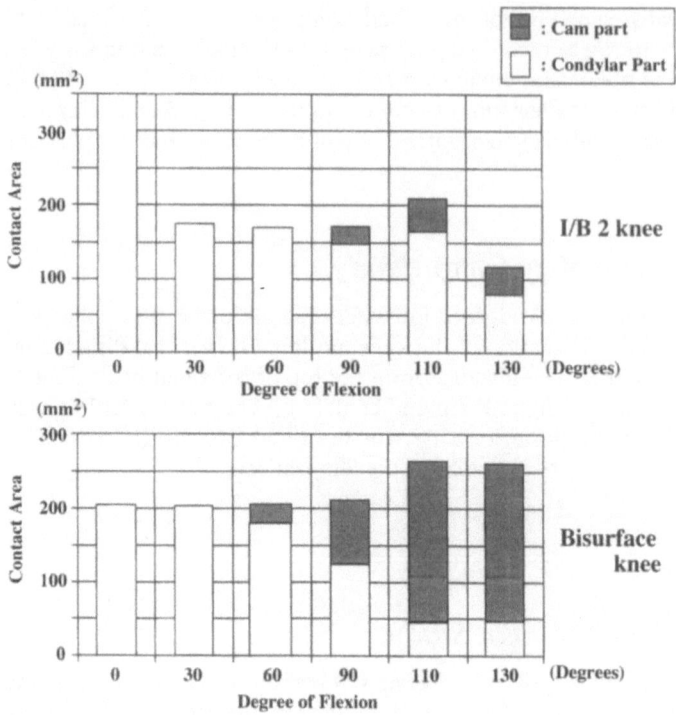

FIG. 2. Measurement of total contact area of cam and condyle

Contact Area Study Based on In Vivo Contact Point Data

Total contact area of the I/B 2 was more than 300 mm² at 0° of flexion but decreased with increasing flexion. Total contact area of the Bisurface knee was about 200 mm² from 0° to 90° of flexion, but increased to more than 250 mm² in deep flexion because the ball-and-socket joint works as a bearing surface (Fig. 2). Figure 3 shows results of the measurements of high contact stress area. Although there was no area over 20 Mpa at 0° of flexion, high contact stress area, more than 40 Mpa, was noticeable in deep flexion in the I/B 2 knee. In the Bisurface knee, the high contact stress area, more than 40 Mpa, was less noticeable than in the I/B 2 knee, especially in deep flexion because the ball-and-socket joint works as a bearing surface.

Intrinsic Stability Test

The intrinsic stability test (Fig. 4) demonstrated that, in the I/B 2 knee, mild posterior stability by the posterior slope of the tibial articular surface was noted at early and midflexion, and the cam mechanism works from 90° of flexion. The ball-and-socket joint of the Bisurface knee works as a posterior stabilizer from 60° of flexion. The Bisurface prosthesis showed sufficient posterior stabilizing ability compared to the I/B 2 under this experimental condition.

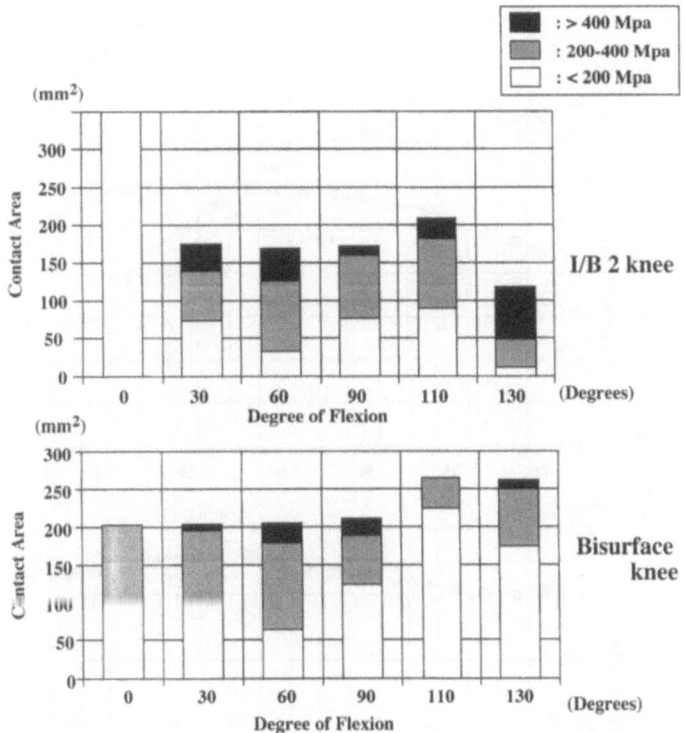

FIG. 3. Measurements of high contact stress areas

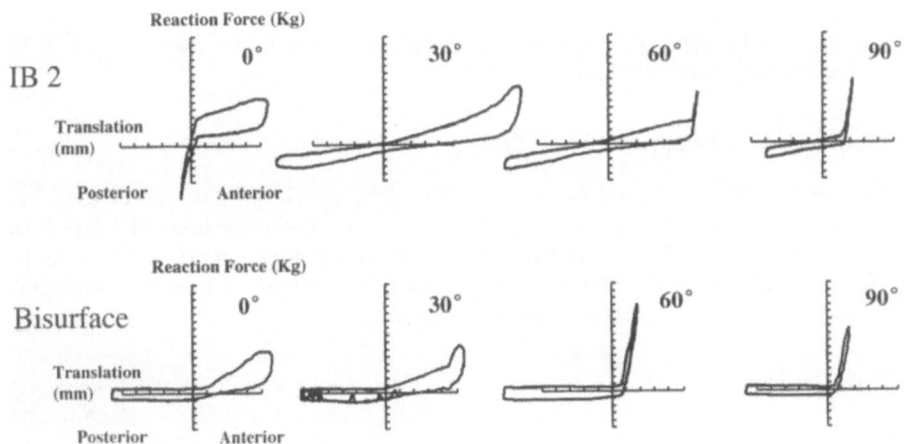

FIG. 4. Intrinsic stability test

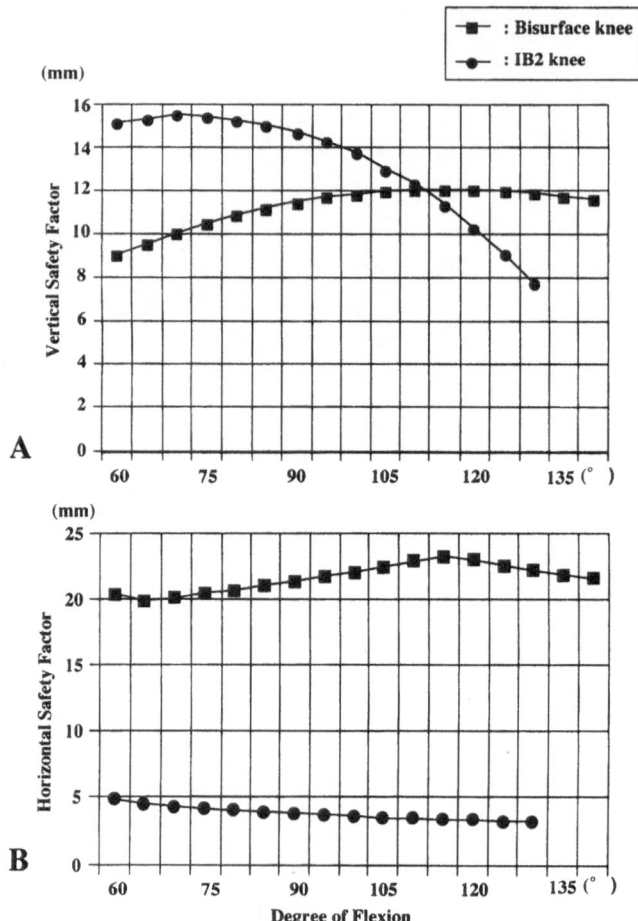

FIG. 5A,B. Dislocation safety factor study. A The vertical dislocation safety factor. B The horizontal dislocation safety factor

Dislocation Safety Factor Study

The vertical dislocation safety factor of I/B 2 (Fig. 5) was gradually decreased from 15 to 8 mm during flexion from 60° to 130°. In the Bisurface knee, the factor was gradually increased from 9 to 12 mm. The horizontal dislocation safety factor was less than 5 mm in the I/B 2. However, the factor in the Bisurface knee was more than 20 mm through range of flexion from 60° to 140°.

Discussion

Advantages of the posterior stabilizing knee include absolute posterior stability provided by the cam, improved range of motion, increased lever arm of quadriceps power, excellent exposure during surgery, easily accomplished ligamentous balance, and easy correction of severe deformities [8]. On the other hand, disadvantages of posterior stabilizing knee include removal of the large piece of bone for the cam, posterior dislocation of the cam, patellar clunk syndrome, restricted axial rotation caused by the tibial post and the femoral box, and polyethylene wear of the cam [8–10]. New designs of the PCL-substituting prosthesis include low height of the femoral box to preserve bone stock of the intercondylar region, anterior setting of the tibial post to avoid posterior dislocation of the cam, and curved articulating surface of the cam to provide axial rotational freedom. However, there are trade-offs between range of motion and stability; the range of flexion decreases by setting the tibial post anteriorly due to posterior impingement of the femur and the tibia [6].

The Bisurface knee has a unique cam mechanism for posterior stability, that is, the ball-and-socket joint in the midposterior portion of the FT joint. The unique cam mechanism was devised by upside-down inversion of the post-and-cam mechanism of the ordinary PS knee, which can work not only as the posterior stabilizing cam but also as a weight-bearing surface and a center of axial rotation in deep flexion. The present study demonstrated that the Bisurface knee has a sufficient rollback to improve range of flexion, wide contact area and low contact stress in flexion position, and sufficient posterior stabilizing ability. We believe that this new posterior stabilizing prosthesis could overcome some disadvantages inherent in the ordinary PS knee, including intercondylar bone removal for the cam, the posterior dislocation of the cam, patellar clunk syndrome, and polyethylene wear in the cam.

References

1. Stiehl JB, Komistek RD, Dennis DA, et al (1995) Fluoroscopic analysis of kinematics after posterior-cruciate-retaining knee arthroplasty. J Bone Joint Surg (Br Vol) 77:884–889
2. Akagi M, Ueo T, Matsusue Y, et al (1997) Improved range of flexion after total knee arthroplasty. The total condylar knee versus the KU knee. Bull Hosp Jt Dis 56:225–232
3. Akagi M, Nakamura T, Matsusue Y, et al (2000) The bisurface total knee replacement: A unique design for flexion. Four-to-nine-year follow-up study. J Bone Joint Surg (Am Vol) 82:1626–1633
4. Insall JN, Lachiewicz PF, Burstein AH (1982) The posterior stabilized condylar prosthesis: A modification of the total condylar design. Two to four-year clinical experience. J Bone Joint Surg (Am Vol) 64:1317–1323
5. Stern SH, Insall JN (1992) Posterior stabilized prosthesis. Results after follow-up of nine to twelve years. J Bone Joint Surg (Am Vol) 74:980–986
6. Delp SL, Kocmond JH, Stern SH (1995) Tradeoffs between motion and stability in posterior substituting knee arthroplasty design. J Biomech 28:1155–1166
7. Kocmond JH, Delp SL, Stern SH (1995) Stability and range of motion of Insall-Burstein condylar prostheses. A computer simulation study. J Arthroplasty 10:383–388
8. Vince KG (1993) Principles of condylar knee arthroplasty: Issues evolving. In: Instructional course lectures, Vol 42. American Academy of Orthopaedic Surgeons, Rosemont, IL, pp 315–324
9. Hozack WJ, Rothman RH, Booth RE Jr, et al (1989) The patellar clunk syndrome. A complication of posterior stabilized total knee arthroplasty. Clin Orthop 241:203–208
10. Puloski S, McCalden R, MacDonald S, et al (2000) Post wear in posterior stabilized TKA: An unrecognized source of polyethylene debris. Trans ORS 25:444

Part 9 Total Knee Arthroplasty for Charcot Joint

Long-Term Results After TKA for Charcot Disease

Tae Seong Kim, Hideshige Moriya, Toyomistu Tsuchida, Masahiko Suzuki, Kimio Masuda, Hiroshi Tamai, Hajime Yamanaka, and Eiichirou Watanabe

Summary. The clinical results of 8 patients (12 knees) with Charcot disease (mean age, 63.6 years) who had undergone total knee arthroplasty (TKA) were studied retrospectively 6–13 years after the operation. All the procedures had been performed using cementless fixation of the femoral and tibial components, except for 4 joints. Revision had been the reason for 3 patients, tibial polyethlene insert delamination for 1, and tibial component loosening for 2 patients. None of the patients who underwent cementless TKA required revision. Survival rate was 91.7% at 5 years and 70.7% at 10 years. Cementless TKA was shown to be a reliable and effective means of treating the Charcot knee.

Key words. Charcot disease, TKA, Cementless, Long-term results, Revision

Introduction

As it was Charcot who reported in 1868 on the central nerve and articular disorders caused by tabes dorsalis, neuropathic arthropathy came to be called Charcot disease. The pathology of this disease concerns the disorder in the reflective defense function, resulting in a loose joint and joint mutilation. Due to the loose joint, the treatment of a Charcot knee is often very difficult [1,2]. For the surgical treatment method, arthrodesis was indicated in the past, but several cases of total knee arthroplasty (TKA) in Charcot disease have recently been reported [3–5]. However, these were all short-term and medium-term results, which were variable; that is, some reported on the necessity of revision soon after operation while others reported favorable results. Therefore, no fixed view has been established on TKA in Charcot disease for the time being. In this connection, we were able to observe patients with Charcot disease during many years after TKA. The clinical results and problems in these patients are reported here.

Department of Orthopedic Surgery, School of Medicine, Chiba University, 1-8-1 Inohana, Chuo-ku, Chiba 260-8677, Japan

Subjects and Methods

TKA was performed in 12 cases with Charcot disease (15 joints) from 1986 to 1993. Of these cases, we were able to follow 12 joints from 8 cases, including 5 joints from 3 men and 7 joints from 5 women. Their age at the time of surgery ranged from 52 years to 78 years old, with a mean of 63.6 years. The primary disease was tabes dorsalis in 11 joints and diabetes mellitus in 1 joint. These patients were placed under observation for 6–13 years and 3 months (mean, 8 years and 10 months).

The prostheses used were Whiteside Ortholoc II (Whiteside) in 10 joints, and PCA and Miller/Galante type I (MGI) in 1 joint each. Cement was used in 3 joints and 1 joint by Whiteside and PCA, respectively. Excluding one Whiteside joint, posterior cruciate ligament (PCL) retention type (CR [cruciate-retaining] type) was used in all the cases. In the investigation, the presence or absence of revision was investigated first. Then, the surviving cases were clinically assessed by Japanese Orthopedic Association Knee Evaluation Score (JOA score); that is, time-course comparison of the JOA score was done before surgery, 4 years after surgery, and at the time of final observation. X-ray findings were investigated for changes in component fixation alignment and radiolucent lines.

Results

Of the 12 joints, revision was done in 3 from 2 cases, both of which were men. Their mean age was 58.0 years. Eight joints from women and 1 joint from a man survived; their mean age was 65.4 years. No revision occurred in any of the 8 cementless cases, whereas 3 of the 4 joints in which cement was used required revision. Those who received revision were engaged in jobs such as a plant worker, a carpenter, etc., requiring considerable physical movement. The duration to revision was 50–95 months, with a mean of 6 years and 11 months. Revision was needed because of tibial component loosening in 2 joints and tibial insert delamination in joint.

The survival rates calculated using the revision assessed by the Kaplan–Meier method as the endpoint were 91.7% and 70.7% after 5 years and 10 years, respectively, after the surgery (Fig. 1).

As to the nine joints that did not require revision, the JOA score improved from a mean of 35.6 points before operation to 80.8 points after 4 years from surgery. However, a decrease to 74.4 points was observed at the final observation time point (Fig. 2). The factors resulting in a decrease in points included hydroarthrosis in two joints as well as decreased movement, such as the stair function, and pain.

As to range of motion, extension, which was 0.5° after 4 years from surgery, decreased to 2.8° at the final observation point, and flexion changed from 101.7° to 108.3°, respectively, demonstrating an increase from the preoperative status (Fig. 3).

Femorotibial angle (FTA) improved from 187° before surgery to 174.4° after surgery. It was 176.2° at the final observation point, demonstrating a slight tendency to varus. When the component fixation angle was investigated, the tibial prosthesis angle (TPA) went up to 92.1° at the final time point, indicating an increase of varus by 3.1°, which seemed to have been partially responsible for an increase in FTA (Fig. 4).

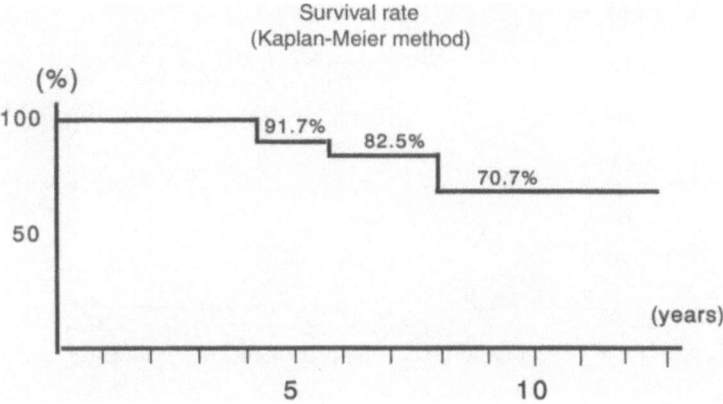

FIG. 1. Survival rate

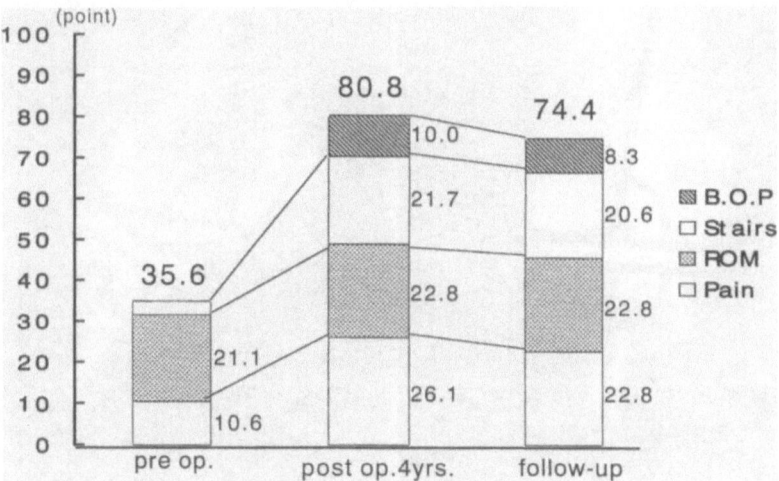

FIG. 2. The time-course comparison of JOA (Japanese Orthopaedic Association) score

The loose joint is a problem in Charcot knee joint cases. In this regard, the PCL function was assessed on the basis of stress-loaded X-ray findings using Telos. The results indicated functional failure of PCL in three joints (group II). When the JOA score was compared by PCL function at the final observation time point, the score was as low as 71.7 points in functionally PCL failure cases and 75.8 points in functionally PCL good cases (group I). The factor causing the decrease was the difference of pain (Fig. 5).

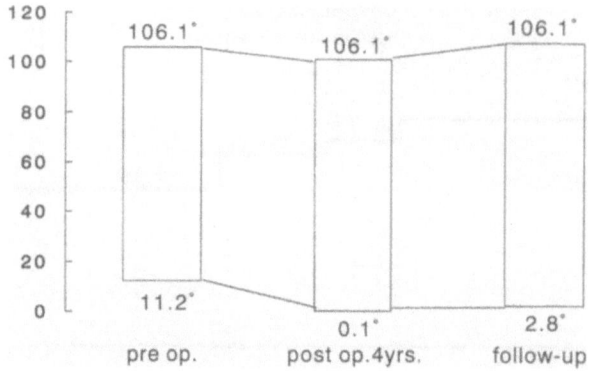

FIG. 3. The time-course comparison of range of motion

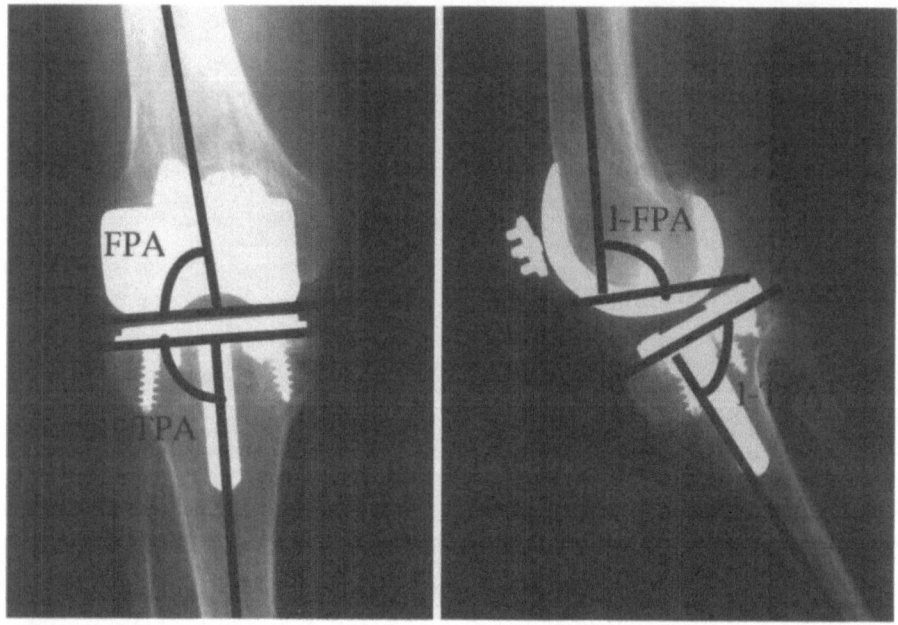

FIG. 4. Prosthesis angle. *FPA*, femoroprosthesis angle; *TPA*, tibioprosthesis angle; *l-FPA*, lateral femoroprosthesis angle; *l-TPA*, lateral tibioprosthesis angle

As the complications observed in the nine joints that did not require revision, hydroarthrosis and tibial component sinking were observed in two joints each (two cases each). Although there was no loosening, radiolucent lines were observed in 22.6% (two cases of nine) at the femoral component and pedestal formation in 55.6% (five cases of nine), indicating the need for continuous observation in the future.

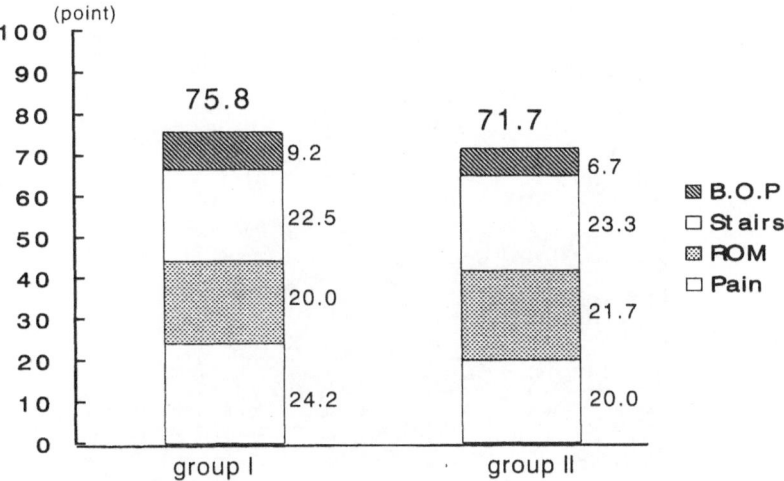

FIG. 5. The comparison of JOA score by PCL function

Case 1

This 72-year-old woman (Fig. 6) had subjective right knee joint pain for 1.5 years before she visited this department at the first time in June 1991. X-ray findings already indicated marked mutilation of the joint, which was in stage II by Eichenholt classification. Using Whiteside (CR type), TKA of the right knee was conducted in November of the same year. Bone graft was done in the deficient site in the lateral tibia plateau without using cement. The JOA score was 85 points after 4 years from surgery, but decreased to 75 points after 8 years. However, the patient does not need any help in getting on and off transportation, and her gait has been maintained with a crutch.

Case 2

For this 70-year-old man (Fig. 7), the lesion seen in the preoperative X-ray was assessed to be in stage II by Eichenholt classification. Right TKA with Whiteside was done using cement in November 1990. He was rehabilitated to work, and the early clinical results were favorable. However, collapse gradually occurred in the bone graft part in the lateral tibia plateau during the course of time. Tibial prosthesis angle (TPA) deteriorated, and the tibial prosthesis gradually deviated to varus. Revision was done in November 1998. According to the findings obtained during the surgery, marked delamination of the tibial insert (5 mm thick) was noted in addition to synovitis in the periphery of the patella. Revision of the tibial prosthesis, patellar component, and a 20-mm-thick tibial insert was necessary.

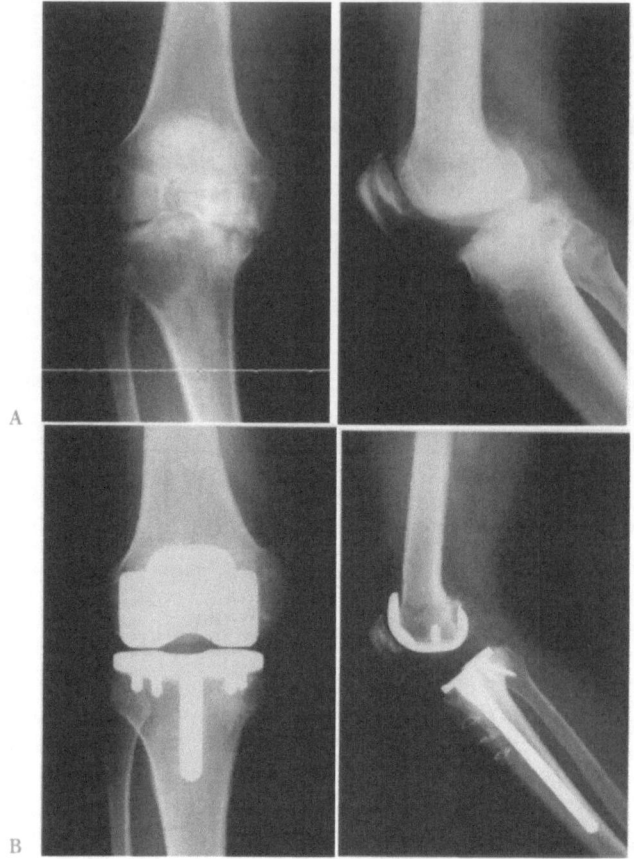

FIG. 6A,B. Case 1: 72-year-old woman. **A** Before operation (stage II). **B** Eight years after operation

Discussion

Considering that a loose joint due to disturbed reflective defense function is involved in the pathology of Charcot disease and that the knee joint is a loaded joint, it is not easy to treat a knee with this disorder. Arthrodesis has been the first choice in surgical treatment, but the bone union rate is not necessarily high, requiring solid fixation [6].

Because of Charcot disease, loosening of the ligament and subluxation were anticipated in the long-term observation of our cases. However, the stress-loaded X-ray findings indicated functional failure of PCL in three of the nine joints while PCL function was maintained in the remaining six joints. As to the long-term TKA results with retained PCL (CR, cruciate retention type), no report has been made on the PCL function. However, considering that the function was maintained in six of the nine joints

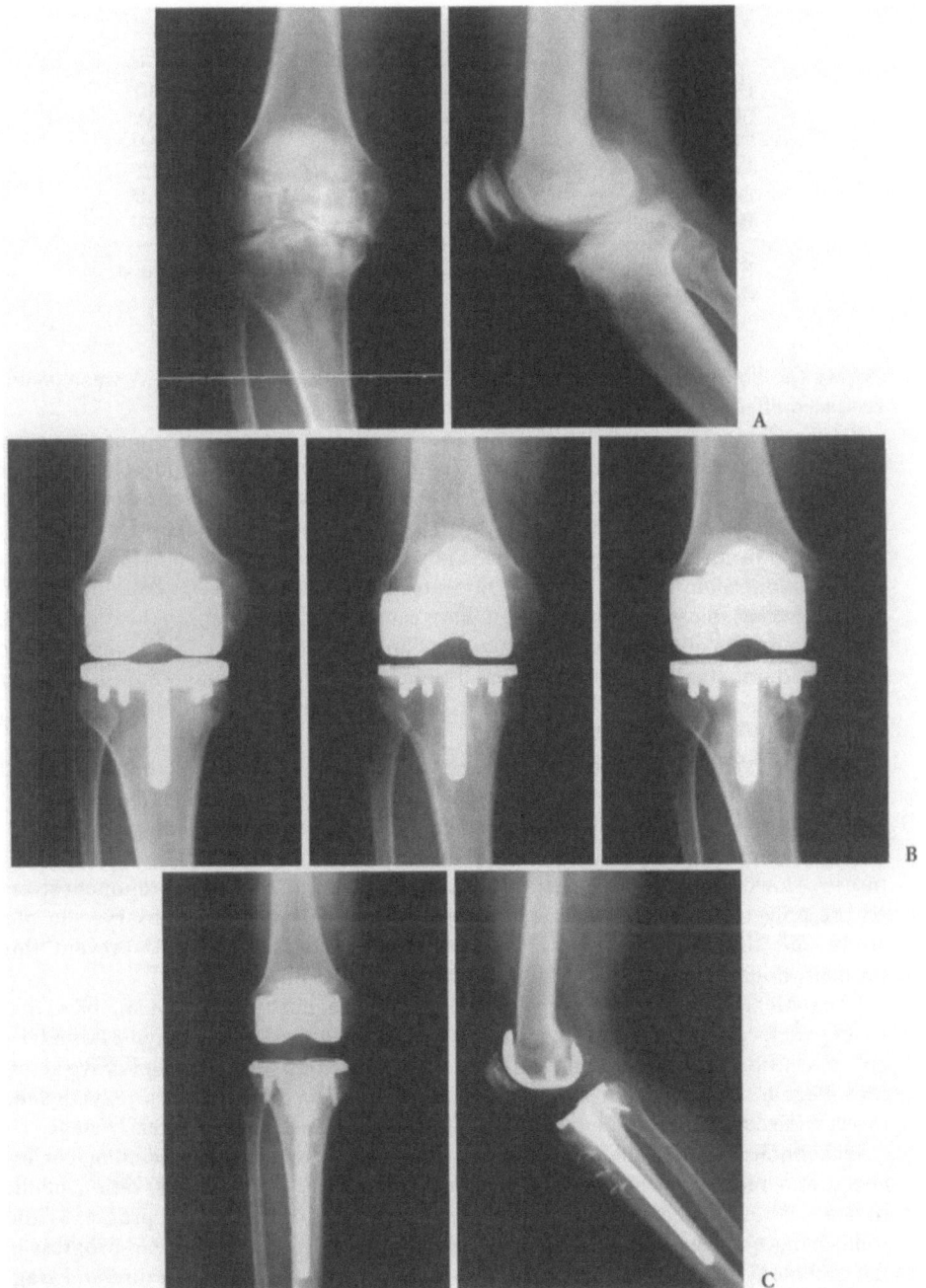

FIG. 7A–C. Case 2: 70-year-old man. **A** Before operation (stage II). **B** Change of the TKA alignment. *Left*, 2 years after TKA (TPA, 92°); *middle*, 5 years after TKA (TPA, 95°); *right*, 8 years after
TKA (TPA 99°). **C** Revision TKA

TABLE 1. Prosthesis alignment

	Five years after operation	Follow-up
FTA	174.7° ± 1.4°	176.2° ± 3.2°
FPA	83.7° ± 1.4°	83.9° ± 1.4°
TPA	89.0° ± 2.9°	92.1° ± 1.5°
Lateral FPA	87.2° ± 1.9°	87.7° ± 2.7°
Lateral TPA	88.4° ± 3.2°	88.6° ± 2.8°
Patella tilt angle	4.1° ± 2.6°	5.0° ± 5.4°

FTA, femorotibial angle; FPA, femoroprosthesis angle; TPA, tibial prosthesis angle

during the observation period of 8 years and 10 months, CR-type TKA was considered also effective as a treatment method of Charcot disease.

Of the Charcot disease patients who underwent TKA, reports were made on early component loosening when hinge-type TKA began to be employed [3]. On the other hand, Soundry et al. reported on favorable midterm results in the cases in which surface revision type was employed [4]. Hinge-type TKA was used to depend on an artificial joint for support because the Charcot knee is a loose joint. However, even though a long stem was used, stress concentrated on the interface of component and bone as well as micromotion seemed to have caused the loosening. On the other hand, favorable results obtained with surface revision-type TKA seemed to be attributable to diffusion of stress on the femoral and tibial components through the tibial insert and cementless biological fixation of the component because of the porous coating, which resulted in bone ingrowth [7].

When we were able to observe patients for the long term (mean, 8 years and 10 months), 9 of the 12 joints were surviving. Considering that cement was used in all the 3 cases that needed revision, cementless TKA, which achieved biological fixation, was considered to be useful over the long term as a treatment method of Charcot disease. However, excessive concentration of femoral bone and tibial component stress on the polyethylene insert may cause insert delamination, as was observed in our study, and this may cause secondary osteolysis and loosening. To prevent this problem, appropriate ligament balance was considered important.

The patients who received revision had general prognosis risk factors of TKA; that is, they were comparatively young and had jobs that required much activity. It is advisable to caution the patients aggressively in this risk group about postoperative activities. Regular checkup by X-rays is also necessary. When abrasion of a polyethylene insert is discovered, revision of the insert should be considered at an early stage.

Eichenholt classified the Charcot disease into three stages of development, coalescence, and reconstruction based on X-ray findings [8]. Careful observation of the patient's status is necessary in the development stage, during which progress from mild changes to fracture and fragmentation may occur, indicating a rapid progress in the pathology in this stage [9]. Our cases were all in stage 1, but fracture and fragmentation did not develop in any of them. As no advanced deformity such as subluxation was observed in our series, the flat-surface type of polyethylene insert was employed in all cases. However, a constrain type or posterior stabilizer type of insert is indicated for advanced deformity cases that demonstrate ligament loosening. In this regard, it is necessary to accurately judge the pathology of patient in selecting the prosthesis to be employed in TKA.

Conclusion

TKA was performed in patients with Charcot disease and the long-term results were investigated. The mean observation period was 8 years and 10 months. Revision was conducted in 3 of the 12 knees, and the survival rate was 70.7%. When stress-loaded X-rays were taken in the surviving group, PCL function decrease was observed in 3 of the 9 joints. No revision was necessary in the cementless cases, indicating the usefulness of cementless TKA in Charcot disease cases.

References

1. Johnson JTH (1967) Neuropathic fractures and joint injuries: pathogenesis and rationale of prevention and treatment. J Bone Joint Surg 49A:1–30
2. Norman A, Robbins H, Milgram JE (1968) The acute neuropathic arthropathy: a rapid severely disorganizing form of arthritis. Radiology 90:1159–1164
3. Hirohata K (1987) Clinical significance of neuropathic arthropathy (in Japanese). Rinsho Seikei Saigai 22:238–252
4. Soundry M, Binazzi R, Johanson NA, et al (1985) Total knee artroplasty in Charcot and Charcot-like knee joints. Clin Orthop 208:199–204
5. Suguro T, et al (1991) Clinical results of TKA for Charcot joint (in Japanese). Kotsu Kansetsu Jintai 4:1797–1802
6. Drennan DB, Fahey JJ, Maylahn DJ (1971) Important factors in achieving arthrodesis of the Charcot knee. J Bone Joint Surg 53A:1180–1185
7. Whiteside LA (1994) Cementless total knee replacement: nine to 11 year results and 10-year survivorship analysis. Clin Orthop 309:185–192
8. Eichenholt SN (1966) Charcot joints. Thomas, Springfield
9. Kats I, Rabinowits JG, Dziachiv R (1961) Early changes in Charcot's joints. AJR 86:965–974

Total Knee Arthroplasty for Charcot Knees: Two Cases Followed Up for More than 10 Years

YOICHI TANEDA, NOBUO MATSUI, YUKIO YOSHIDA,
MASAAKI KOBAYASHI, TOSHIYUKI KAWANISHI, and YUKO NAGATANI

Summary. We report two patients with Charcot knees, caused by tabes dorsalis, who showed satisfactory postoperative results for more than 10 years after kinematic rotating-hinge total knee arthroplasty. Surface-replacing total knee arthroplasty in a Charcot knee with massive tibial defect or inadequate ligamentous balancing may leave knee instability after surgery, possibly causing prosthetic loosening during the early postoperative period. It is particularly difficult to treat a Charcot knee if knee instability, especially genu recurvatum, is present before operation. Thus, we performed kinematic rotating-hinge total knee arthroplasty on Charcot knees with severe genu recurvatum, and very satisfactory clinical results were obtained for more than 10 years although we had been concerned about a possibility of stem breakage. Total knee arthroplasty can be recommended for Charcot knees as a choice of surgical procedures.

Key words. Charcot joint, Total knee arthroplasty, Kinematic rotating hinge

Introduction

Arthrodesis has been most widely recognized for the treatment of Charcot joints, whereas arthroplasty has been generally considered to be contraindicated for this disorder. However, knee joints are recently included as candidates for arthroplasty among Charcot joints, and there are a number of reports describing satisfactory results of arthroplasty for Charcot knee joints. Because Charcot joints arise from various diseases, issues of the indications for arthroplasty are still conflicting. We observed satisfactory postoperative results in two cases of Charcot knees with marked knee instability, caused by tabes dorsalis, for more than 10 years following kinematic rotating-hinge total knee arthroplasty, and these cases are herein reported.

Department of Orthopedic Surgery, Nagoya City University Medical School, 1 Kawasumi, Mizuho-cho, Mizuho-ku, Nagoya 467-8601, Japan

Case Reports

Case 1

A woman aged 63 years at surgery had arthralgia in the right knee since 1973, which was treated by a nearby clinic. She visited our department in April 1987 for the first time because of aggravation of the arthralgia in the right knee. Radiographic findings of the medial aspect of the knee were characteristic of the Charcot knee joint, including bone destruction, osteosclerosis, and fragmentations (Fig. 1). In the standing position, the knee showed a medial inclination and hyperextension. (TPHA) was 2+. Charcot arthropathy also involved the lumbar vertebrae and left ankle. Total knee arthroplasty was done on the right knee in December 1987 (Fig. 2). After surgery, the patient could walk with a T-cane while wearing knee braces to prevent hyperextension and a short leg brace in the left ankle joint. Radiographs obtained 6 months after surgery and thereafter revealed thickening and hypertrophy of the posterior tibial cortex, probably caused by hyperextension stress. The patient became incapable of walking due to severe leg pain, probably the result tabes dorsalis, and she began to use a wheelchair in 1996. A radiograph obtained 10 years after surgery disclosed no radiolucent lines or evidence of loosening, and the hypertrophy of the posterior tibial cortex was slightly reduced because of her inability to walk (Fig. 3). The range of motion in the knee was 5° to 145°. This patient died of alimentary tract hemorrhage in December 1997.

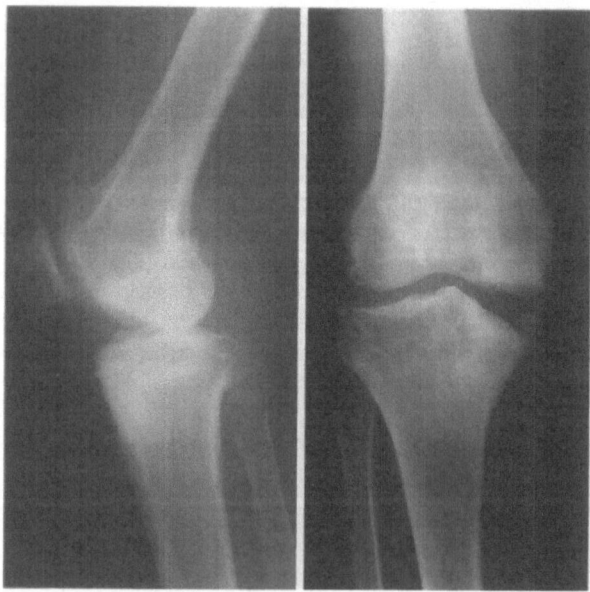

FIG. 1. Case 1. Radiographs of a 63-year-old woman at surgery showed typical Charcot changes in the right knee

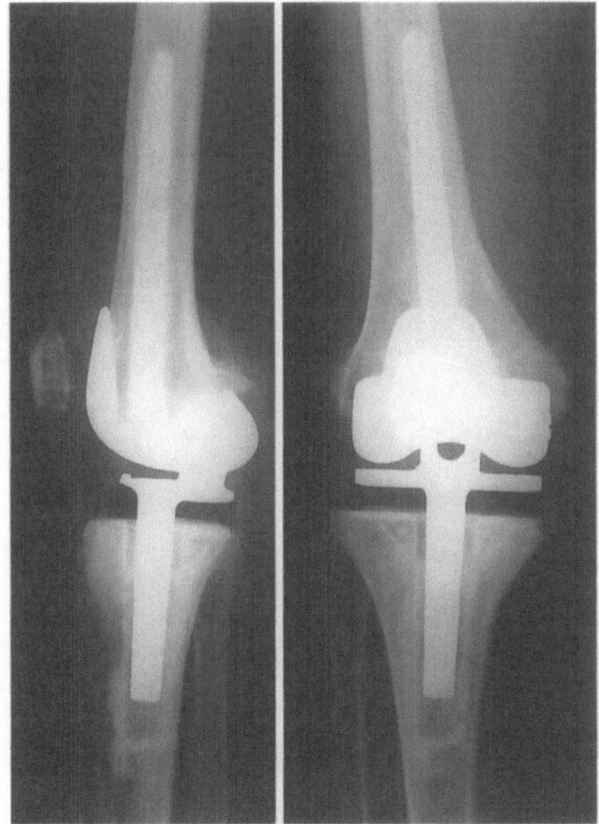

FIG. 2. Case 1. Immediately after operation. A kinematic rotating-hinge knee prosthesis was used with bone cement

Case 2

Case 2 was a woman aged 59 years at surgery whose left knee became unstable in about 1977, and she used a T-cane. Arthralgia, swelling, and hemarthrosis occurred in the left knee in July 1987, and a knee brace was prescribed by a nearby clinic. She visited our department in November 1987 for the first time. At that time, TPHA was 2+. Hyperextension and valgus/varus instability were remarkable in both knees, and the patient could walk only with knee braces and crutches. Plain radiographs showed only mild osteoarthritic changes, but radiographs in the standing position revealed joint space narrowing and marked genu recurvatum (Fig. 4).

Total knee arthroplasty was performed on the left knee in November 1988 and on the right knee in February 1989 (Fig. 5). After surgery, she could walk with a crutch while wearing knee braces to prevent hyperextension, or even without the aid of a crutch indoors. Radiographs obtained 6 months after surgery and thereafter revealed a thickening and hypertrophy of the posterior tibial cortex, as with case 1 (Fig. 5).

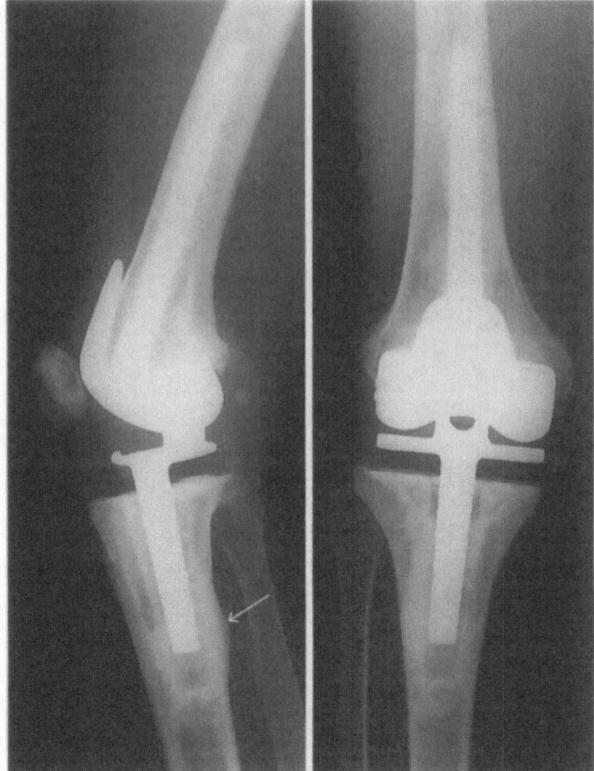

FIG. 3. Case 1. Ten months after operation. Thickening of the posterior tibial cortex, probably resulting from hyperextension stress, was observed

After March 1994, low back pain due to Charcot spine and disturbance of deep sensitivity were aggravated; she became incapable of walking and needed the aid of crutches, even for indoor walking, and used a wheelchair outdoors. However, radiographs obtained 12 years after surgery disclosed no radiolucent lines or evidence of loosening (Fig. 6), and the knee range motion was 0° to 145° on both sides.

Discussion

Arthroplasty has been considered to be contraindicated for Charcot joint, and this is true for many cases of Charcot joints. However, Charcot knee joints have different aspects, and arthroplasty is now considered one of the treatments for this disorder as a result of the availability of verious kinds of knee prostheses and advances in surgical techniques. Total knee arthroplasty has been used for Charcot knee joints, probably since a report was released by Saudry et al. in 1986 [1]. These authors obtained satisfactory results after surface-replacing total knee arthroplasty, and they stated that

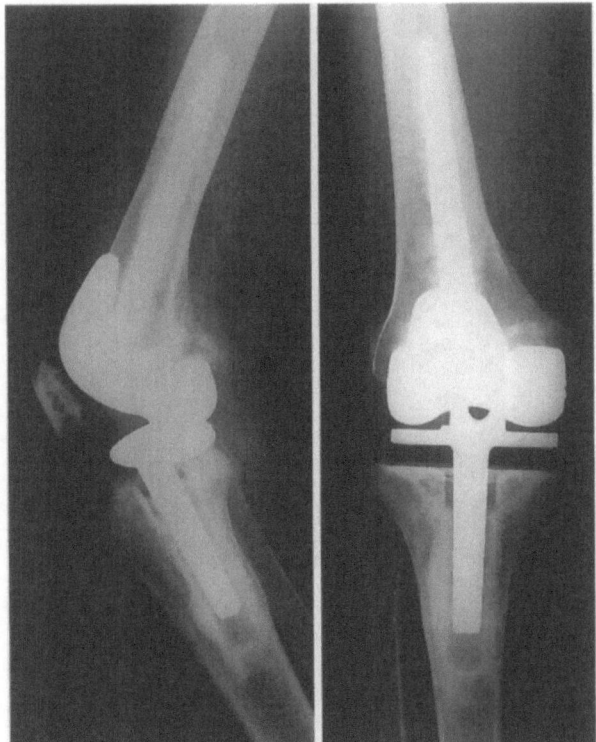

FIG. 4. Case 1. Ten years after operation. There was no radiolucent line or loosening, and thickening of the posterior tibial cortex was slightly reduced

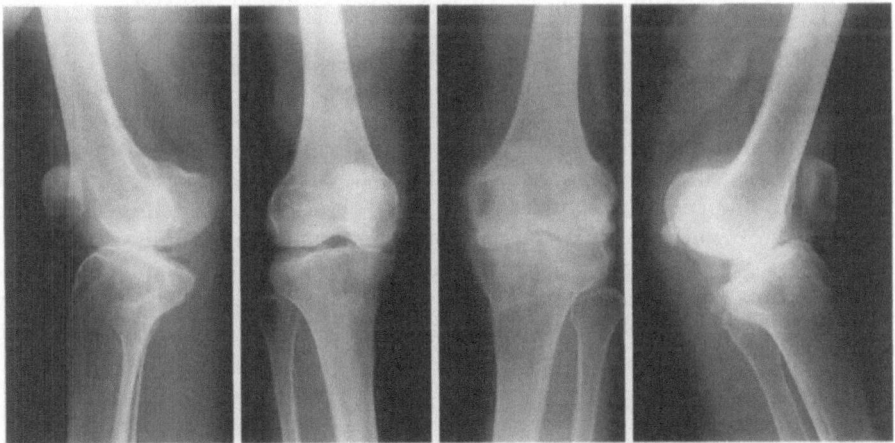

FIG. 5. Case 2. Radiographs of a 59-year-old woman at surgery. Both knees showed joint-space narrowing and marked hyperextension in the standing position

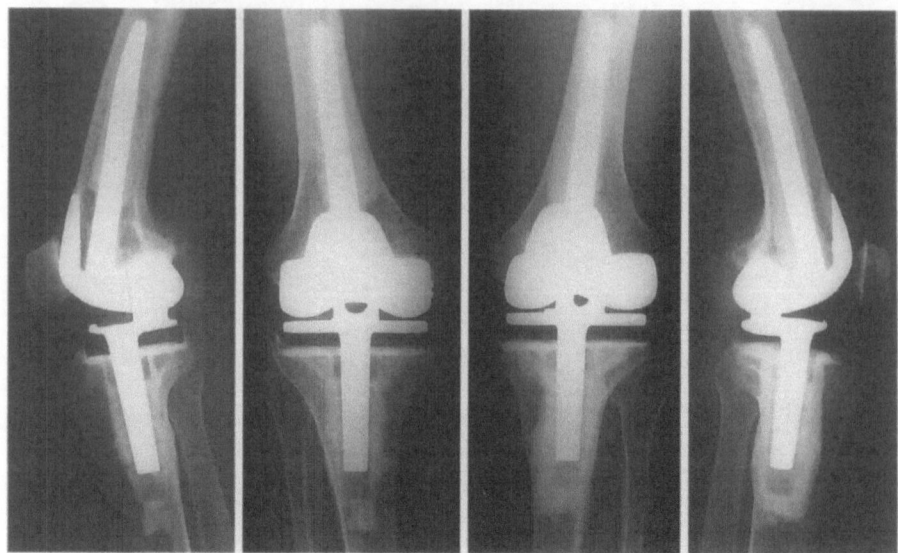

FIG. 6. Case 2. Immediately after operation. Kinematic rotating-hinge knee prostheses were used in both knees with bone cement

Charcot knees can be treated by total knee arthroplasty if ligamentous balancing is adequately secured. However, the period of their follow-up was short, 2–4.25 years, and no long-term follow-up was made. In a report by Yoshino et al. in 1993 [2], the authors followed up three cases of Charcot knee joints for more than 8 years after total knee arthroplasty, and they observed satisfactory results in two cases who did not develop postoperative fractures.

We performed kinematic rotating-hinge total knee arthroplasty in our two cases because surface-replacing total knee arthroplasty could not control their instability, caused by genu recurvatum in both cases. Our patients showed satisfactory postoperative results for more than 10 years because they fortunately had no fractures. However, some orthopedic surgeons insist that total knee arthroplasty should not be performed on patients categorized as the ataxic phase on Eichenholtz's classification because the disturbance of deep sensitivity is severe in patients with tabes dorsalis, and the risk of falling down is much higher in those patients. We think that indications for total knee arthroplasty and the choice of prosthesis in Charcot knee joints should be discussed with overall consideration of the disease pathology, affected joint, and Eichenholtz's stage.

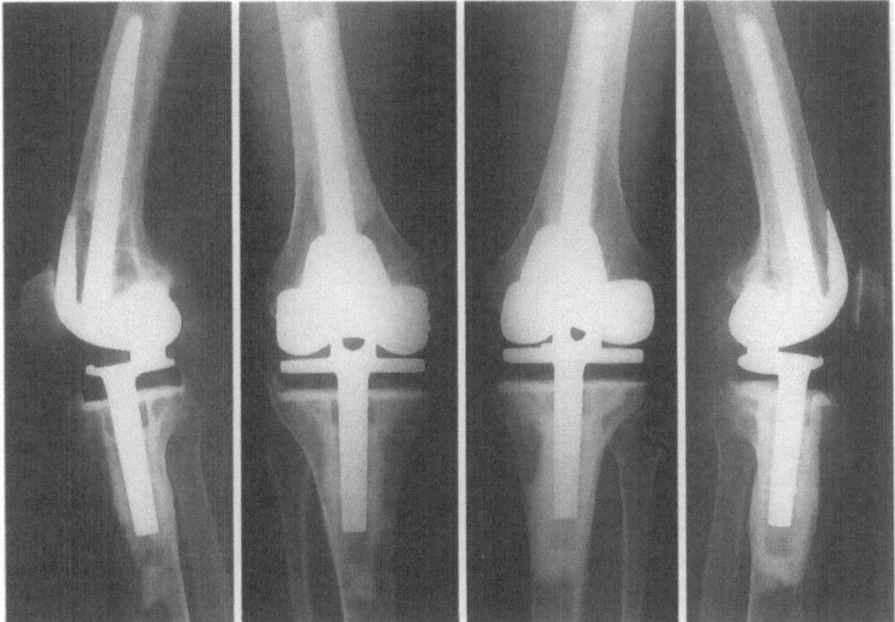

FIG. 7. Case 2. Twelve years after operation. There was no radiolucent line or evidence of loosening in either knee

Conclusion

1. Kinematic rotating-hinge total knee arthroplasty in Charcot knee joints caused by tabes dorsalis provided satisfactory radiographic findings and good clinical results for more than 10 years.
2. Total knee arthroplasty was thought to provide satisfactory postoperative results for Charcot knee joints caused by tabes dorsalis, if performed at an early stage.

References

1. Soudry M, Binazzi R, Johanson NA, et al (1986) Total knee arthroplasty in Charcot and Charcot-like joints. Clin Orthop 208:199–204
2. Yoshino S, Fujimori J, Kajino A, et al (1993) Total knee arthroplasty in Charcot's joint. J Arthroplasty 8:335–340

Total Knee Arthroplasty in Charcot's Knees

Masami Tokunaga, Toshihiro Ohdera, Akira Kobayashi, and
Shiro Hiroshima

Summary. We describe here the treatment of three cases of Charcot's knee (caused by tabes dorsalis) with total knee arthroplasty. At the time of surgery, the average age of the patients was 72.6 years (range, 69–77 years). The average follow-up interval was 6.3 years (range, 9 months–12 years). Five total knee arthroplasties in three cases were performed. Three of these joints were followed for more than 6 years. The results were good knee joint function, with no evidence of instability or pain over 6 years. At the time of follow-up, however, all these patients required the use of a wheelchair because of either neglected supracondylar periprosthetic fracture, severely migrated ipsilateral hip hemiarthroplasty, or ataxia and subsequent joint instability. Knee replacement appears to be a feasible treatment for Charcot's knee if strict patient selection is carried out.

Key words. Neuropathic joint disease, Charcot's knee, Total knee arthroplasty, Ataxia, Tabes dorsalis

Introduction

Total joint replacement for Charcot's joint is controversial and represents a technical challenge. Total joint replacement is generally contraindicated in neuropathic joint disease because initial pain relief is followed by subluxation or loosening [1,2]. However, there have been some reports of successful arthroplasties of neuropathic joints [3–6]. We report here three cases of Charcot's knee joint treated with total knee arthroplasty (TKA).

Subjects

Three cases (one man and two women) with neuropathic arthropathy of the knee underwent five TKAs between 1988 and 1998 at Fukuoka Orthopaedic Hospital. Two cases had bilateral procedures. At the time of surgery, the average age of the patients

Fukuoka Orthopaedic Hospital, 2-10-50 Yanagouchi, Minami-ku, Fukuoka 815-0063, Japan

was 72.6 (range, 69–77) years. The average follow-up interval was 6.3 years; three of the five TKAs were followed for more than 6 years. All cases were caused by tabes dorsalis.

Standard screening serum tests for syphilis were positive in all cases. On neurological examination, Romberg's sign was positive in one case, Westphal's sign present in two cases, and Argyll–Robertson pupil was evident in all cases. In one case, ataxic gait was noted. No patient had evidence of dementia paralytica.

Knee joint examination in all cases revealed varus deformity, instability, and gonalgia and marked joint effusion. All cases suffered from moderate pain, but less than would be expected from the degree of joint destruction and deformity.

According to the roentogenographic classification of Eichenholz [7], the stage of development was seen in one knee, the stage of coalescence in three knees, and the stage of reconstruction in one knee. A high tibial osteotomy (HTO) had been performed in one knee 10 months before TKA, and another knee had undergone osteosynthesis for a medial tibial plateau fracture a month before TKA.

All three cases had bilateral neuropathic knee joints. Neuropathic arthropathy and pathological spontaneous fractures of the calcaneus, distal tibia and fibula, and supracondylar femur were noted in case 1; involvement of hip, spine, and talus was noted in case 2, and a lumbar lesion was noted in case 3. The prostheses used were of the surface replacement semiconstrained type. All implants except one were inserted using bone cement. Three blocked bone grafts and a morselized bone graft were utilized.

Case Reports

Case 1

A 69-year-old woman complained of acute pain in her right knee in July 1987. Six weeks later she visited our hospital. Right knee roentgenograms demonstrated marked collapse and sclerotic change of medial tibial plateau (Fig. 1a) (in retrospect, they demonstrated Eichenholz's stage of development). Standard serum screening tests for syphilis were positive. As the initial diagnosis was necrosis of the right medial tibial condyle, she underwent HTO in September 1987 (Fig. 1b). Seven months after surgery, she suffered from a medial tibial plateau compression fracture (Fig. 1c). In July 1988, right TKA was performed with the use of bone grafting for the medial tibial plateau defect (Fig. 1d). At the time of the second operation, right knee roentgenograms showed Eichenholz's stage of coalescence.

The patient developed swelling in her left knee in December 1988. A month later, she complained of severe knee pain, and left knee hemarthrosis was diagnosed. Although roentgenograms of her left knee were normal in July 1987 (Fig. 2a), by December 1988 they demonstrated Eichenholz's stage of development (Fig. 2b). Roentgenograms taken in January 1989 showed evidence of coalescence (Fig. 2c). Subsequently, in February 1989, left TKA was performed, with bone grafting for a defect of the left medial tibial plateau (Fig. 2d).

On review in 1995, 6 years after TKA, knee joint function appeared to be preserved bilaterally with no evidence of instability or pain. From 1995 she was treated at a hospital nearer to her home. In October 1995 she complained of pain in her right knee following a fall. Although initial roentgenograms were reported as showing no frac-

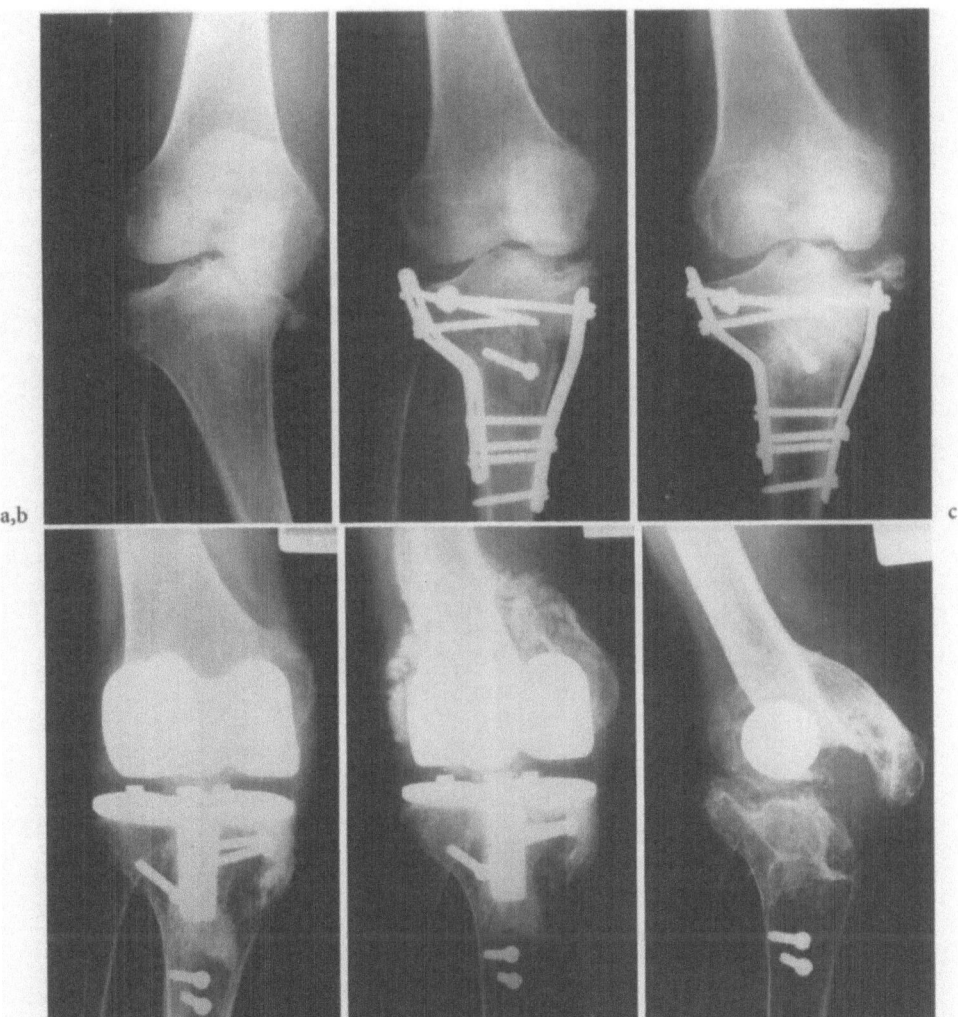

a,b

c

d,e

f

FIG. 1a–f. Case 1: 69-year-old woman, right knee. **a** Preoperative roentgenogram. **b** Postoperative roentgenogram following high tibial osteotomy. **c** Seven months after high tibial osteotomy, a medial tibial plateau fracture was noted. **d** Postoperative roentgenogram following a total knee arthroplasty. **e** Roentgenogram demonstrated a supracondylar fracture of the right femur. **f** Twelve years after the primary total knee arthroplasty, after removal of both prostheses

ture, further films demonstrated a supracondylar fracture of the right femur (Fig. 1e). In view of her persistent knee pain, it was decided to perform revision surgery with osteosynthesis of her right knee. Unfortunately only removal of the femoral and tibial components was carried out, and reimplantation was not successful (Fig. 1f).

Postoperatively, despite the use of a long leg brace on her right knee, she was unable to walk unassisted and required the use of a wheelchair. Approximately 10 years after

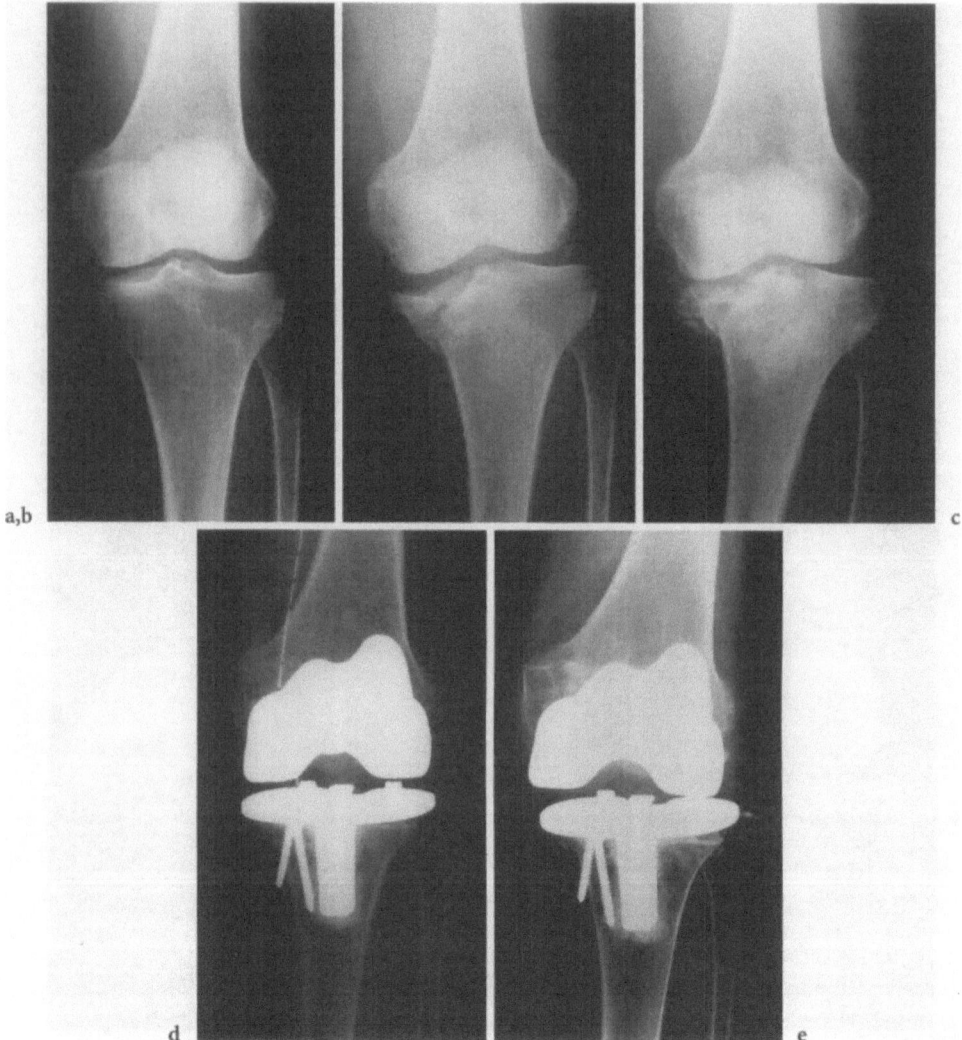

FIG. 2a–e. Case 1: 69-year-old woman, left knee. **a** Roentgenogram taken in 1987. **b** Roentgenogram in 1988. **c** Preoperative roentgenogram. **d** Postoperative roentgenogram following total knee arthroplasty. **e** Eleven years after total knee arthroplasty

left TKA, follow-up roentgenograms showed no evidence of loosening in her left knee (Fig. 2e).

Case 2

A 73-year-old woman was referred to us in July 1987 with a 6-month history of pain and swelling of the right knee and gait disturbance due to knee instability. Roentgenograms demonstrated Eichenholz's stage of development (Fig. 3a). Standard

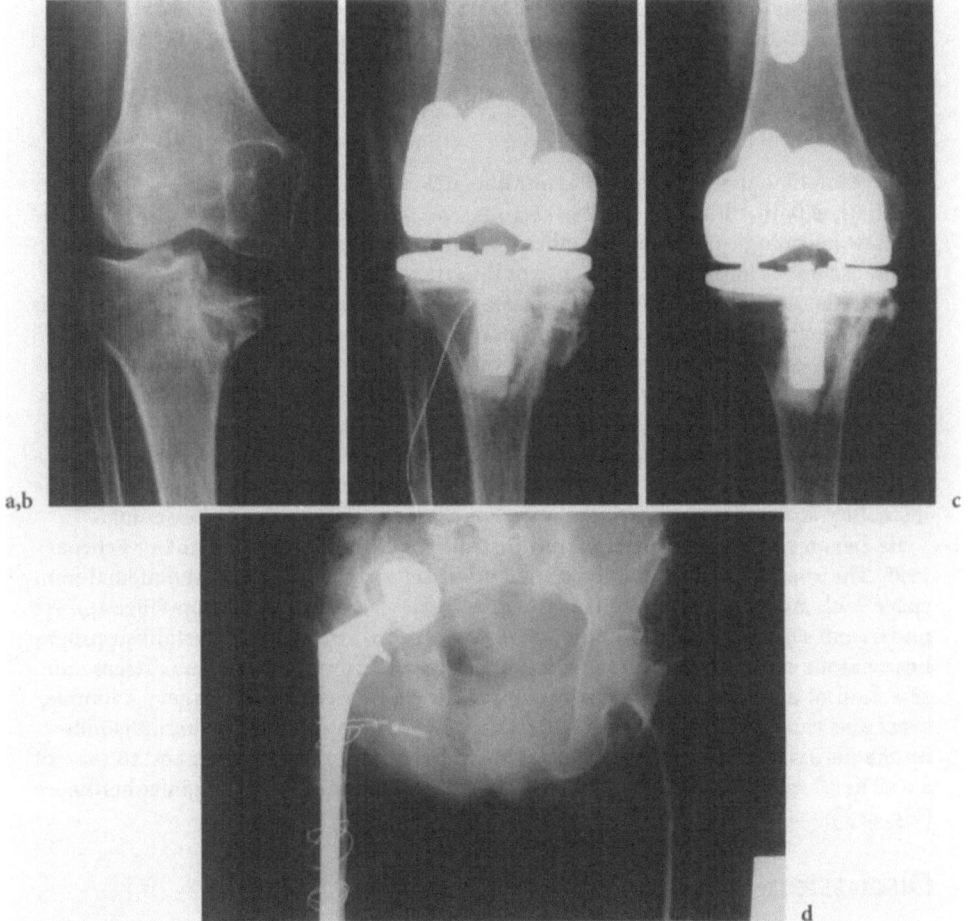

a,b   c

                                                                                        d

FIG. 3a–d. Case 2: 73-year-old woman, right knee. **a** Preoperative roentgenogram. **b** Postoperative roentgenogram following total knee arthroplasty. **c** Seven years after total knee arthroplasty. **d** The outer femoral head had migrated into the pelvis

serum screening tests for syphilis were positive. Because repeat roentgenograms in June 1988 showed progression to the stage of coalescence, she underwent right TKA with blocked bone grafting for the tibial defect (Fig. 3b).

In 1986, before onset of her neuropathic joint disease, she had undergone a bipolar hemiarthroplasty of her right hip as treatment for an intracapsular right femoral neck fracture. Roentgenograms in 1988 revealed marked radiolucency around the femoral stem. Consequently, she had a revision hip hemiarthroplasty. Unfortunately, a fall 4 months after the revision surgery resulted in a periprosthetic femoral shaft fracture, and the patient underwent a further revision surgery with insertion of a long stem prosthesis in August 1988.

Approximately 7 years after TKA, roentgenograms showed no evidence of loosening in her right knee (Fig. 3c). Her right knee joint function was relatively good and she could walk outdoors using a T-cane. However, the outer right femoral head had migrated into the pelvis (Fig. 3d), and consequent disruption of the hip joint caused some gait disability.

Case 3

A 74-year-old man was admitted to our hospital in October 1995 with a 9-year history of left knee pain. Although standard serum screening test for syphilis was positive, he had few neurological findings of tabes dorsalis. Roentgenograms showed bicompart-mental sclerosis and marked collapse of the left medial tibial plateau (Fig. 4a) (in ret-rospect, the X-ray showed Eichenholz's stage of reconstruction). The initial diagnosis was osteoarthritis of the left knee joint, and he underwent left TKA in November 1995 (Fig. 4b). Two months postoperatively, however, joint instability was apparent in the replaced knee, and the patient had developed signs and symptoms of tabes dorsalis. Argyll–Robertson pupil was evident, Westphal's sign was present, deep sensation was impaired, and Romberg's sign was positive. He had an ataxic gait and had to use a walker. A long leg brace was required for his left lower extremity because of soft tissue instability. Roentgenograms of the left TKA showed no evidence of loosening.

He began to complain of pain and instability of his right knee joint in February 1998. The roentgenogram demonstrated sclerosis and narrowing of the medial joint space with no evidence of collapse of the right medial tibial plateau (Fig. 4e). He underwent right TKA in December 1998. Special care was taken to establish proper ligamentous balancing and bony alignment, by performing ligamentous release and resection of an adequate amount of bone. However, 4 weeks after surgery a long leg brace was required for his right leg because of worsening ataxia. At 9 months follow-up the patient was able to walk indoors with bilateral long leg braces and the use of a wall hand railing. Roentgenograms showed no evidence of loosening in either knees (Fig. 4c,f).

Discussion

We have analyzed the causes that led to gait disability in these three cases. In case 1, knee joint function was preserved in both knees, with no instability or pain evident for up to 7 years after surgery. At this point, however, the patient had a fall and the resulting right supracondylar femoral fracture was initially missed. Thus, she lost an opportunity of undergoing conservative treatment for this fracture. If consolidation of the femoral supracondylar fracture had been achieved with correct alignment, removal of the prosthesis would have been unnecessary, and she would have continued to retain good knee joint function.

In case 2, severe migration of an ipsilateral hip hemiarthroplasty was the sole cause of her gait disability. Eight years after TKA, knee joint function had been preserved.

In case 3, although evidence of tabes dorsalis was not detected before the first left TKA, ataxia was apparent before the right TKA. Therefore, ataxia and the consequent joint instability were the cause of this patient's gait disability. As Sprenger [5] and other authors have noted, TKA should not be performed in ataxic patients.

One of the most important factors that must be taken into consideration when performing TKA for Charcot's joint is the roentgenographic stage [3,6]. It is essential that

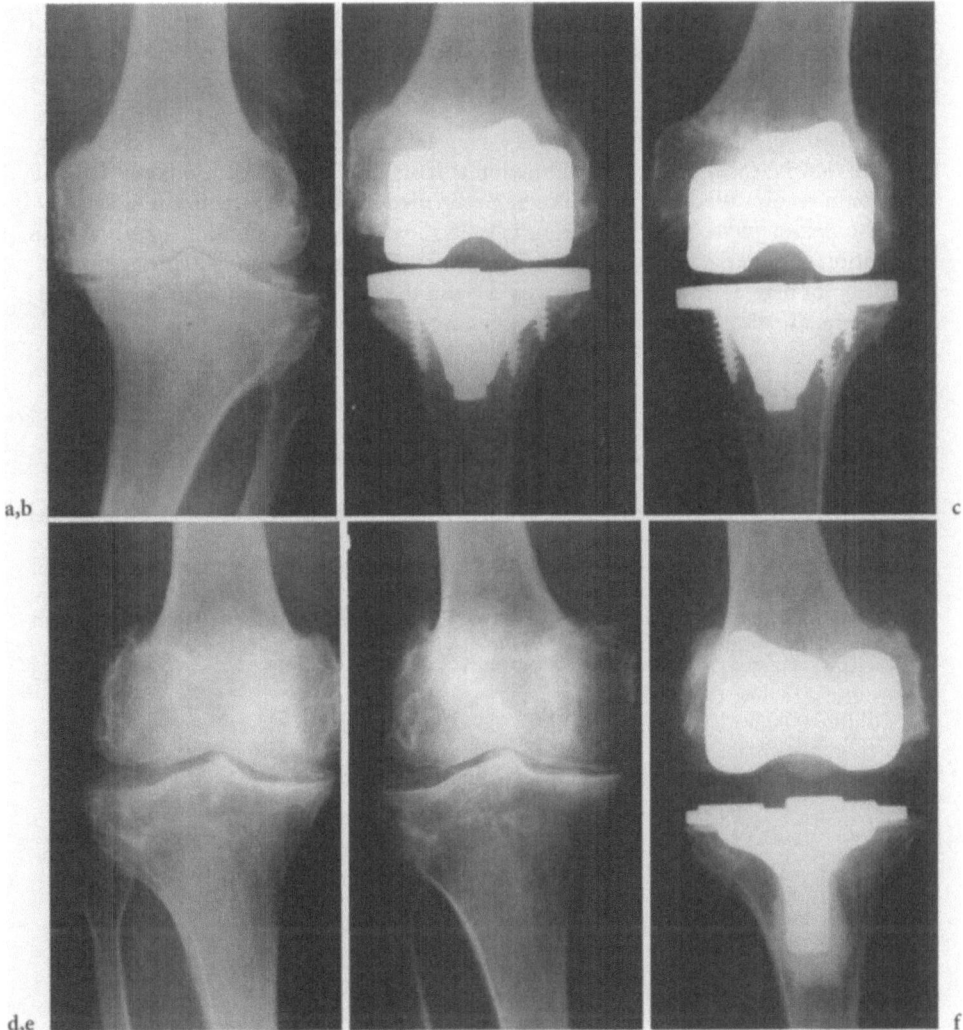

a,b

c

d,e

f

Fig. 4a–f. Case 4: 74-year-old man. a Preoperative roentgenogram, left knee. b Postoperative roentgenogram following left total knee arthroplasty. c At 3.7 years after the left knee arthroplasty. d Roentgenogram taken in 1985. e Preoperative roentgenogram, right knee. There was few developments of X-ray staging from d to e. f Nine months after right knee arthroplasty

the osteolytic/destructive phase of the disease has ceased and that bone reconstruction has begun before surgical intervention.

Soudry et al. [4] reported nine TKAs in seven patients with neuropathic joint disease. Excellent results were obtained in eight knees and good results in one with an average follow-up of 3 years. The histological and radiologic findings were diagnostic of neuropathic joint disease, but four patients with clinically apparent neurological abnormalities had no definable neurological disease. He concluded that if either bone grafting or a custom-augmented prosthesis corrects severe bone loss, and if ligamentous balancing is adequately secured, neuropathic knees can be treated by TKA.

Based on the literature and the cases we have described, we would suggest that successful TKA is feasible for neuropathic joints if strict patient selection is carried out. We would recommend the procedure be performed in elderly patients with low activity who retain some pain sensation, have no loss of deep sensation, and have no indication of either ataxia or dementia paralytica. Evidence of consolidation or reconstruction of osteolytic areas before surgery and the use of surgical techniques as outlined here, are also important.

References

1. Ellman MH (1989) Neuropathic joint disease. In: Arthritis and allied conditions, 11th edn. Lea & Febiger, Philadelphia, pp 1255–1272
2. Edmonson AS, Crenshaw AH (1980) Campbell's operative orthopedics. Mosby, St. Louis, p 1108
3. Fullerton BD, Browngoehl LA (1997) Total knee arthroplasty in a patient with bilateral Charcot's knees. Arch Phys Med Rehabil 78:780–782
4. Soudry M, Binszzi R, Johanson NA, et al (1986) Total knee arthroplasty in Charcot's and Charcot-like joints. Clin Orthop 208:199–204
5. Sprenger TR, Foley CJ (1982) Hip replacement in a Charcot's joint: a case report and historical review. Clin Orthop 165:191–194
6. Yoshino S, Fujimori J, Kajino A, et al (1993) Total knee arthroplasty in Charcot's joint. J Arthroplasty 8:335–340
7. Eichenholz SN (1966) Charcot's joints. Thomas, Springfield

Key Word Index